AMERICAN ACADEMY OF OPHTHALMOLOGY®
Protecting Sight. Empowering Lives.

MW01701681

11 | Lens and Cataract

Last major revision 2020–2021

2022–2023

BCSC

Basic and Clinical Science Course™

EB Published after collaborative review with the European Board of Ophthalmology subcommittee

The American Academy of Ophthalmology is accredited by the Accreditation Council for Continuing Medical Education (ACCME) to provide continuing medical education for physicians.

The American Academy of Ophthalmology designates this enduring material for a maximum of 10 *AMA PRA Category 1 Credits*™. Physicians should claim only the credit commensurate with the extent of their participation in the activity.

CME expiration date: June 1, 2023. *AMA PRA Category 1 Credits*™ may be claimed only once between June 1, 2020, and the expiration date.

BCSC® volumes are designed to increase the physician's ophthalmic knowledge through study and review. Users of this activity are encouraged to read the text and then answer the study questions provided at the back of the book.

To claim *AMA PRA Category 1 Credits*™ upon completion of this activity, learners must demonstrate appropriate knowledge and participation in the activity by taking the posttest for Section 11 and achieving a score of 80% or higher. For further details, please see the instructions for requesting CME credit at the back of the book.

The Academy provides this material for educational purposes only. It is not intended to represent the only or best method or procedure in every case, nor to replace a physician's own judgment or give specific advice for case management. Including all indications, contraindications, side effects, and alternative agents for each drug or treatment is beyond the scope of this material. All information and recommendations should be verified, prior to use, with current information included in the manufacturers' package inserts or other independent sources, and considered in light of the patient's condition and history. Reference to certain drugs, instruments, and other products in this course is made for illustrative purposes only and is not intended to constitute an endorsement of such. Some material may include information on applications that are not considered community standard, that reflect indications not included in approved FDA labeling, or that are approved for use only in restricted research settings. **The FDA has stated that it is the responsibility of the physician to determine the FDA status of each drug or device he or she wishes to use, and to use them with appropriate, informed patient consent in compliance with applicable law.** The Academy specifically disclaims any and all liability for injury or other damages of any kind, from negligence or otherwise, for any and all claims that may arise from the use of any recommendations or other information contained herein.

Cover image: From BCSC Section 12, *Retina and Vitreous*. Confocal scanning laser ophthalmoscopy multicolor fundus image (30° field of view) of a healthy eye. (*Courtesy of Lucia Sobrin, MD.*)

FSC
www.fsc.org
MIX
Paper from responsible sources
FSC® C001701

Printed in China.

Basic and Clinical Science Course

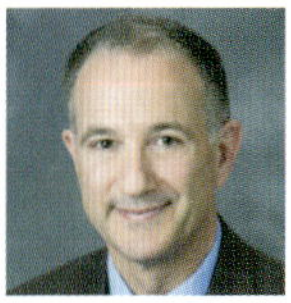

Christopher J. Rapuano, MD, Philadelphia, Pennsylvania
Senior Secretary for Clinical Education

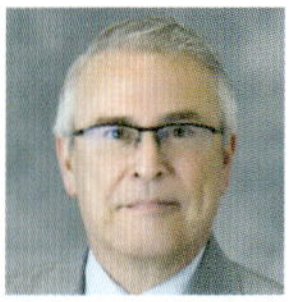

J. Timothy Stout, MD, PhD, MBA, Houston, Texas
Secretary for Lifelong Learning and Assessment

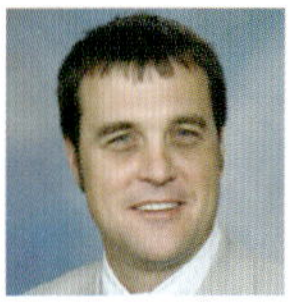

Colin A. McCannel, MD, Los Angeles, California
BCSC Course Chair

Section 11

Faculty for the Major Revision

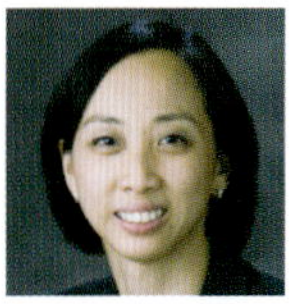

Linda M. Tsai, MD
Chair
St Louis, Missouri

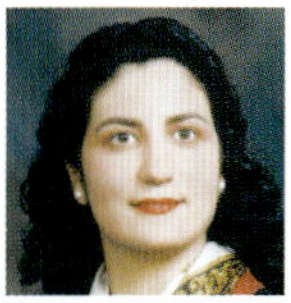

Natalie A. Afshari, MD
San Diego, California

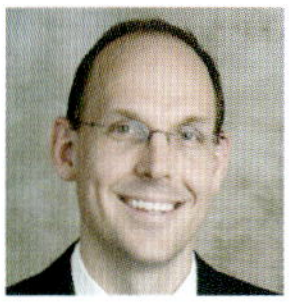

Chadwick R. Brasington, MD
Burlington, North Carolina

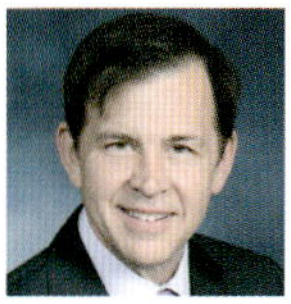

Charles Cole, MD
New York, New York

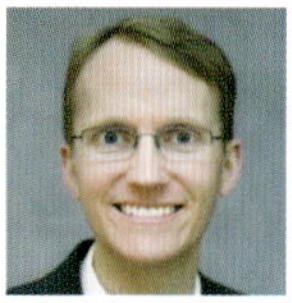

Benjamin D. Currie, MD
Holland, Michigan

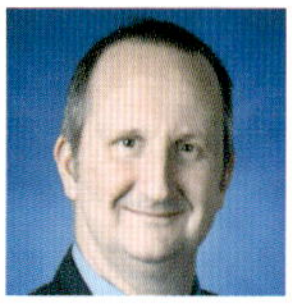

Bryan D. Edgington, MD
Portland, Oregon

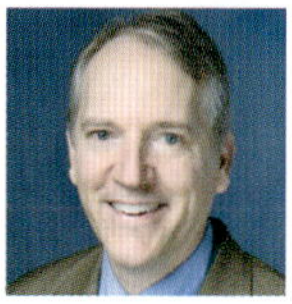

Erich P. Horn, MD, MBA
Gainesville, Florida

The Academy acknowledges the *American Society of Cataract and Refractive Surgery* and the *Contact Lens Association of Ophthalmologists* for recommending faculty members to the BCSC Section 11 committee.

The Academy also acknowledges the following committees for review of this edition:

Committee on Aging: Suzann Pershing, MD, Palo Alto, California

Vision Rehabilitation Committee: Linda M. Lawrence, MD, Salina, Kansas

BCSC Resident/Fellow Reviewers: Sharon L. Jick, MD, *Chair*, St Louis, Missouri; Michael P. Ellis, MD; Angela Jiang, MD; Grace L. Paley, MD, PhD; Daniel M. Vu, MD

Practicing Ophthalmologists Advisory Committee for Education: Cynthia S. Chiu, MD, *Primary Reviewer,* Oakland, California; Bradley D. Fouraker, MD, *Chair,* Tampa, Florida; George S. Ellis Jr, MD, New Orleans, Louisiana; Stephen R. Klapper, MD, Carmel, Indiana; Gaurav K. Shah, MD, Town and Country, Missouri; Rosa A. Tang, MD, MPH, MBA, Houston, Texas; Troy M. Tanji, MD, Waipahu, Hawaii; Michelle S. Ying, MD, Ladson, South Carolina

The Academy also acknowledges the following committee for assistance in developing Study Questions and Answers for this BCSC Section:

Resident Self-Assessment Committee: Robert A. Beaulieu, MD, Royal Oak, Michigan; Benjamin W. Botsford, MD, Pittsburgh, Pennsylvania; Olga M. Ceron, MD, Worcester, Massachusetts; Ian P. Conner, MD, PhD, Pittsburgh, Pennsylvania; Kimberly A. Crowder, MD, Jackson, Missouri; James Andrew David, MD, New Orleans, Louisiana; Claire E. Fraser, MD, PhD, Lexington, Kentucky; Kevin Halenda, MD, Augusta, Georgia; Rola N. Hamam, MD, Beirut, Lebanon; Amanda D. Henderson, MD, Baltimore, Maryland; Joshua Hendrix, MD, Dalton, Georgia; Matthew B. Kaufman, MD, Portland, Oregon; Sangeeta Khanna, MD, St Louis, Missouri; Chandrasekharan Krishnan, MD, Boston, Massachusetts; Ajay E. Kuriyan, MD, Pittsford, New York; Kevin E. Lai, MD, Indianapolis, Indiana; Kenneth C. Lao, MD, Temple, Texas; Ken Y. Lin, MD, Irvine, California; Kelly T. Mitchell, MD, Lubbock, Texas; Yasha S. Modi, MD, New York, New York; Matthew S. Pihlblad, MD, McDonald, Pennsylvania; Lorraine A. Provencher, MD, Cincinnati, Ohio; Jamie B. Rosenberg, MD, New York, New York; Syed Mahmood Shah, MD, Pittsburgh, Pennsylvania; Ann Shue, MD, Palo Alto, California; Misha F. Syed, MD, Galveston, Texas; Parisa Taravati, MD, Seattle, Washington; Sarah Van Tassel, MD, New York, New York; Evan L. Waxman, MD, PhD, Pittsburgh, Pennsylvania; Jules A. Winokur, MD, Great Neck, New York

In addition, the Academy recognizes the important contributions of David Beebe, PhD, in the development of Chapter 2.

EB

European Board of Ophthalmology: Béatrice Cochener-Lamard, MD, PhD, *Chair,* Brest, France; Marie-José Tassignon, MD, PhD, *Liaison,* Edegem, Belgium; Roberto Bellucci, MD, Salò, Italy; Simonetta Morselli, MD, Verona, Italy; Zoltan Nagy, MD, Budapest, Hungary

Financial Disclosures

Academy staff members who contributed to the development of this product state that within the 24 months prior to their contributions to this CME activity and for the duration of development, they have had no financial interest in or other relationship with any entity that produces, markets, resells, or distributes health care goods or services consumed by or used in patients, or with any competing commercial product or service.

The authors and reviewers state that within the 24 months prior to their contributions to this CME activity and for the duration of development, they have had the following financial relationships:*

Dr Afshari: Aescula Tech (C, O), Alpine Biotherapeutics (C, O), Dompé Pharmaceuticals (C), Shire (C), SPARK Therapeutics (C), Trefoil (C,O)

Dr Bellucci: Bausch + Lomb Surgical (C), Physiol (C), Sifi (C)

Dr Cochener-Lamard: Abbott Medical Optics (C, L), Alcon Laboratories (C, L), Bausch + Lomb (S), Horus (C, L), Physiol (C, L), ReVision Optics (C, L), Santen (C, L), Théa (C, L)

Dr Conner: Ocugenix (C, O, P)

Dr. Crowder: Gore (C), Medtronic (C), Phillips (C)

Dr Fouraker: Addition Technology (C, L), Alcon Laboratories (C, L), OASIS Medical (C, L)

Dr Hamam: Abbvie (C, L, S)

Dr Klapper: AdOM Advance Optical Technologies (O)

Dr Kuriyan: Alimera Sciences (C), Allergan (C), Regeneron (C), Second Sight (S) Valeant (C)

Dr Lin: Johnson & Johnson (C)

Dr Modi: Alimera (C), Allergan (C), Genentech (C), Novartis (C)

Dr Nagy: Alcon Laboratories (C, L)

Dr Pershing: Acumen, LLC (C)

Dr Gaurav Shah: Allergan (S, C), Bausch + Lomb (L), DORC International, bv/Dutch Ophthalmic, USA (S), Johnson & Johnson (L), QLT Phototherapeutics (C, L), Regeneron (C, L)

Dr Syed Shah: Quantum Analytics (O), Quantum Ophthalmic (O), Quantum Vision (O)

Dr Tang: EMD Serono (L), Horizon (C, S), Immunovant (S), Quark (C, S), Regenera (S), Sanofi (L), Zeiss (L)

Dr Tassignon: Morcher GmbH (P)

Dr Van Tassel: New World Medical (L)

The other authors and reviewers state that within the 24 months prior to their contributions to this CME activity and for the duration of development, they have had no financial interest in or other relationship with any entity that produces, markets, resells, or distributes health care goods or services consumed by or used in patients, or with any competing commercial product or service.

*C = consultant fee, paid advisory boards, or fees for attending a meeting; E = employed by or received a W2 from a commercial company; L = lecture fees or honoraria, travel fees or reimbursements when speaking at the invitation of a commercial company; O = equity ownership/stock options in publicly or privately traded firms, excluding mutual funds; P = patents and/or royalties for intellectual property; S = grant support or other financial support to the investigator from all sources, including research support from government agencies, foundations, device manufacturers, and/or pharmaceutical companies

Recent Past Faculty

Thomas L. Beardsley, MD
Carlos Buznego, MD
Richard J. Grostern, MD
Sharon L. Jick, MD
Lisa Park, MD
Timothy V. Roberts, MD

In addition, the Academy gratefully acknowledges the contributions of numerous past faculty and advisory committee members who have played an important role in the development of previous editions of the Basic and Clinical Science Course.

American Academy of Ophthalmology Staff

Dale E. Fajardo, EdD, MBA, *Vice President, Education*
Beth Wilson, *Director, Continuing Professional Development*
Denise Evenson, *Director, Brand & Creative*
Ann McGuire, *Acquisitions and Development Manager*
Stephanie Tanaka, *Publications Manager*
Susan Malloy, *Acquisitions Editor and Program Manager*
Jasmine Chen, *Manager, E-Learning*
Lana Ip, *Senior Designer*
Beth Collins, *Medical Editor*
Eric Gerdes, *Interactive Designer*
Lynda Hanwella, *Publications Specialist*
Debra Marchi, *Permissions Assistant*

American Academy of Ophthalmology
655 Beach Street
Box 7424
San Francisco, CA 94120-7424

Contents

Introduction to the BCSC

The Basic and Clinical Science Course (BCSC) is designed to meet the needs of residents and practitioners for a comprehensive yet concise curriculum of the field of ophthalmology. The BCSC has developed from its original brief outline format, which relied heavily on outside readings, to a more convenient and educationally useful self-contained text. The Academy updates and revises the course annually, with the goals of integrating the basic science and clinical practice of ophthalmology and of keeping ophthalmologists current with new developments in the various subspecialties.

The BCSC incorporates the effort and expertise of more than 100 ophthalmologists, organized into 13 Section faculties, working with Academy editorial staff. In addition, the course continues to benefit from many lasting contributions made by the faculties of previous editions. Members of the Academy Practicing Ophthalmologists Advisory Committee for Education, Committee on Aging, and Vision Rehabilitation Committee review every volume before major revisions, as does a group of select residents and fellows. Members of the European Board of Ophthalmology, organized into Section faculties, also review volumes before major revisions, focusing primarily on differences between American and European ophthalmology practice.

Organization of the Course

The Basic and Clinical Science Course comprises 13 volumes, incorporating fundamental ophthalmic knowledge, subspecialty areas, and special topics:

1 Update on General Medicine
2 Fundamentals and Principles of Ophthalmology
3 Clinical Optics and Vision Rehabilitation
4 Ophthalmic Pathology and Intraocular Tumors
5 Neuro-Ophthalmology
6 Pediatric Ophthalmology and Strabismus
7 Oculofacial Plastic and Orbital Surgery
8 External Disease and Cornea
9 Uveitis and Ocular Inflammation
10 Glaucoma
11 Lens and Cataract
12 Retina and Vitreous
13 Refractive Surgery

References

Readers who wish to explore specific topics in greater detail may consult the references cited within each chapter and listed in the Additional Materials and Resources section at the back of the book. These references are intended to be selective rather than exhaustive, chosen by the BCSC faculty as being important, current, and readily available to residents and practitioners.

Multimedia

This edition of Section 11, *Lens and Cataract,* includes videos related to topics covered in the book. Selected by members of the BCSC faculty, the videos are available to readers of the print and electronic versions of Section 11 (www.aao.org/bcscvideo_section11). Mobile-device users can scan the QR code below (you may need to install a QR-code reader on the device) to access the video content.

Self-Assessment and CME Credit

Each volume of the BCSC is designed as an independent study activity for ophthalmology residents and practitioners. The learning objectives for this volume are given on page 1. The text, illustrations, and references provide the information necessary to achieve the objectives; the study questions allow readers to test their understanding of the material and their mastery of the objectives. Physicians who wish to claim CME credit for this educational activity may do so by following the instructions given at the end of the book.*

Conclusion

The Basic and Clinical Science Course has expanded greatly over the years, with the addition of much new text, numerous illustrations, and video content. Recent editions have sought to place greater emphasis on clinical applicability while maintaining a solid foundation in basic science. As with any educational program, it reflects the experience of its authors. As its faculties change and medicine progresses, new viewpoints emerge on controversial subjects and techniques. Not all alternate approaches can be included in this series; as with any educational endeavor, the learner should seek additional sources, including Academy Preferred Practice Pattern Guidelines.

The BCSC faculty and staff continually strive to improve the educational usefulness of the course; you, the reader, can contribute to this ongoing process. If you have any suggestions or questions about the series, please do not hesitate to contact the faculty or the editors.

The authors, editors, and reviewers hope that your study of the BCSC will be of lasting value and that each Section will serve as a practical resource for quality patient care.

*This activity meets the Self-Assessment CME requirements defined by the American Board of Ophthalmology (ABO). Please be advised that the ABO is not an accrediting body for purposes of any CME program. ABO does not sponsor this or any outside activity, and ABO does not endorse any particular CME activity. Complete information regarding the ABO Self-Assessment CME Maintenance of Certification requirements is available at https://abop.org/maintain-certification/cme-self-assessment/.

Objectives

Upon completion of BCSC Section 11, *Lens and Cataract,* the reader should be able to

- describe the normal anatomy, embryologic development, physiology, and biochemistry of the crystalline lens
- identify congenital anomalies of the lens
- list types of congenital and acquired cataracts
- describe the association of cataracts with aging, trauma, medications, and systemic and ocular diseases
- describe the evaluation and management of patients with cataract and other lens abnormalities
- state the principles of cataract surgery techniques and associated surgical technology
- describe an appropriate differential diagnosis and management plan for intraoperative and postoperative complications of cataract surgery
- identify special circumstances in which cataract surgery techniques should be modified, and describe appropriate treatment plans

Introduction to Section 11

The ancient Greeks and Romans believed that the lens was the part of the eye responsible for the faculty of seeing. They theorized that the optic nerves were hollow channels through which "visual spirits" traveled from the brain to meet visual rays from the outside world at the lens, which they thought was located in the center of the globe. The visual information would then flow back to the brain. This concept was known as the *emanation theory of vision*. Celsus (25 BC–AD 50) drew the lens in the center of the globe, with an empty space called the *locus vacuus* anterior to it, in AD 30 (Fig I-1).

These erroneous ideas about lens position and function persisted through the Middle Ages and into the Renaissance, as shown by the drawing of the Belgian anatomist Andreas Vesalius in 1543 (Fig I-2). The true position of the crystalline lens was illustrated by the Italian anatomist Fabricius ab Aquapendente in 1600 (Fig I-3), and the Swiss physician Felix Plater (1536–1614) was the first to postulate that the retina, not the lens, was the part of the eye responsible for sight.

Today, many areas of lens physiology and biochemistry are still subjects of active research. Lens regeneration has been studied since the 18th century. This regeneration, from epithelial cells from the lens, cornea, or iris, has succeeded repeatedly in several vertebrate species, especially newts and rabbits. In 2016, an experimental trial in children with congenital cataracts was able to regenerate working lenses from intact lens epithelial

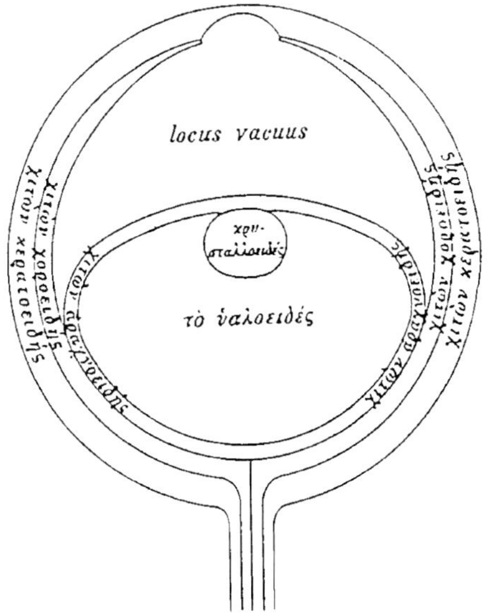

Figure I-1 The eye, after Celsus. *(From Gorin G.* History of Ophthalmology. *Wilmington: Publish or Perish, Inc; 1982.)*

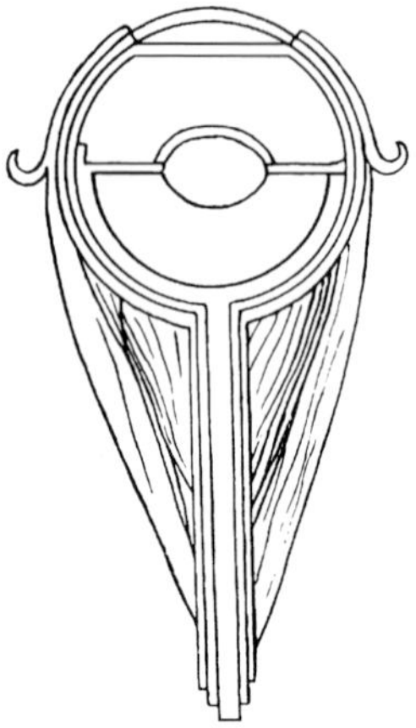

Figure I-2 Schematic eye from *De fabrica corporis humani* of Andreas Vesalius (1514–1564). *(Reproduced with permission from the Ophthalmic Publishing Company. Feigenbaum A. Early history of cataract and the ancient operation for cataract.* Am J Ophthalmol. *1960;49:307.)*

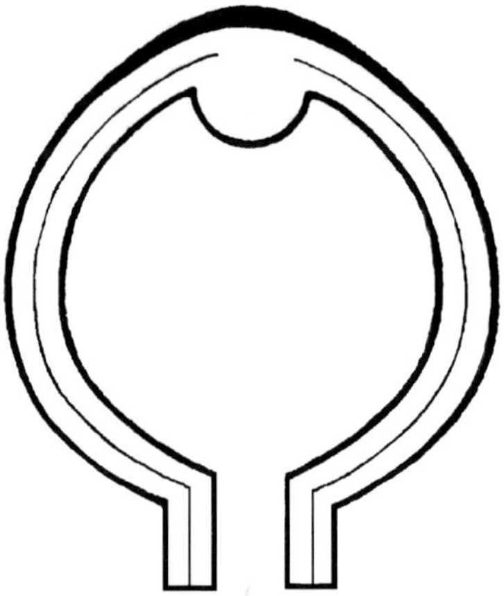

Figure I-3 Sketch from *De oculo* of Fabricius ab Aquapendente (1537–1619), showing the correct position of the lens within the eyeball. *(Reproduced with permission from the Ophthalmic Publishing Company. Feigenbaum A. Early history of cataract and the ancient operation for cataract.* Am J Ophthalmol. *1960;49:307.)*

stem cells within six to eight months. However, no medical treatment can yet prevent the formation or progression of cataract in the lens of the otherwise healthy adult eye, and theories about cataract formation and innovative forms of management continue to be controversial. Although various risk factors for cataract development have been identified (discussed in Chapter 1), data to develop guidelines for reducing the risk of cataract remain inconclusive.

The prevalence of lens disorders and continuing developments in their management make the basic and clinical science of this structure a vital component of ophthalmology training. The goal of Section 11 is to provide a curriculum for the study of the structure and function of the normal lens, the features of diseases involving the lens, and the surgical management of cataract.

Lin H, Ouyang H, Zhu J, et al. Lens regeneration using endogenous stem cells with gain of visual function. *Nature.* 2016;531(7594):323–328.

CHAPTER 1

Epidemiology of Cataract

Highlights

- Cataracts are a growing world health problem and a leading cause of blindness and visual impairment.
- The risk of developing cataracts is strongly correlated with older age, tobacco use, diabetes mellitus, and ultraviolet exposure. Other associated risk factors include hypertension, prolonged corticosteroid use, genetic predisposition, ocular trauma, high myopia, and female gender. The role of various diets and nutritional supplements for preventing cataract development has not been consistently proven.
- The global rate of cataract surgery is increasing and can be correlated to the economic availability of health care. Cataract surgery is cost-effective and associated with improved morbidity.

Introduction

Cataract is the leading cause of vision loss in the world. The World Health Organization (WHO) has estimated that more than 20 million people are blind due to cataract and that the condition causes 51% of blindness worldwide. The majority of cases (up to 90%) of blindness due to cataract are found in developing areas. Cataract is also the leading cause of visual impairment, with 33% of the world's population experiencing decreased vision because of this disorder; only refractive error has a greater impact in this regard.

Cataracts may be congenital, metabolic, age-related, or traumatic in origin. Cataracts affected 24.4 million individuals in the United States in 2015, and the Centers for Disease Control and Prevention (CDC) Vision Health Initiative estimates that this number is expected to rise to almost 39 million by 2030. Age-related cataracts are presumed to have the greatest socioeconomic impact because of their high prevalence. Congenital cataracts are responsible for 5%–20% of cases of blindness in children worldwide.

Pascolini D, Mariotti SP. Global estimates of visual impairment: 2010. *Br J Ophthalmol.* 2012;96(5):614–618.

Cataract Prevalence and Distribution of Subtypes

While the adverse impact of cataract on vision worldwide is undeniable, the lack of a widely accepted, standardized classification for lens opacities makes it difficult to precisely determine the incidence and prevalence of cataract. Most estimates of the frequency of age-related cataract are based on data from select groups rather than from the general population. These population-based studies had differences in methodology, disease definition, and study participants.

According to data published by the National Institute of Health (NIH) in 2010, the risk of developing cataract in the United States increases with each decade of life starting around age 40. By age 75, half of White individuals in the United States have cataract. By age 80, 70% of White individuals have cataract, compared with 53% of Black individuals and 61% of Hispanic American individuals. Among all people with cataracts in the United States, the vast majority (80%) were White, 8% were Black, and 7% were Hispanic; 61% were women and 39% were men.

The Beaver Dam Eye Study conducted in the late 1980s reported that 38.8% of men and 45.9% of women older than 74 years had visually significant cataracts. For this study, "visual significance" was determined by photographic grading of lens opacities and a specified best-corrected visual acuity of 20/32 (logarithm of the minimum angle of resolution [logMAR] equivalent closest to the 20/30 Snellen fraction), excluding individuals with severe age-related maculopathy.

A follow-up to the Beaver Dam Eye Study in the early 1990s found incident nuclear cataract occurred in 13.1%, cortical cataract in 8.0%, and posterior subcapsular cataract (PSC) in 3.4% in the study cohort. The incidence of all types of lens opacities rose with increasing age.

The 1998 Salisbury Eye Evaluation project was a prospective population-based cohort study designed to identify racial differences in the prevalence of cataracts in a group of Americans older than 65 years. Nuclear cataract was noted in 50.7% of White participants versus 33.5% of Black participants. Conversely, cortical cataract was more than 4 times more likely to be identified in Black individuals than in White individuals. PSC was found at roughly the same rate in both groups, between 5% and 10%.

The Barbados Eye Study provided prevalence data on lens opacities in a predominantly Black population. Cortical opacities were the most frequent type of cataract, and women had a higher frequency of opacification than did men.

Studies of Asian populations evaluating the incidence of different cataract subtypes include the Singapore Malay Eye Study and the Handan Eye Study. These studies suggest a higher rate of cortical cataract in Asian individuals than in White individuals. In 1994, the Italian-American Cataract Study Group conducted a study based in Parma, Italy. In this study's subgroup of participants aged 65–74, the cataract incidence was 18% cortical, 6% nuclear, and 6% PSC.

The prevalence of congenital cataract varies from country to country. Retrospective studies have shown a rate of 3 to 4 visually significant cataracts per 10,000 live births in the United States. Infantile cataracts can be unilateral or bilateral and can vary in size, morphology, and opacification. Affected vision, as well as the course of treatment and prognosis, is widely variable and is described in more detail in BCSC Section 6, *Pediatric Ophthalmology and Strabismus.*

The Italian-American Cataract Study Group. Incidence and progression of cortical, nuclear, and posterior subcapsular cataracts. *Am J Ophthalmol.* 1994;118(5):623–631.

Kahn HA, Leibowitz HM, Ganley JP, et al. The Framingham Eye Study. I. Outline and major prevalence findings. *Am J Epidemiol.* 1977;106(1):17–32.

Klein BE, Klein R, Lee KE. Incidence of age-related cataract: The Beaver Dam Eye Study. *Arch Ophthalmol.* 1998;116(2):216–225.

Livingston PM, Carson CA, Stanislavzky YL, Lee SE, Guest CS, Taylor HR. Methods for a population-based study of eye disease: The Melbourne Visual Impairment Project. *Ophthalmic Epidemiol.* 1994;1(3):139–148.

Leske MC, Connell AM, Wu SY, Hyman L, Schachat A. Prevalence of lens opacities in the Barbados Eye Study. *Arch Ophthalmol.* 1997;115(1):105–111.

Varma R, Richter GM, Torres M, et al; Los Angeles Eye Study Group. Four-year incidence and progression of lens opacities: the Los Angeles Latino Eye Study. *Am J Ophthalmol.* 2010;149(5):728–734.

West SK, Duncan DD, Muñoz B, et al. Sunlight exposure and risk of lens opacities in a population-based study: The Salisbury Eye Evaluation project. *JAMA.* 1998;280(8):714–718.

Wu R, Wang JJ, Mitchell P, et al. Smoking, socioeconomic factors, and age-related cataract: The Singapore Malay Eye Study. *Arch Ophthalmol.* 2010;128(8):1029–1035.

Risk Factors for the Development of Cataract

Correlations for cataract development have been found, some stronger than others, within various populations and geographic locations. Increasing age was a consistent risk factor across all studies. Smoking increases the risk for nuclear sclerotic cataract and PSC. The Beaver Dam Eye Study and the Blue Mountains Eye Study, among others, concluded that there was a higher and dose-related risk of cataract development for study participants who smoked. Some smoking-related damage to the lens may be reversible upon cessation. Diabetes mellitus and exposure to ultraviolet light are also well-established and consistent risk factors for cataract development.

Additional studies have suggested hypertension, prolonged corticosteroid use (systemic, inhaled, and topical), ocular trauma (including prior ocular surgery), genetic predisposition, and high myopia as a risk factors for cataract development. Although high myopia was clearly associated with an increased incidence of nuclear cataract, all forms of myopia (low, moderate, and high) were associated with increased incidence of cataract surgery.

Studies have inconsistently associated certain other risk factors with cataract development. These factors include exogenous estrogen use, increased body mass index, and alcohol consumption. Heavy alcohol consumption increased the risk of cataract development, whereas moderate consumption may be protective.

The role of nutrition in cataract prevention (specifically, the potential benefit of antioxidant supplementation) has long been a subject of interest and controversy.

Although some initial studies suggested that increased intake of vitamins C and E could be beneficial in cataract prevention, in the Age-Related Eye Disease Study 1 (AREDS1), a formulation of vitamin C, vitamin E, beta carotene, zinc, and copper did not reduce the risk of progression to cataract surgery. In a large Italian trial, use of a multivitamin and mineral supplement benefited individuals with nuclear sclerotic cataract but increased the risk of PSC development. The Age-Related Eye Disease Study 2 (AREDS2) concluded that lutein/zeaxanthin supplements had no significant overall effect on rates of progression to cataract surgery, although patients in the lowest quintile of dietary lutein/zeaxanthin intake did have a reduced risk of cataract development following supplementation.

Age-Related Eye Disease Study Research Group. Risk factors associated with age-related nuclear and cortical cataract: a case-control study in the Age-Related Eye Disease Study, AREDS Report No. 5. *Ophthalmology.* 2001;108(8):1400–1408.

Chew EY, SanGiovanni JP, Ferris FL, et al; Age-Related Eye Disease Study 2 (AREDS2) Research Group. Lutein/zeaxanthin for the treatment of age-related cataract: AREDS2 randomized trial report no. 4. *JAMA Ophthalmol.* 2013;131(7):843–850.

Mitchell P, Cumming RG, Attebo K, Panchapakesan. Prevalence of cataract in Australia: The Blue Mountains Eye Study. *Ophthalmology*. 1997;104(4):581–588.

Cataract Surgery Rate and Outcomes

Globally, over 10 million cataract operations are performed each year. Cataract surgical rate and economic indicators have been shown to be closely associated to each other, indicating the strong influence of resource availability on health care delivery. In developed areas, the rate of cataract surgery can reach up to 10,000 surgeries per million population per year. The highest rates have been reported in Malta, Japan, Suriname, Hungary, Croatia, Australia, Argentina, and the United States. In most developing areas in the Asia-Pacific region, and in many countries in Africa, the surgery rate is less than 500 surgeries per million. In some developing areas, the number may be as low as 150 surgeries per million. The WHO has determined that due to population growth and increasing longevity, the number of cataract surgeries performed worldwide has to triple to keep pace with need, with a goal of 3000 surgeries per million population annually.

Cataract surgery is correlated with reduced morbidity. A 2004 prospective study by Harwood, et al found that first-eye cataract surgery was statistically significant in reducing the rate of falling, thereby reducing the risk of fractures, as well as improving visual function and general health status in women over the age of 70. In 2012, a study of over 1.1 million US Medicare beneficiaries aged 65 and older determined that patients who had been diagnosed with cataracts had a reduced risk of hip fracture within 1 year after surgery compared with patients who had not undergone cataract surgery. Patients who have undergone cataract surgery also receive higher scores on standardized cognition assessments after the procedure.

A 2013 follow-up of the Blue Mountains Eye Study showed that cataract surgical correction was associated with significantly better long-term survival of older persons. However, in 2018, a large prospective cohort study conducted by the Women's Health Initiative showed that in women participants aged 65 and older, cataract surgery was associated with an increased risk for all-cause mortality and mortality attributed to vascular, cancer-related, accidental, pulmonary, and infectious causes. It is unclear whether the results were related to the surgical procedure itself, or to the individual participants postponing the surgery until the hazard rates increased.

Cataract surgery is the most common surgery performed on an outpatient basis in the United States; approximately 3.5 million cataract surgeries are performed each year. The direct medical cost related to the treatment of cataract in the United States, including office visits, surgery, and prescriptions, is approximately $6.8 billion annually. The rate of cataract surgery has increased steadily over the last 3 decades, and so has the rate of second-eye surgeries within 3 months of the first. Although initial studies suggested second-eye cataract surgery had no effect on fall risk, a 2018 prospective study found that second-eye surgery provided additional benefits (73% fall reduction) compared to the number of falls before the first surgery, most likely due to increased binocular visual acuity and increased contrast sensitivity. Cataract surgery has been demonstrated to be a cost-effective intervention for visual improvement in the United States, with an estimated cost per-quality-adjusted life-year gain of $2020 for the first eye and $2727 for the second eye.

Feng YR, Meuleners LB, Fraser ML, Brameld KJ, Agramunt S. The impact of first and second eye cataract surgeries on falls: a prospective cohort study. *Clin Interv Aging.* 2018;13: 1457–1464.

Fong CS, Mitchell P, Rochtchina E, Teber ET, Hong T, Wang JJ. Correction of visual impairment by cataract surgery and improved survival in older persons: The Blue Mountains Eye Study cohort. *Ophthalmology.* 2013;120(9):1720–1727.

Gollogly HE, Hodge DO, St Sauver JL, Erie JC. Increasing incidence of cataract surgery: population-based study. *J Cataract Refract Surg.* 2013;39(9):1383–1389.

Harwood RH, Foss AJ, Osborn F, Gregson RM, Zaman A, Masud T. Falls and health status in elderly women following first eye cataract surgery: a randomised controlled trial. *Br J Ophthalmol.* 2005;89(1):53–59.

Tseng VL, Chlebowski RT, Yu F, et al. Association of cataract surgery with mortality in older women: findings from the Women's Health Initiative. *JAMA Ophthalmol.* 2018;136(1): 3–10.

Tseng VL, Yu F, Lum F, Coleman AL. Risk of fractures following cataract surgery in Medicare beneficiaries. *JAMA.* 2012;308(5):493–501.

Wang W, Yan W, Fotis K, et al. Cataract surgical rate and socioeconomics: a global study. *Invest Ophthalmol Vis Sci.* 2016;57(14):5872–5881.

CHAPTER 2

Anatomy

This chapter includes a related video. Go to www.aao.org/bcscvideo_section11 or scan the QR code in the text to access this content.

Highlights

- The lens contributes approximately 20.00 diopters (D) of the 60.00 D of power of an average eye.
- The anterior curvature of the lens increases with age, causing increased myopia. At the same time, the index of refraction decreases, which may make the eye more hyperopic.
- The central pole of the posterior lens capsule measures 2–4 μm thick.

See BCSC Section 2, *Fundamentals and Principles of Ophthalmology,* for additional discussion and illustrations of the topics covered in this chapter.

Normal Crystalline Lens

The crystalline lens is a transparent, biconvex structure located posterior to the iris and anterior to the vitreous body (Fig 2-1). The lens is suspended by numerous fibers that together are called the zonule. Collectively, this ring of fibers (zonule of Zinn) attaches the lens to the ciliary body and can be considered a ligament. Components of the lens include the capsule, the epithelium, the cortex, and the nucleus (Fig 2-2).

An imaginary line called the *optic axis* joins the anterior and posterior poles of the lens, passing through them. Hypothetical lines on the lens surface that pass from one pole to the other are referred to as *meridians.* The *equator* of the lens is its greatest circumference.

The functions of the lens are

- to maintain its own clarity
- to refract light
- to provide accommodation, in conjunction with the zonule and the ciliary body

Lacking a blood supply and innervation after fetal development, the lens depends entirely on the aqueous humor to meet its metabolic requirements and also to remove its wastes.

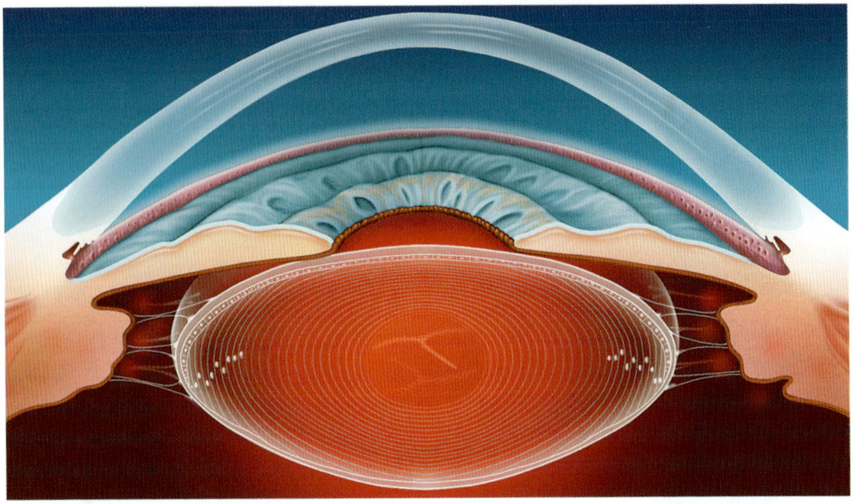

Figure 2-1 Cross section of the human crystalline lens, showing the relationship of the lens to surrounding ocular structures. *(Illustration by Christine Gralapp.)*

The lens is able to refract light because its index of refraction—normally about 1.4 in the center and 1.36 in the periphery—is different from that of the aqueous and vitreous humors surrounding it. In its nonaccommodative state, the lens contributes approximately 20.00 D of the approximately 60.00 D of convergent refractive power of the average human eye; the air–cornea interface provides the rest, about 40.00–45.00 D.

The lens continues to grow throughout an individual's life. At birth, it measures about 6.4 mm equatorially and 3.5 mm anteroposteriorly and weighs approximately 90 mg. The lens of an adult typically measures 9–10 mm equatorially and about 5 mm anteroposteriorly and weighs approximately 255 mg. With increasing age, the relative thickness of the cortex increases; the lens also adopts an increasingly curved shape, so that older lenses have more refractive power. However, the index of refraction of the lens decreases with increasing age, probably as a result of the increasing presence of insoluble protein particles. Thus, with increasing age, the eye may become either more hyperopic or more myopic, depending on the balance of these opposing changes.

Capsule

The lens capsule is an elastic, transparent basement membrane that is composed of type IV collagen and other matrix proteins and laid down by the epithelial cells. The capsule contains the lens substance and is capable of molding it during accommodative changes. The outer layer of the lens capsule, the *zonular lamella,* also serves as the point of attachment for the zonular fibers. The lens capsule is thickest in the anterior and posterior preequatorial zones and thinnest at the central posterior pole, where it may measure only 2–4 µm (Fig 2-3). At birth, the anterior lens capsule is considerably thicker than the posterior capsule; its thickness increases throughout a person's life.

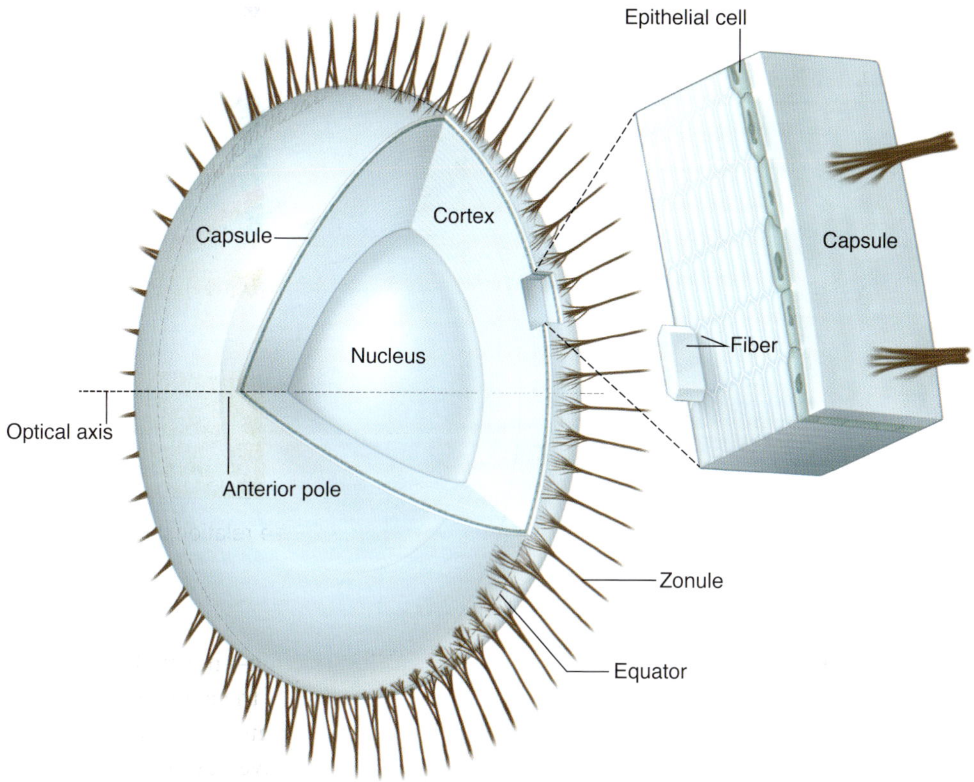

Figure 2-2 Structure of the normal human lens. *(Illustration by Mark Miller.)*

Zonular Fibers

As mentioned, the lens is supported by a system of fibers (the zonule) that originate from the basal lamina of the nonpigmented epithelium of the pars plana and pars plicata of the ciliary body. These zonular fibers, which are located in the valleys between the ciliary processes, consist of microfibrils composed of elastic tissue. They insert at discrete points on the lens capsule 1.5 mm anterior to the equator and 1.25 mm posterior to the equator (Fig 2-4). With increasing age, the equatorial zonular fibers regress, leaving separate anterior and posterior layers that appear in a triangular shape on cross section of the zonular ring. The fibers are 5–30 µm in diameter; on light microscopy, they are revealed as eosinophilic structures that have a positive periodic acid–Schiff (PAS) reaction. Ultrastructurally, the strands, or microfibrils, composing the fibers are 8–10 nm in diameter, with 12–14 nm of banding (Video 2-1).

VIDEO 2-1 Endoscopic view of ciliary body, zonular fibers, and lens capsule.
Courtesy of Charles Cole, MD.
Go to www.aao.org/bcscvideo_section11 to access all videos in Section 11.

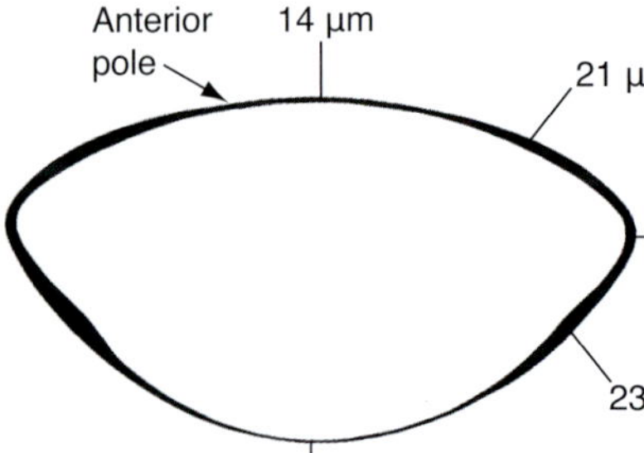

Figure 2-3 Schematic of the adult lens capsule showing the relative thickness of the capsule in different zones. *(Illustration by Christine Gralapp.)*

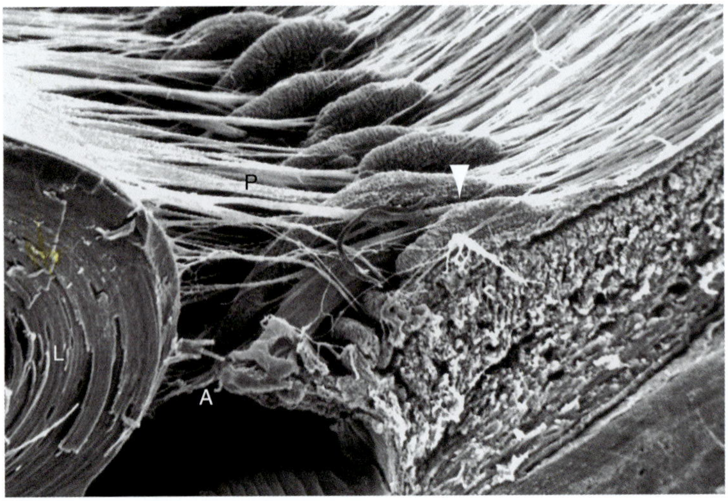

Figure 2-4 Scanning electron micrograph of a sagittally cut specimen of the ciliary body, zonular fibers, and lens *(L)* of the eye of a 4-year old rhesus monkey. The anterior *(A)* and posterior *(P)* zonules are attached to the zonular plexus *(arrowhead)* posteriorly in the valleys between the ciliary processes. *(Courtesy of Johannes W. Rohen, MD, PhD, and Cassandra Flügel-Koch, MD, PhD.)*

Lens Epithelium

Immediately posterior to the anterior lens capsule is a single layer of epithelial cells. These cells are metabolically active and carry out all normal cell activities, including biosynthesis of DNA, RNA, protein, and lipid. They also generate adenosine triphosphate to meet the energy demands of the lens. The epithelial cells are mitotic; the greatest activity of premitotic (replicative, or S phase) DNA synthesis occurs in a ring around the anterior lens known as the *germinative zone.* The newly formed cells migrate toward the equator, where they differentiate into fibers. This area, called the bow region, is where the epithelial cells begin the process of terminal differentiation into lens fibers (Fig 2-5).

During this differentiation, perhaps the most dramatic morphologic change occurs when the epithelial cells elongate to form lens fiber cells. This elongation is associated with a tremendous increase in the mass of cellular proteins in the fiber cell membrane. At the same time, the cells lose organelles, including nuclei, mitochondria, and ribosomes. The

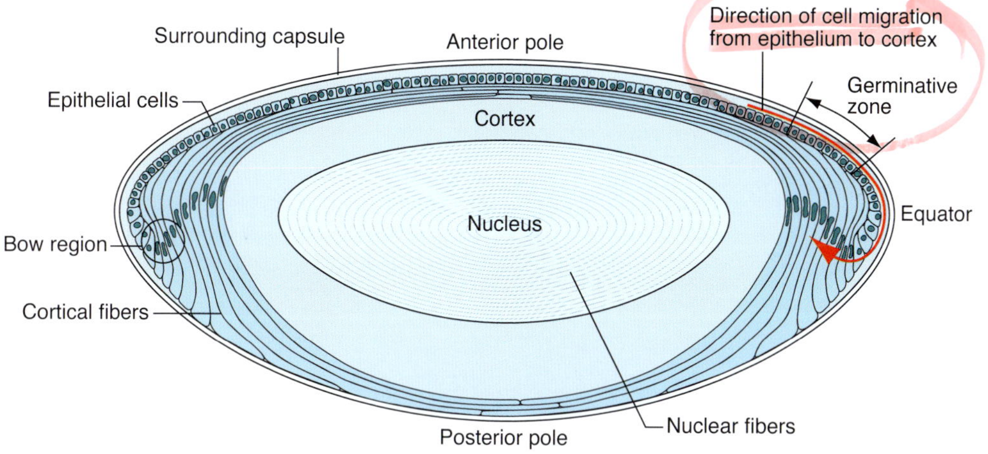

Figure 2-5 Schematic of the mammalian lens in cross section. *Arrow* indicates the direction of cell migration from the epithelium to the cortex. *(Illustration by Mark Miller.)*

loss of these organelles is optically advantageous, because light passing through the lens is no longer absorbed or scattered by these structures. However, because these new lens fiber cells lack the metabolic functions previously carried out by the organelles, they are now dependent on glycolysis for energy production (see Chapter 3 in this volume).

Nucleus and Cortex

As new fibers are laid down, no cells are lost from the lens. The new fibers crowd and compact the previously formed fibers; the older layers are located toward the center. The oldest layers, the *embryonic and fetal lens nuclei,* were produced during embryogenesis and persist in the center of the lens (see Chapter 4, Fig 4-1). The outermost fibers are the most recently formed and make up the cortex of the lens.

Lens sutures (see Chapter 4, Fig 4-1) are formed by the interdigitation of the anterior and posterior tips of the spindle-shaped fibers. Multiple optical zones, as well as Y-shaped sutures located within the lens nucleus, are visible on slit-lamp biomicroscopy. (See Chapter 4 in this volume for further discussion of the embryonic nucleus and lens sutures.)

Strata of epithelial cells with differing optical densities are laid down throughout life, creating the zones of demarcation between the cortex and the nucleus. However, there is no morphologic distinction between the cortex and the nucleus; rather, the transition between these regions is gradual. Although some surgical texts and this volume make distinctions between the nucleus, epinucleus, endonucleus, and cortex, these terms relate only to potential differences in the behavior and appearance of the material during surgical procedures.

Kuszak JR, Clark JI, Cooper KE, et al. Biology of the lens: lens transparency as a function of embryology, anatomy and physiology. In: Albert D, Miller J, Azar D, Blodi B, eds. *Albert & Jakobiec's Principles and Practice of Ophthalmology.* 3rd ed. Saunders; 2008: vol 1, chapter 104.

Snell RS, Lemp MA. *Clinical Anatomy of the Eye.* 2nd ed. Blackwell Science; 1998: 197–204.

CHAPTER 3

Biochemistry and Physiology

This chapter includes a related video. Go to www.aao.org/bcscvideo_section11 or scan the QR code in the text to access this content.

Highlights

- The human lens is composed of 66% water and 33% protein.
- Water-soluble proteins make up 80% of a young lens; water-insoluble proteins increase with both increasing age and opacification and make up as much as 90% of a brunescent cataract.
- Anaerobic glycolysis produces most of the ATP used in lens metabolism.
- High glucose levels in an individual result in elevated sorbitol and fructose within the lens.
- Accommodation increases the curvature of the central anterior lens surface and the dioptric power of the eye.

See BCSC Section 2, *Fundamentals and Principles of Ophthalmology,* for additional discussion of several of the topics discussed in this chapter.

Molecular Biology

Crystallin Proteins

The human lens has a protein concentration of 33% of its wet weight, which is at least twice the concentration found in most tissues. Lens proteins are commonly divided into 2 groups, based on water solubility (Fig 3-1); the ratio of these 2 groups changes with increasing age. Water-soluble proteins account for approximately 80% of lens proteins in a young lens; with increasing age, the percentage of water-insoluble proteins increases. The water-soluble group consists mainly of a group of proteins called *crystallins.* The crystallins can be divided into 2 major groups, α-crystallins and β,γ-crystallins.

α-Crystallins are the largest of the crystallins. In their native state, their molecular mass ranges between 600 and 800 kilodaltons (kDa); they represent about one-third of the lens proteins by mass. They may also combine with other crystallins, yielding complexes greater than 2×10^6. There are 2 α-crystallin subunits, αA and αB, each with a molecular mass of approximately 20 kDa, which form heteromeric complexes containing about 30 subunits. The α-crystallins are members of the family of small heat-shock proteins;

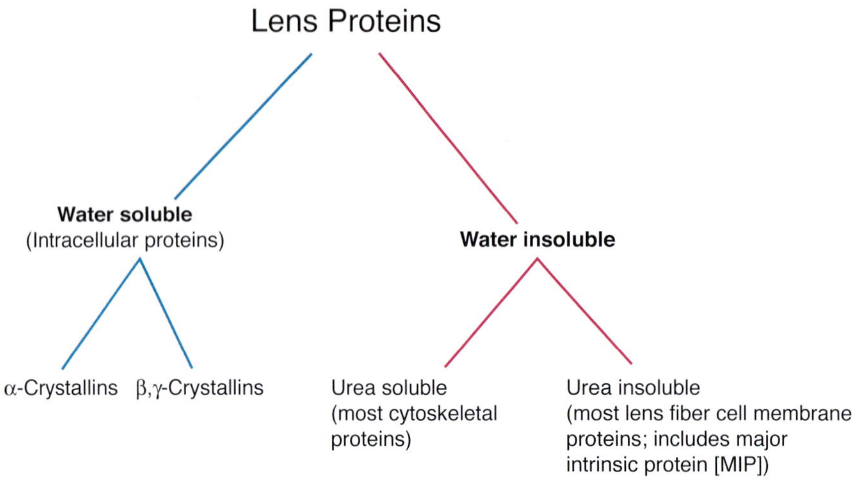

Figure 3-1 Overview of lens proteins.

their complexes bind to partially denatured proteins and prevent them from aggregating. Their primary function in lens fiber cells appears to be to inhibit the complete denaturation and insolubilization of the other crystallins.

The basic structure of the β-crystallins and γ-crystallins has been maintained through hundreds of millions of years of vertebrate evolution. X-ray studies have demonstrated fourfold repetition of a core 3-dimentional structural motif, suggesting that the β,γ-crystallins might have arisen from double duplication and fusion of a gene for a 40-residue polypeptide. β,γ-Crystallins are subdivided into 2 groups, based on molecular mass and isoelectric points.

The β-crystallins, a complex group of oligomers composed of polypeptides, are encoded by 7 genes. Their molecular masses range from 23 to 32 kDa. The individual polypeptides associate with each other, forming dimers and higher-order complexes in their native state. By gel chromatography, the β-crystallins can be separated into βH (β high-molecular-mass) and βL (β low-molecular-mass) fractions.

The γ-crystallins are the smallest of the crystallins, with a molecular mass in the range of 20 kDa or less. In humans, the gamma family is encoded by 4 genes. Because the native γ-crystallins do not associate with each other or with other proteins, they have the lowest molecular mass of the crystallin fractions.

Membrane Structural Proteins and Cytoskeletal Proteins

The water-insoluble fraction of lens proteins can be divided into 2 fractions based on solubility in an 8 molar (M) solution of urea:

- The *urea-soluble fraction* of the young lens contains cytoskeletal proteins that provide the structural framework of the lens cells.
- The *urea-insoluble fraction* of the young lens contains the plasma membranes of the lens fiber cells.

In the urea-soluble fraction of the lens, the microfilaments and microtubules found are similar to those found in other cell types. However, the lens contains 2 types of intermediate filaments that are unusual: 1 class is made from the protein *vimentin,* which is not usually found in epithelial cells; the other class, the *beaded filaments,* is composed of the proteins phakinin and filensin, which are specific to the lens. Genetic disruption of the structure of the beaded filaments leads to disruption of the structure of the lens fiber cells and ultimately to the formation of a cataract.

In the urea-insoluble fraction of the lens, several proteins are associated with the fiber-cell plasma membranes. One of these makes up nearly 50% of the membrane proteins and is known as the *major intrinsic protein* (*MIP;* also known as *aquaporin 0*), a member of a class of proteins called *aquaporins.* Other members of the aquaporin family are found throughout the body, where they serve predominantly as water channels. MIP first appears in the lens just as the fibers begin to elongate. With increasing age, this protein, which has a molecular mass of 28 kDa, undergoes proteolytic cleavage, forming a protein fragment with a molecular mass of 22 kDa. When an individual reaches 20–30 years of age, the relative proportions of these 2 proteins become about equal. Over time, the protein fragment that started with the molecular mass of 22 kDa predominates in the lens nucleus.

Hejtmancik JF, Piatigorsky J. Lens proteins and their molecular biology. In: Albert D, Miller J, Azar D, Blodi B, eds. *Albert & Jakobiec's Principles and Practice of Ophthalmology.* 3rd ed. Saunders; 2008: vol 1, chapter 105.

Increase of Water-Insoluble Proteins With Age

As the lens ages, its proteins aggregate, forming very large particles. These particles become water-insoluble and scatter light, increasing the opacity of the lens. Even if the lens remains relatively transparent, the water-insoluble protein fraction increases with age. Although conversion of the water-soluble proteins into water-insoluble proteins appears to be a natural process in lens fiber maturation, it may occur more quickly in cataractous lenses.

In cataracts with significant browning of the lens nucleus *(brunescent cataracts),* the increase in the amount of water-insoluble protein is directly correlated to the degree of opacification. In markedly brunescent cataracts, up to 90% of the nuclear proteins may be insoluble. Associated oxidative changes, including protein-to-protein and protein-to-glutathione disulfide bond formation, result in decreased levels of the reduced form of glutathione and increased levels of glutathione disulfide (oxidized glutathione) in the cytoplasm of the nuclear fiber cells. Glutathione is generally considered essential to maintain a reducing environment in the lens cytoplasm. Depletion of the reduced form of glutathione accelerates protein crosslinking, protein aggregation, and light scattering.

In addition to the increased formation of disulfide bonds, nuclear proteins are highly crosslinked by nondisulfide bonds. This insoluble protein fraction contains yellow-to-brown pigments that are found in higher concentration in nuclear cataracts. Increased fluorescence is generated by the nondisulfide crosslinks that form in brunescent nuclear cataracts.

Carbohydrate Metabolism

See Figure 3-2 for an overall diagram of glucose metabolism in the lens.

Clinical considerations Lens metabolism maintains a clear lens and derives most of its energy from anaerobic glycolysis. In high-glucose conditions, hexokinase becomes inhibited by products of glycolysis, and aldose reductase becomes relatively increased, converting more glucose to sorbitol. Sorbitol is poorly permeable, and elevated levels of both sorbitol and fructose increase the osmotic pressure within the lens, resulting in myopic shift, disruption of normal cytoskeletal architecture, and opacification of the lens.

Glycolysis and Hexose Monophosphate Shunt

The goal of lens metabolism is the maintenance of lens transparency. In the lens, energy production largely depends on glucose metabolism. Glucose enters the lens from the aqueous humor both by *simple diffusion* and by a mediated transfer process called *facilitated diffusion*. Most of the glucose transported into the lens is phosphorylated to glucose-6-phosphate (G6P) by the enzyme hexokinase. This reaction is 70–100 times slower than that of other enzymes involved in lens glycolysis and is, therefore, rate-limited. Once formed, G6P enters 1 of 2 metabolic pathways:

- *Anaerobic glycolysis*. The more active of the 2 pathways, anaerobic glycolysis provides most of the high-energy phosphate bonds required for lens metabolism. In anaerobic glycolysis, substrate-linked phosphorylation of adenosine diphosphate (ADP) to adenosine triphosphate (ATP) occurs at 2 steps along the pathway from glucose metabolism to lactate. The rate-limiting step in the glycolytic pathway itself occurs at the level of the enzyme phosphofructokinase, which is regulated via feedback control by metabolic products of the glycolytic pathway. This pathway is much less efficient than the aerobic citric acid cycle (also called the tricarboxylic acid cycle or the Krebs cycle), because only 2 net molecules of ATP are produced for each glucose molecule utilized, whereas the aerobic citric acid cycle produces an additional 36 molecules of ATP from each metabolized glucose molecule (oxidative metabolism). Because of the low oxygen tension in the lens, only about 3% of the lens glucose passes through the citric acid cycle to produce ATP; however, even this low level of aerobic metabolism produces approximately 25% of the ATP of the lens.
- *The hexose monophosphate (HMP) shunt*. Also known as the *pentose phosphate pathway*, the HMP shunt is the less active pathway for utilization of G6P in the lens—on average, less than 5% of lens glucose is metabolized by this route. This pathway, which is stimulated in the presence of elevated levels of glucose, is involved in the generation of NADPH or reducing power.

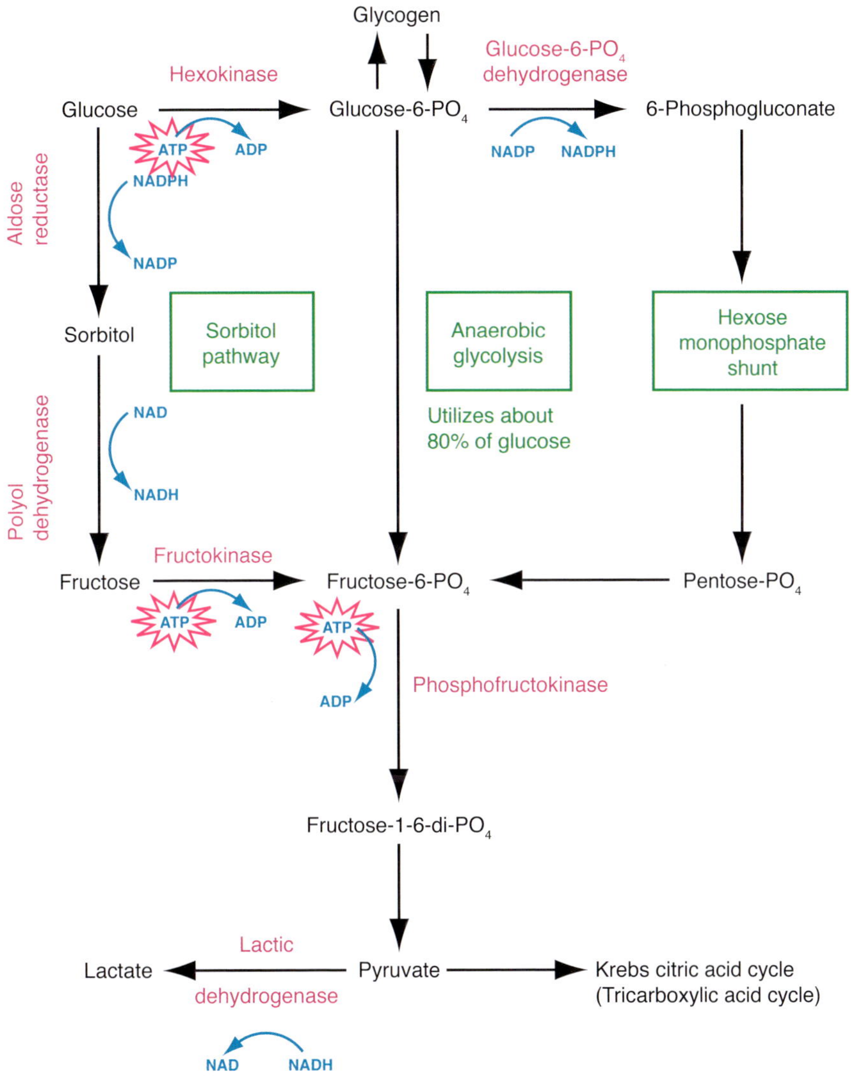

Figure 3-2 Simplified scheme of glucose metabolism in the lens. *(Adapted with permission from Hart WM Jr, ed.* Adler's Physiology of the Eye: Clinical Application. *9th ed. St Louis: Mosby; 1992:362.)*

Sorbitol Pathway

The glucose that is not phosphorylated to G6P enters the *sorbitol pathway,* which is yet another pathway for lens glucose metabolism, or it is converted into gluconic acid. The key enzyme in the sorbitol pathway is aldose reductase; this enzyme has been found to play a pivotal role in the development of "sugar" cataracts. In comparison with hexokinase, aldose reductase has a very low affinity for glucose. Less than 4% of lens glucose is normally converted to sorbitol.

As noted in the previous section, the hexokinase reaction is rate-limited in phosphorylating glucose in the lens and is inhibited by the feedback mechanisms of the products of glycolysis. When the amount of glucose increases in the lens (as occurs in individuals in hyperglycemic states), the sorbitol pathway is activated relatively more than the glycolytic pathway, and sorbitol accumulates (Fig 3-3).

Sorbitol is metabolized to fructose by the enzyme polyol dehydrogenase. Unfortunately, this enzyme has a relatively low affinity (high K_m [Michaelis constant; the apparent affinity constant]), meaning that considerable sorbitol will accumulate before being further metabolized. This characteristic, combined with the poor permeability of the lens to sorbitol, results in retention of sorbitol in the lens.

A high ratio of NADPH/NADH drives the reaction in the direction of sorbitol accumulation. The accumulation of NADP that occurs as a consequence of activation of the

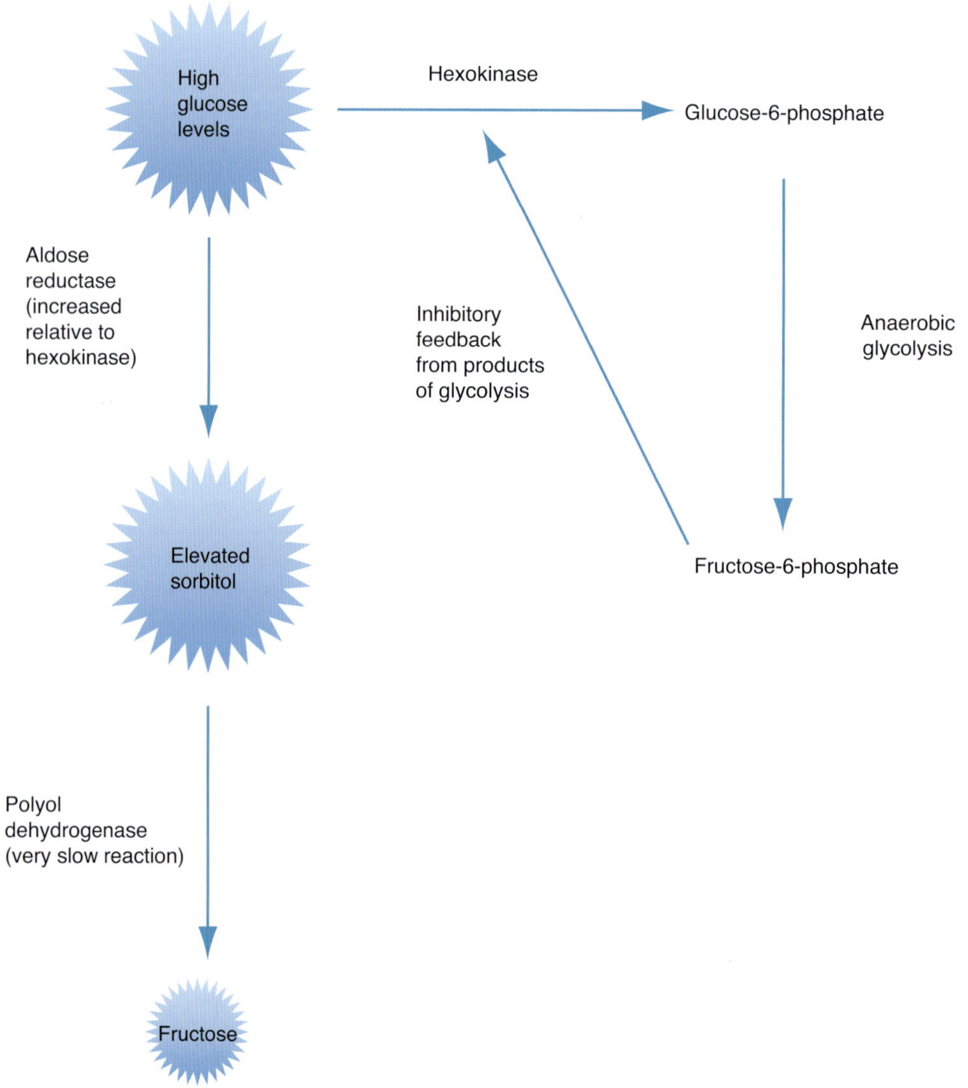

Figure 3-3 Sorbitol pathway in hyperglycemic state. *(Courtesy of Charles Cole, MD.)*

sorbitol pathway may cause the HMP shunt stimulation that is observed in the presence of an elevated lens glucose level. In addition to sorbitol, fructose levels increase in a lens incubated in a high-glucose environment. Together, the 2 sugars increase the osmotic pressure within the lens, drawing in water. At first, the energy-dependent pumps of the lens are able to compensate, but ultimately, they are overwhelmed, resulting in swelling of the fibers, disruption of the normal cytoskeletal architecture, and opacification of the lens.

Studies of cataract development in various hyperglycemic animal species demonstrate the pivotal role of aldose reductase in cataractogenesis in animals. Those species that have high aldose reductase activities develop lens opacities, whereas those lacking aldose reductase do not. In addition, specific inhibitors of this enzymatic activity, applied either systemically or topically to 1 eye, decrease the rate of onset and the severity of glucose cataracts in experimental studies.

Clinical considerations The lens is able to sustain normal metabolism in a nitrogen environment. Provided with ample glucose, the anoxic in vitro lens remains completely transparent, has normal levels of ATP, and maintains its ion and amino acid pump activities. However, when deprived of glucose, the lens cannot maintain these functions and becomes hazy after several hours, even in the presence of oxygen.

Oxidative Damage and Protective Mechanisms

Free radicals are generated in the course of normal cellular metabolic activities and may also be produced by external agents such as radiant energy. These free radicals, which are highly reactive, can damage lens fibers. Peroxidation of lens fiber plasma or plasma membrane lipids has been suggested as a factor contributing to lens opacification.

Because oxygen tension in and around the lens is normally low, free radical reactions may not involve molecular oxygen; instead, the free radicals may react directly with molecules. DNA is easily damaged by free radicals. Although some of the damage to the lens is reparable, some of it may be permanent. Free radicals can also attack the proteins or membrane lipids in the lens cortex. No repair mechanisms are known to ameliorate such damage. In lens fibers, where protein is no longer synthesized, free radical damage may lead to polymerization and crosslinking of lipids and proteins, resulting in an increase in the water-insoluble protein content.

The lens is equipped with several enzymes that work together to destroy the superoxide anion, O_2^-, thus protecting against free radical or oxidative damage (Fig 3-4):

- Superoxide dismutase catalyzes the destruction of the superoxide anion, O_2^-.
- Catalase breaks down the hydrogen peroxide produced by superoxide dismutase.
- Glutathione peroxidase catalyzes a reaction that results in the formation of glutathione disulfide (GSSG), which is then reconverted to glutathione (GSH) by glutathione reductase, using the pyridine nucleotide NADPH. The primary source of erythrocyte NADPH, the HMP shunt provides NADPH as the reducing agent. Thus, glutathione acts indirectly as a major free radical scavenger in the lens.

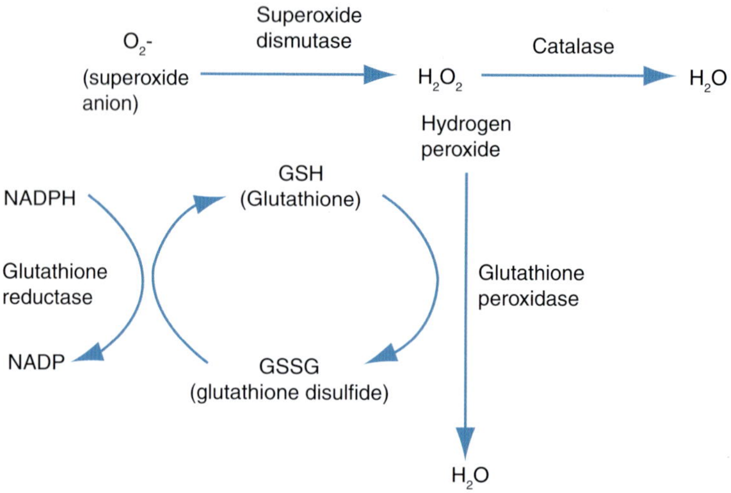

Figure 3-4 Free radical scavenger pathway in the lens. *(Courtesy of Charles Cole, MD.)*

Additionally, both vitamin E and ascorbic acid are present in the lens. Each of these substances can act as a free radical scavenger and thus protect against oxidative damage.

Clinical considerations Increased oxygen levels in the eye may have a role in cataract formation. Long-term hyperbaric oxygen therapy leads to myopic shift, increased opacification of the lens nucleus, and often nuclear cataracts. The lens is also exposed to increased oxygen acutely during retina procedures and chronically after vitrectomy. Because vitrectomy is associated with high rates of nuclear cataract formation, it has been suggested that the low oxygen level created by the gel structure of the vitreous body protects the lens from oxidative damage.

Beebe DC. The lens. In: Kaufman PL, Alm A, eds. *Adler's Physiology of the Eye: Clinical Application.* 11th ed. Mosby; 2011:131–163.

Lens Physiology

Throughout life, lens epithelial cells at the equator divide and develop into lens fibers, resulting in continual growth of the lens (see Chapter 2, Figs 2-2 and 2-5, in this volume). The lens cells with the highest metabolic rate are found in the epithelium and outer cortex. These superficial cells utilize oxygen and glucose for the active transport of electrolytes, carbohydrates, and amino acids into the lens. Because the lens is avascular, the task of maintaining transparency poses several challenges. The older cells, found toward the center of the lens, must be able to communicate with the superficial cells and the environment outside the lens. This communication is accomplished through low-resistance gap junctions that facilitate the exchange of small molecules from cell to cell. Lens fiber cells also have abundant water channels in their membranes, made up of MIP. It is not yet certain whether MIP serves primarily in the lens as a water channel, as an adhesion molecule that minimizes the extracellular space between fiber cells, or as both. Minimizing the extracellular space between fiber cells is important in reducing the scattering of light as it passes through the lens.

Maintenance of Lens Water and Cation Balance

The normal human lens contains approximately 66% water and 33% protein, and this proportion changes very little with aging. The lens cortex is more hydrated than the lens nucleus. About 5% of the lens volume is the water found between the lens fibers in the extracellular spaces. Within the lens, sodium and potassium concentrations are maintained at 20 millimolar (mM) and 120 mM, respectively.

Perhaps the most important aspect of lens physiology is the mechanism that controls water and electrolyte balance, which is critical to lens transparency. Because transparency is highly dependent on the structural and macromolecular components of the lens, perturbation of cellular hydration can readily lead to opacification. It is noteworthy that disruption of water and electrolyte balance is not a feature of nuclear cataracts. In cortical cataracts, however, the water content rises significantly.

Lens epithelium: site of active transport

The lens is less hydrated and has higher levels of potassium ions (K^+) and amino acids than the surrounding aqueous and vitreous humors. Conversely, the lens contains lower levels of sodium ions (Na^+), chloride ions (Cl^-), and water than its surrounding environment. The cation balance between the inside and outside of the lens is the result both of the permeability properties of the lens cell membranes and of the activity of the sodium-potassium pumps, which reside within the cell membranes of the lens epithelium and each lens fiber. The mechanism of the sodium-potassium pumps, namely pumping sodium ions out while taking potassium ions in, relies on the breakdown of ATP and is regulated by the enzyme Na^+,K^+-ATPase. Inhibition of Na^+,K^+-ATPase leads to loss of cation balance and elevated water content in the lens.

Pump–leak theory

The combination of active transport and membrane permeability is often referred to as the pump–leak system of the lens (Fig 3-5). According to the *pump–leak theory,* potassium and various other molecules, such as amino acids, are actively transported into the lens anteriorly via the epithelium. They then passively diffuse out with the concentration gradient through the back of the lens, where there are no active-transport mechanisms. Conversely, sodium flows in through the back of the lens with the concentration gradient and then is actively exchanged for potassium by the epithelium.

In support of the pump–leak theory, an anteroposterior gradient was found for both ions: potassium was concentrated in the anterior lens; sodium, in the posterior lens. Most of the Na^+,K^+-ATPase activity is found in the lens epithelium and the superficial cortical fiber cells. The active-transport mechanisms are lost if the capsule and attached epithelium are removed from the lens but not if the capsule alone is removed by enzymatic

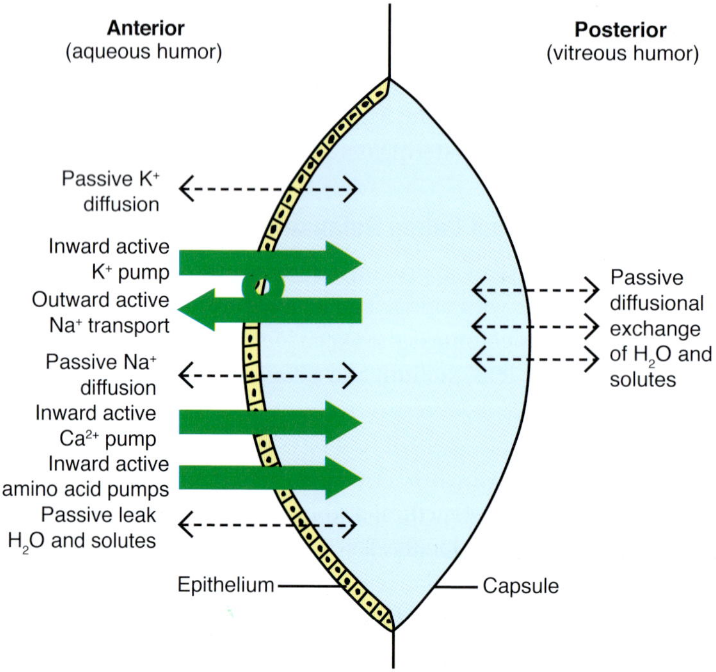

Figure 3-5 The pump–leak hypothesis of pathways of solute movement in the lens. The major site of active-transport mechanisms is the anterior epithelium, whereas passive diffusion occurs over both surfaces of the lens. *(Modified with permission from Paterson CA, Delamere NA. The lens. In: Hart WM Jr, ed.* Adler's Physiology of the Eye. *9th ed. Mosby; 1992:365.)*

degradation with collagenase. These findings support the hypothesis that the epithelium is the primary site for active transport in the lens.

Accommodation and Presbyopia

Accommodation, the mechanism by which the eye changes focus from distant to near images, occurs when the action of the ciliary muscle on the zonular fibers changes the lens shape. The lens substance is most malleable during childhood and the young-adult years, progressively losing its ability to change shape with increasing age.

According to the Helmholtz theory of accommodation, most of the accommodative change in lens shape occurs at the central anterior lens surface. The central anterior capsule is thinner than the peripheral capsule (see Chapter 2, Fig 2-3), and the anterior zonular fibers insert slightly closer to the visual axis than do the posterior zonular fibers, resulting in a central anterior bulge during accommodation. The curvature of the posterior lens surface changes minimally with accommodation. The central posterior capsule, which is the thinnest area of the capsule, maintains the same curvature regardless of zonular tension.

The ciliary muscle is a ring-shaped muscle that, on contraction, has the opposite effect from what one intuitively expects of a sphincter. When a sphincter muscle contracts,

Table 3-1 Changes With Accommodation

	With Accommodation	Without Accommodation
Ciliary muscle action	Contraction	Relaxation
Ciliary ring diameter	Decreases	Increases
Zonular tension	Decreases	Increases
Lens shape	More spherical	Flatter
Lens equatorial diameter	Decreases	Increases
Axial lens thickness	Increases	Decreases
Central anterior lens capsule curvature	Steepens	Flattens
Central posterior lens capsule curvature	Minimal change	Minimal change
Lens dioptric power	Increases	Decreases

it usually tightens its grip. However, when the ciliary muscle contracts, the diameter of the muscle ring is reduced, thereby relaxing the tension on the zonular fibers and allowing the lens to become more spherical. Thus, when the ciliary muscle contracts, the axial thickness of the lens increases, the equatorial diameter of the lens decreases, and the dioptric power of the lens increases, resulting in accommodation. When the ciliary muscle relaxes, the zonular tension increases, the lens flattens, and the dioptric power of the eye decreases (Table 3-1; Video 3-1).

VIDEO 3-1 Changes with accommodation.
Courtesy of Charles Cole, MD.
Go to www.aao.org/bcscvideo_section11 to access all videos in Section 11.

The accommodative response may be stimulated by the known or apparent size and distance of an object or by blur, chromatic aberration, or a continual oscillation of ciliary tone. Accommodation is mediated by the parasympathetic fibers of cranial nerve III (the oculomotor nerve). Parasympathomimetic drugs (eg, pilocarpine) induce accommodation, whereas parasympatholytic medications (eg, atropine) block accommodation. Drugs that relax the ciliary muscle are called *cycloplegics.*

The *amplitude of accommodation* is the amount of change in the eye's refractive power that is produced by accommodation. It diminishes with age and may be affected by some medications and diseases.

CLINICAL PEARL

In adolescents, the accommodative power is generally 12.00–16.00 diopters (D); by age 40 years, the power has decreased to 4.00–8.00 D. After age 50, the average accommodative power decreases to less than 2.00 D.

Presbyopia is the gradual loss of accommodative response, resulting from reduced elasticity of the crystalline lens. Once an individual is approximately 40 years of age or older, the rigidity of the lens nucleus reduces accommodation, as contraction of the ciliary muscle no longer results in increased convexity and dioptric power of the anterior surface of the lens. This decreased accommodation then becomes clinically significant. Studies have shown that, throughout life, the hardness or stiffness of the human lens increases more than 1000-fold. (See also BCSC Section 3, *Clinical Optics and Vision Rehabilitation.*)

Glasser A. Accommodation. In: Kaufman PL, Alm A, eds. *Adler's Physiology of the Eye: Clinical Application.* 11th ed. Mosby; 2011:40–69.

CHAPTER 4

Embryology and Developmental Defects

This chapter includes a related video. Go to www.aao.org/bcscvideo_section11 or scan the QR code in the text to access this content.

Highlights

- The lens is derived from surface ectoderm.
- Approximately one-third of congenital cataracts are a component of a syndrome, one-third are an isolated inherited trait, and one-third result from undetermined causes.
- Most hereditary cataracts are inherited in an autosomal dominant pattern, and they are almost always bilateral.
- Trauma is the most common cause of acquired lens displacement.
- A subluxated lens is partially displaced from the pupil but remains in the pupillary area; a luxated or dislocated lens is completely displaced from the pupil.

Normal Development of the Lens

The formation of the human crystalline lens begins very early in embryogenesis (Fig 4-1; Video 4-1). At approximately 25 days of gestation, 2 lateral evaginations, called the *optic vesicles,* form from the forebrain, or diencephalon. As the optic vesicles enlarge and extend laterally, they become closely apposed and adherent to the *surface ectoderm,* a single layer of cuboidal cells, in 2 patches on either side of the head. (See BCSC Section 2, *Fundamentals and Principles of Ophthalmology,* for additional discussion and illustrations of ocular development.)

VIDEO 4-1 Lens development.
Courtesy of Charles Cole, MD.
Go to www.aao.org/bcscvideo_section11 to access all videos in Section 11.

Lens Placode

At approximately 27 days of gestation, the ectoderm cells that overlie the optic vesicles become columnar. This area of thickened cells is called the *lens placode.* Growth factors

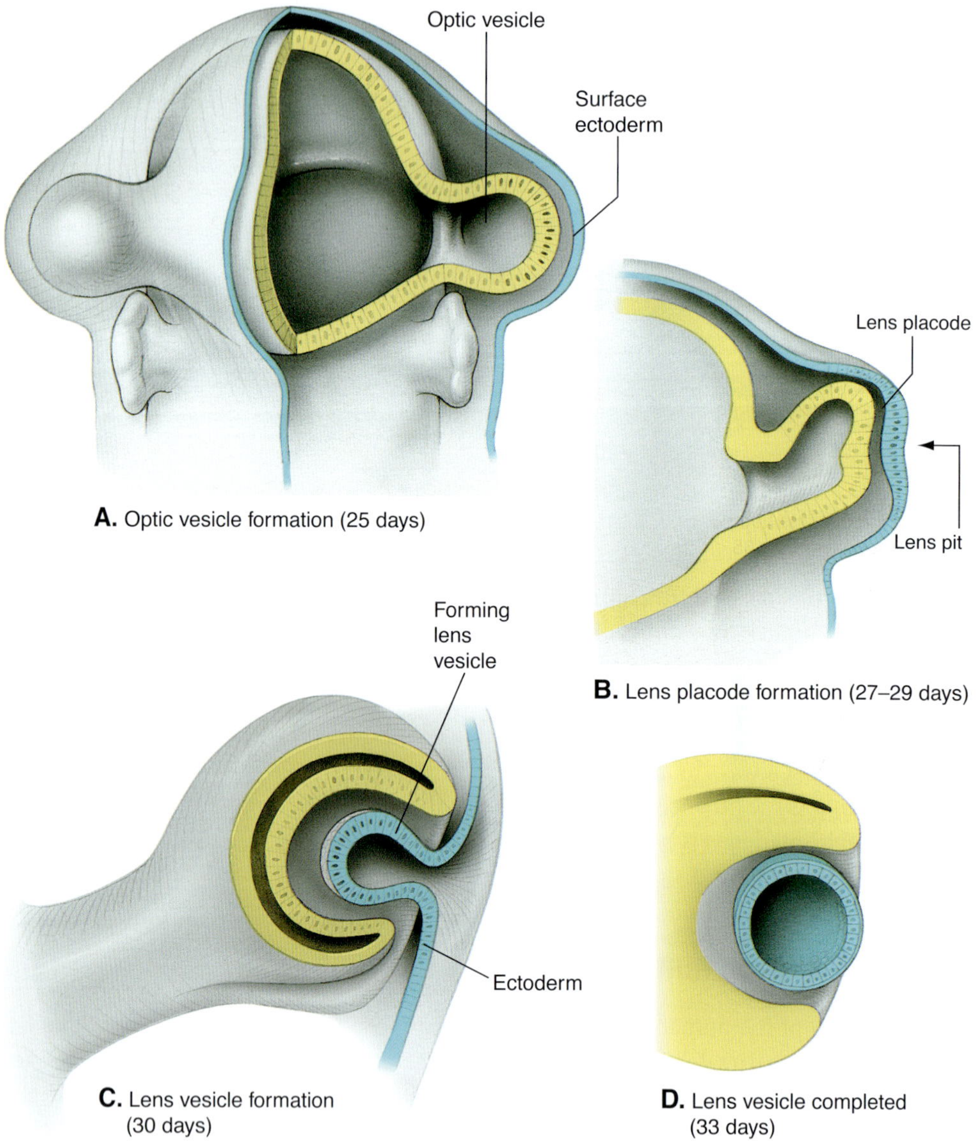

Figure 4-1 Embryologic development of the lens. *(Illustration by Christine Gralapp.)*

(Continued)

of the *bone morphogenetic protein (BMP)* family are required for formation of the lens placode and, subsequently, the lens.

Lens Pit

The lens pit appears at 29 days of gestation as an indentation (infolding) of the lens placode. The lens pit deepens and invaginates to form the lens vesicle.

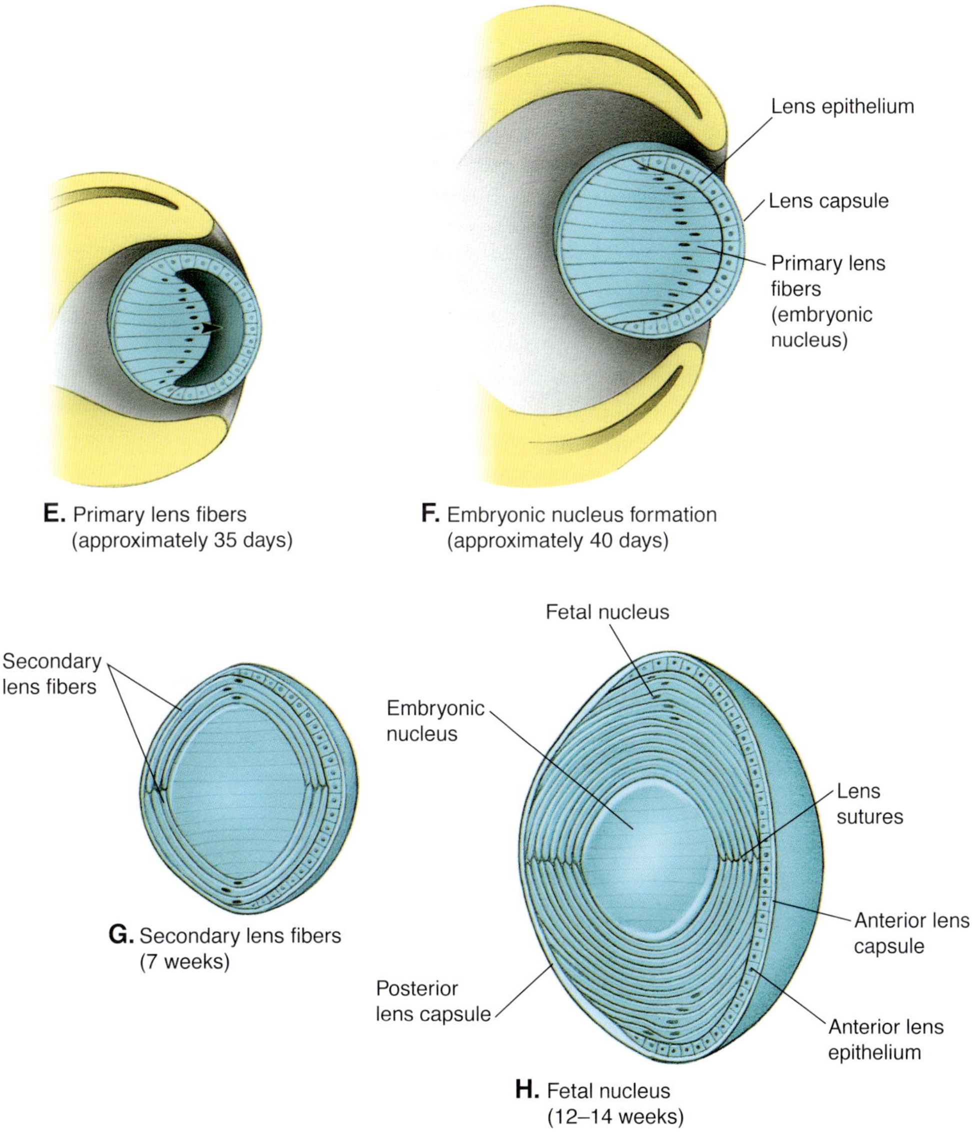

Figure 4-1 *(continued)*

Lens Vesicle

As the lens pit continues to invaginate, the stalk of cells connecting it to the surface ectoderm degenerates by programmed cell death (apoptosis), separating the lens cells from the surface ectoderm. The resultant sphere, a single layer of cuboidal cells encased in a basement membrane (the *lens capsule*), is called the *lens vesicle.* At the time of its formation at 30 days of gestation, the lens vesicle is approximately 0.2 mm in diameter.

Because the lens vesicle was formed through a process of invagination of the surface ectoderm, the apices of the cuboidal cells are oriented toward the lumen of the lens vesicle, with the base of each cell attached to the capsule around the periphery of the vesicle. While the lens vesicle is forming, the optic vesicle is simultaneously invaginating to form the 2-layered *optic cup.*

Primary Lens Fibers and the Embryonic Nucleus

The cells in the posterior layer of the lens vesicle stop dividing and begin to elongate between 33 and 35 days of gestation. As they elongate, they begin to fill the lumen of the lens vesicle. At approximately 40 days of gestation, the lumen of the lens vesicle is obliterated. The elongated cells are called the *primary lens fibers.* As the fiber cells mature, their nuclei and other membrane-bound organelles undergo degradation, a process that reduces light scattering. The primary lens fibers make up the embryonic nucleus that will ultimately occupy the central area of the adult lens.

The cells of the anterior lens vesicle give rise to the *lens epithelium,* a monolayer of cuboidal cells. Proliferation within the epithelium causes subsequent growth of the lens. The *lens capsule* develops as a basement membrane elaborated by the lens epithelium anteriorly and by lens fibers posteriorly.

Secondary Lens Fibers

After they proliferate, the epithelial cells near the lens equator elongate to form secondary lens fibers. The anterior aspect of each developing lens fiber extends anteriorly beneath the lens epithelium, toward the anterior pole of the lens. The posterior aspect of each developing lens fiber extends posteriorly along the capsule, toward the posterior pole of the lens. In this manner, new lens fibers are continually formed, layer upon layer. As each secondary fiber cell detaches from the capsule, it loses its nucleus and membrane-bound organelles. The secondary lens fibers formed between 2 and 8 months of gestation make up the *fetal nucleus.*

Lens Sutures and the Fetal Nucleus

As lens fibers grow anteriorly and posteriorly, a pattern emerges where the ends of the fibers meet and interdigitate with the ends of fibers arising on the opposite side of the lens, near the anterior and posterior poles. These patterns of cell association are known as *sutures.* Y-shaped sutures are recognizable at approximately 8 weeks of gestation; an erect Y-suture appears anteriorly and an inverted Y-suture appears posteriorly (Fig 4-2). As the lens fibers continue to form and the lens continues to grow, the pattern of lens sutures becomes increasingly complex, resulting in 12 or more suture branches in the adult eye. The mechanisms responsible for the precise formation and changing organization of the suture pattern remain obscure.

The human lens weighs approximately 90 mg at birth, and it increases in mass by approximately 2 mg per year throughout life as new fibers form. With increasing age, the central, or oldest, lens fibers gradually become less malleable, and the lens nucleus becomes more rigid. This process progressively reduces the amplitude of accommodation.

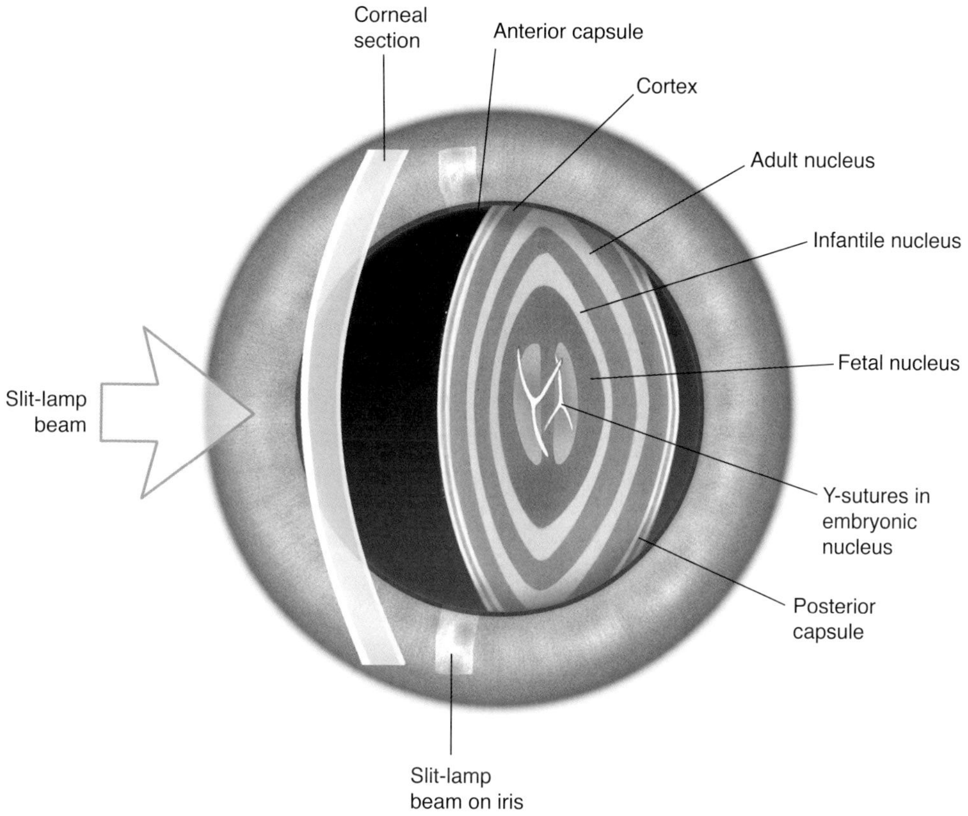

Figure 4-2 Y-shaped sutures, formed during embryogenesis, are visible within the adult lens with the use of the slit lamp. *(Illustration by Christine Gralapp.)*

Tunica Vasculosa Lentis

Around 1 month of gestation, the hyaloid artery, which enters the eye at the optic nerve head (also called the optic disc), branches to form a network of capillaries, the tunica vasculosa lentis, on the posterior surface of the lens capsule (Fig 4-3). These capillaries grow toward the equator of the lens, where they anastomose with a second network of capillaries, called the *anterior pupillary membrane,* which derives from the ciliary veins and covers the anterior surface of the lens. At approximately 9 weeks of gestation, the capillary network surrounding the lens is fully developed; it disappears by an orderly process of programmed cell death shortly before birth. Sometimes a remnant of the tunica vasculosa lentis persists as a small opacity or strand, called a *Mittendorf dot* (discussed later in this chapter), on the posterior aspect of the lens. In other eyes, remnants of the pupillary membrane are often visible as pupillary strands.

The Zonule of Zinn

Experimental evidence suggests that the zonular fibers are secreted by the ciliary epithelium, although how these fibers insert into the lens capsule is not known. The zonular fibers begin to develop at the end of the third month of gestation.

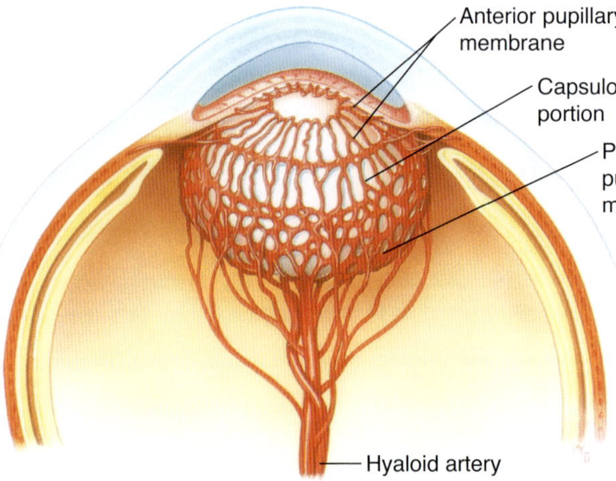

Figure 4-3 Components of the tunica vasculosa lentis. *(Illustration by Christine Gralapp.)*

Congenital Anomalies and Abnormalities

Most significant congenital anomalies of the eye and orbit are apparent on ultrasonography before birth. As a rule, the more profound the abnormality, the earlier in development it occurred. Disorders of the lens include abnormalities in lens shape, size, location, and development, as well as cataract (Table 4-1).

Congenital Aphakia

The lens is absent in congenital aphakia, a very rare anomaly. Congenital aphakia can be classified into 2 types:

- In *primary aphakia,* the lens placode fails to form from the surface ectoderm in the developing embryo.
- In *secondary aphakia,* the more common type, the developing lens is spontaneously absorbed.

Both forms of aphakia are usually associated with other malformations of the eye.

Lenticonus and Lentiglobus

Lenticonus is a localized, cone-shaped deformation of the anterior or posterior lens surface (Fig 4-4). Posterior lenticonus is more common than anterior lenticonus and is usually unilateral and axial in location. Anterior lenticonus is often bilateral and may be associated with Alport syndrome.

In lentiglobus, the localized deformation of the lens surface is spherical. Posterior lentiglobus is more common than anterior lentiglobus and is often associated with posterior polar opacities that vary in density.

Table 4-1 Lens Abnormalities

Abnormality	Disorder	Associated With
Shape	Microspherophakia	Weill-Marchesani syndrome (AR) Peters anomaly type 2
	Lenticonus/lentiglobus	Alport syndrome
	Anterior lenticonus	
	Coloboma	
Lens position	Ectopia lentis	Simple (AD)
		Ectopia lentis et pupillae (AR)
		Trauma
		Marfan syndrome
		Homocystinuria
		Aniridia
		Congenital glaucoma
		Ehlers-Danlos syndrome
		Hyperlysinemia
		Weill-Marchesani syndrome
		Sulfite oxidase deficiency
		Peters anomaly type 2
Extralenticular opacities	Persistent fetal vasculature	—
	Mittendorf dot	
	Epicapsular star	
Lenticular (cataract)	Capsulolenticular	Peters anomaly type 2
	Polar	Aniridia
	Capsular	Persistent fetal vasculature
	Sutural	
	Coronary	
	Cerulean	
	Nuclear	
	Complete	
	Membranous	
	Rubella	

AD = autosomal dominant; AR = autosomal recessive.

Retinoscopy through the center of the lens reveals a distorted and myopic reflex in both lenticonus and lentiglobus. These deformations can also be seen in the *red reflex,* where, by retroillumination, they appear as an "oil droplet." (This condition should not be confused with the "oil droplet" cataract of galactosemia, which is discussed in Chapter 5.) The posterior bulging may progress with initial worsening of the myopia, followed by opacification of the defect. Surrounding cortical lamellae may also opacify.

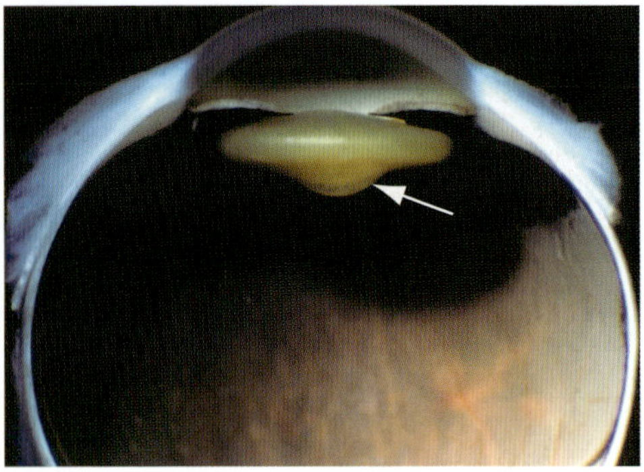

Figure 4-4 Posterior lenticonus *(arrow)*. *(Courtesy of Mission for Vision.)*

Lens Coloboma

A lens coloboma is an anomaly of lens shape (Fig 4-5). *Primary coloboma* is a wedge-shaped defect or indentation of the lens periphery that occurs as an isolated anomaly. *Secondary coloboma* is a flattening or indentation of the lens periphery caused by the lack of ciliary body or zonular development. Lens colobomas are typically located inferonasally and may be associated with colobomas of the iris, optic nerve, or retina. Cortical lens opacification or thickening of the lens capsule may appear adjacent to the coloboma. The zonular attachments in the region of the coloboma are usually weakened or absent.

Mittendorf Dot

Mittendorf dot, mentioned earlier in this chapter, is a common anomaly observed in many healthy eyes. A small, dense white spot generally located inferonasal to the posterior pole of the lens, a Mittendorf dot is a remnant of the posterior pupillary membrane of the tunica vasculosa lentis (Fig 4-6). It marks the place where the hyaloid artery came into

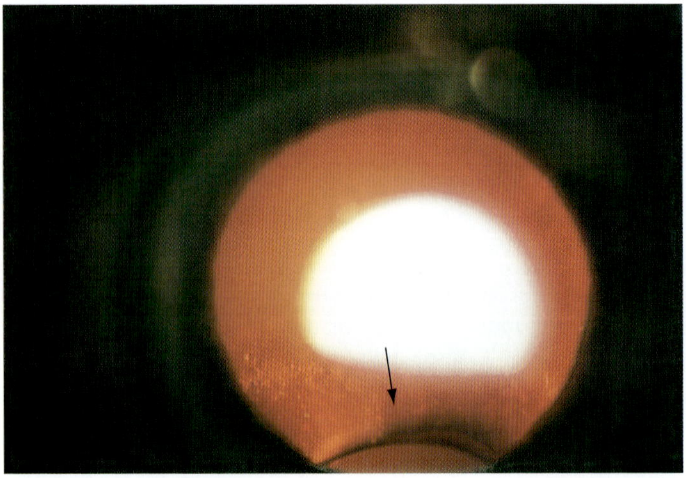

Figure 4-5 Coloboma of the lens *(arrow)* as viewed by retroillumination.

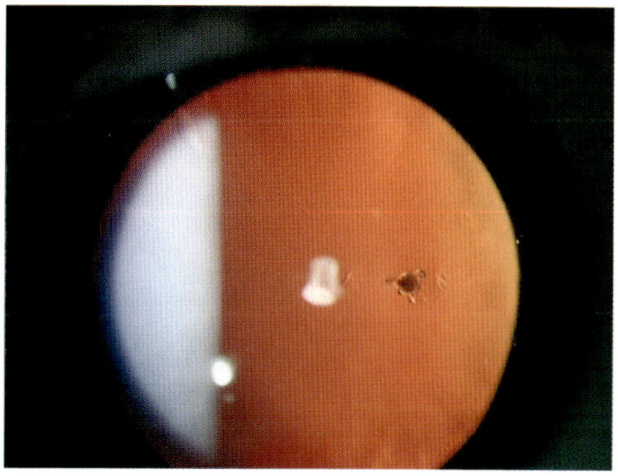

Figure 4-6 Mittendorf dot, as viewed by retroillumination. *(Courtesy of Matt Weed, MD. Photograph by D. Brice Critser, CRA. Used with permission from the University of Iowa and EyeRounds.org.)*

contact with the posterior surface of the lens in utero. Sometimes a Mittendorf dot is associated with a fibrous tail or remnant of the hyaloid artery that projects into the vitreous body.

Epicapsular Star

Another very common remnant of the tunica vasculosa lentis is an epicapsular star (Fig 4-7). As its name suggests, this anomaly is a star-shaped distribution of tiny brown or golden flecks on the central anterior lens capsule. It may be unilateral or bilateral.

Peters Anomaly

Peters anomaly is part of a spectrum of disorders known as *anterior segment dysgenesis syndrome,* also referred to as *neurocristopathy* or *mesodermal dysgenesis.* (See also BCSC Section 6, *Pediatric Ophthalmology and Strabismus.*) Peters anomaly is characterized by a central or paracentral corneal opacity (leukoma) associated with thinning or absence of adjacent endothelium and Descemet membrane. In Peters anomaly type 1, iris strands

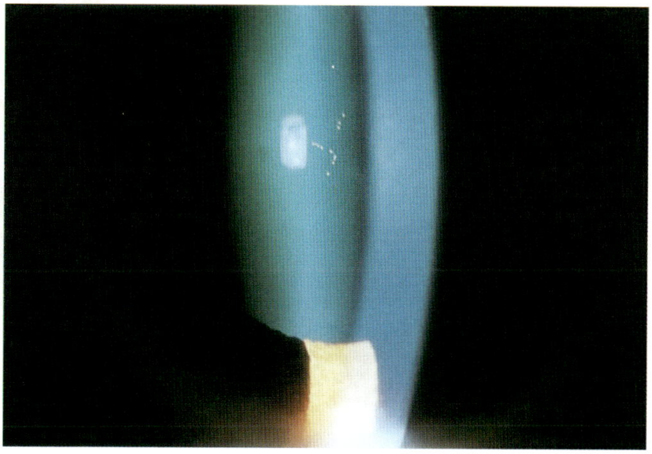

Figure 4-7 Epicapsular star.

adherent to the cornea are often present. In Peters anomaly type 2, the lens is adherent to the posterior cornea. In normal ocular development, the lens vesicle separates from the surface ectoderm (the future corneal epithelium) at approximately 33 days of gestation. Peters anomaly is typically linked with the absence of this separation. It is often associated with mutations in or deletion of 1 allele of the genes normally involved in anterior segment development, including the transcription factors *PAX6, PITX2,* and *FOXC1.* Patients with Peters anomaly type 2 may also display the following lens anomalies:

- anterior cortical or polar cataract
- a misshapen lens displaced anteriorly into the pupillary space and the anterior chamber
- microspherophakia

Microspherophakia

Microspherophakia is a developmental abnormality in which the lens is small in diameter and spherical. The entire lens equator can be visualized at the slit lamp when the pupil is widely dilated (Fig 4-8). The spherical shape of the lens results in increased refractive power, which causes the eye to be highly myopic.

The cause of microspherophakia is believed to be faulty development of the secondary lens fibers during embryogenesis. Microspherophakia is most often seen as a part of Weill-Marchesani syndrome, but it may also occur as an isolated hereditary abnormality or, occasionally, in association with Peters anomaly, Marfan syndrome, Alport syndrome, Lowe syndrome, or congenital rubella. Individuals with Weill-Marchesani syndrome commonly have small stature, short and stubby fingers, and broad hands with reduced joint mobility. Weill-Marchesani syndrome is usually inherited as an autosomal recessive trait.

The spherical lens can block the pupil, causing secondary angle-closure glaucoma. Use of miotics aggravates this condition by increasing pupillary block and allowing additional forward lens displacement. Cycloplegics are the medical treatment of choice to break an attack of angle-closure glaucoma in patients with microspherophakia, because these agents decrease pupillary block by tightening the zonular fibers, decreasing the anteroposterior lens diameter, and pulling the lens posteriorly. A laser iridotomy may also

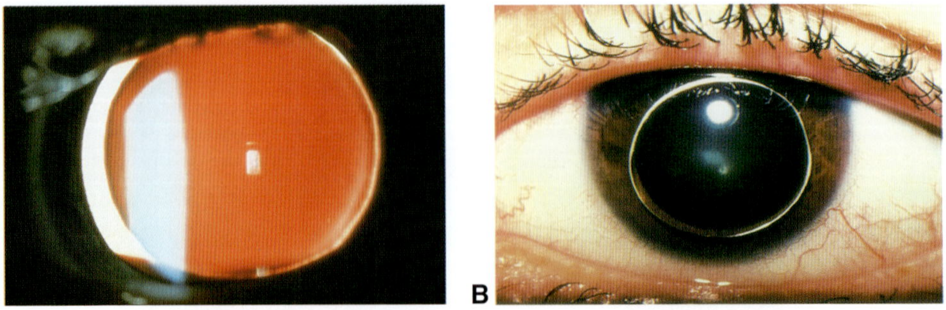

A B

Figure 4-8 Microspherophakia. **A,** When the pupil is dilated, the entire lens equator can be seen at the slit lamp. **B,** Anterior dislocation of a microspherophakic lens. *(Part A courtesy of Karla J. Johns, MD.)*

be useful in relieving angle closure in patients with microspherophakia. (See also BCSC Section 10, *Glaucoma.*)

Aniridia

Aniridia is an uncommon panocular syndrome in which the most dramatic manifestation is partial or nearly complete absence of the iris (Fig 4-9). Aniridia has been linked to the loss of 1 allele of the *PAX6* gene, a transcription factor that is important for the development and function of the cornea, lens, and retina. Associated findings include corneal pannus and epitheliopathy, glaucoma, foveal and optic nerve hypoplasia, and nystagmus. Aniridia is almost always bilateral. Two-thirds of cases are familial; one-third of cases are sporadic. Sporadic cases of aniridia are associated with a high incidence of Wilms tumor and the WAGR complex (*W*ilms tumor, *a*niridia, *g*enitourinary malformations, and mental *r*etardation).

Anterior or posterior polar lens opacities may be present at birth in patients with aniridia. Cortical, subcapsular, or lamellar opacities develop in 50%–85% of patients within the first 2 decades of life. The lens opacities may progress, further impairing vision. Poor zonular integrity and ectopia lentis have also been reported in patients with aniridia.

Persistent Fetal Vasculature

Persistent fetal vasculature (PFV), also known as *persistent hyperplastic primary vitreous (PHPV),* is a congenital, nonhereditary ocular malformation that frequently involves the lens (Fig 4-10). In 90% of patients, it is unilateral. A white, fibrous retrolental tissue is present, often in association with posterior cortical opacification. Progressive cataract formation often occurs, sometimes leading to a complete cataract. Other abnormalities associated with PFV include elongated ciliary processes, prominent radial iris vessels, and persistent hyaloid artery. (See BCSC Section 6, *Pediatric Ophthalmology and Strabismus,* and Section 12, *Retina and Vitreous,* for additional discussion.)

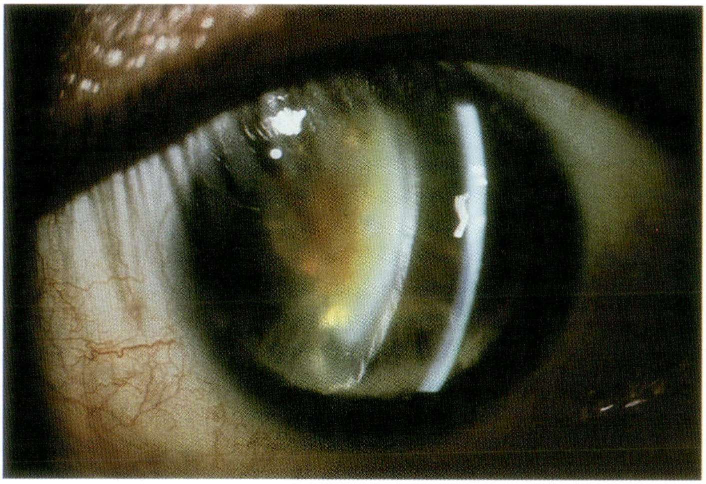

Figure 4-9 Cataract in a patient with aniridia.

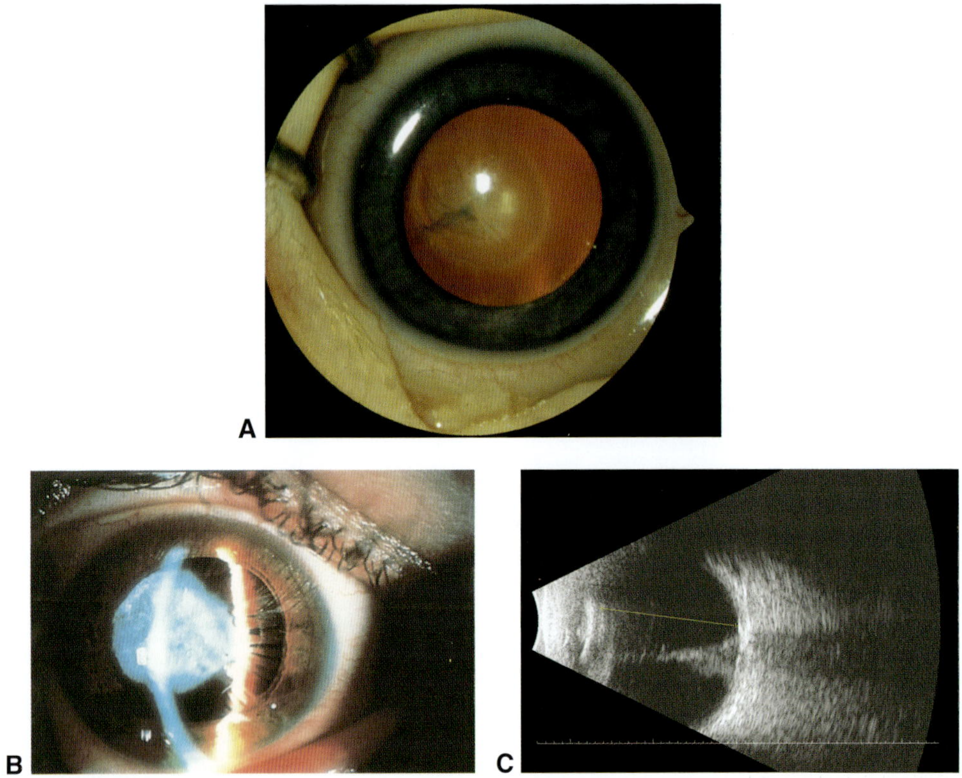

Figure 4-10 Persistent fetal vasculature (PFV). **A,** Mild variant with central retrolental membrane. **B,** Elongated ciliary processes are adherent to the lens. Note the dense fibrous plaque on the posterior lens capsule. **C,** Ultrasonogram of an eye with PFV. Note the dense stalk arising from the optic nerve and attaching to the posterior lens. *(Part A courtesy of David A. Plager, MD; part C courtesy of Edward L. Raab, MD.)*

CLINICAL PEARL

Eyes with persistent fetal vasculature are usually smaller than normal. Although retinoblastoma is included in the differential diagnosis, retinoblastoma is found in microphthalmic eyes only on rare occasions, and cataracts are unusual in eyes with retinoblastoma.

Congenital Cataract

Congenital cataracts are present at birth but may not be identified immediately. Infantile cataracts develop during the first year of life. Because some lens opacities escape detection at birth and are noted only on later examination, these terms are used interchangeably by many physicians. In this book, the term *congenital cataract* is used for both categories of lens opacities. These cataracts are fairly common, occurring in 1 of every 2000 live births, and cover a broad spectrum of severity. While some lens opacities do not progress and are visually insignificant, others can cause profound visual impairment.

Congenital cataracts may be unilateral or bilateral. They can be classified by morphology, presumed or defined genetic etiology, presence of specific metabolic disorders, or associated ocular anomalies or systemic findings (Table 4-2). In general, approximately one-third of congenital cataracts are a component of a more extensive syndrome or disease (eg, cataract resulting from congenital rubella syndrome), one-third occur as an isolated inherited trait, and one-third result from undetermined causes. Metabolic diseases tend to be more commonly associated with bilateral cataracts. (For a discussion of the

Table 4-2 Etiology of Pediatric Cataracts

Type	
Unilateral	**Bilateral**
Idiopathic	Idiopathic
Ocular anomalies	Heredity[a]
Persistent fetal vasculature	Genetic and metabolic diseases
Anterior segment dysgenesis	Down syndrome
Posterior lenticonus	Hallermann-Streiff syndrome
Posterior lentiglobus	Lowe syndrome
Posterior pole tumors	Galactosemia
Retinal detachment (any cause)	Trisomy 13–15
Coloboma	Hypoglycemia
Trauma (rule out child abuse)	Alport syndrome
Masked bilateral cataract	Myotonic dystrophy
Radiation (may be unilateral or bilateral)	Fabry disease
	Hypoparathyroidism
	Conradi-Hünermann syndrome
	Intrauterine infections
	Cytomegalovirus
	Rubella
	Syphilis
	Toxoplasmosis
	Varicella
	Ocular anomalies
	Aniridia
	Anterior segment dysgenesis syndrome
	Toxicity
	Corticosteroids
	Radiation (may be unilateral or bilateral)

[a]Autosomal dominant most common; also autosomal recessive or X-linked.

evaluation of pediatric patients with congenital cataracts, see BCSC Section 6, *Pediatric Ophthalmology and Strabismus.*) Congenital cataracts occur in a variety of morphologic configurations, including lamellar, polar, sutural, coronary, cerulean, nuclear, capsular, complete, membranous, and rubella.

Lamellar

Of the congenital cataracts, lamellar, or *zonular,* cataracts are the most common type (Fig 4-11). They are characteristically bilateral and symmetric, and their effect on vision varies with the size and density of the opacity. Lamellar cataracts may be inherited as an autosomal dominant trait. In some cases, they may occur as a result of a transient toxic influence during embryonic lens development. The earlier this toxic influence occurs, the smaller and deeper is the resulting lamellar cataract.

Lamellar cataracts are opacifications of specific layers or zones of the lens. Clinically, the cataract is visible as an opacified layer that surrounds a clearer center and is itself surrounded by a layer of clear cortex. Viewed from the front, the lamellar cataract has a

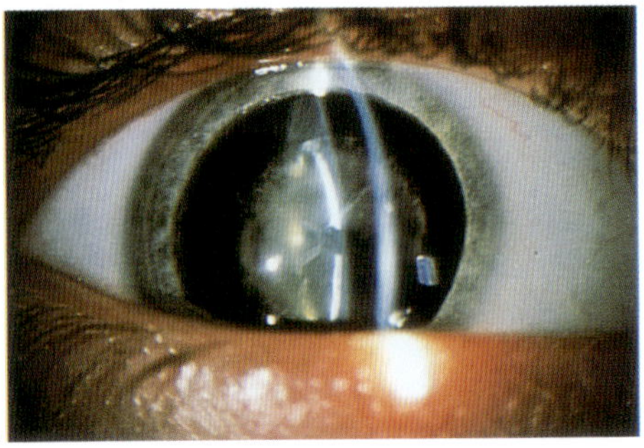

A

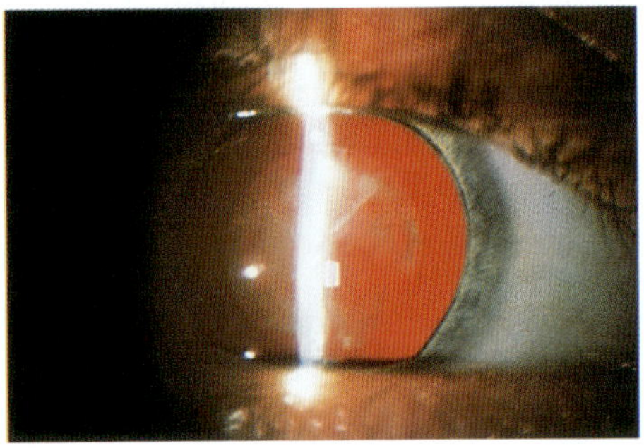

B

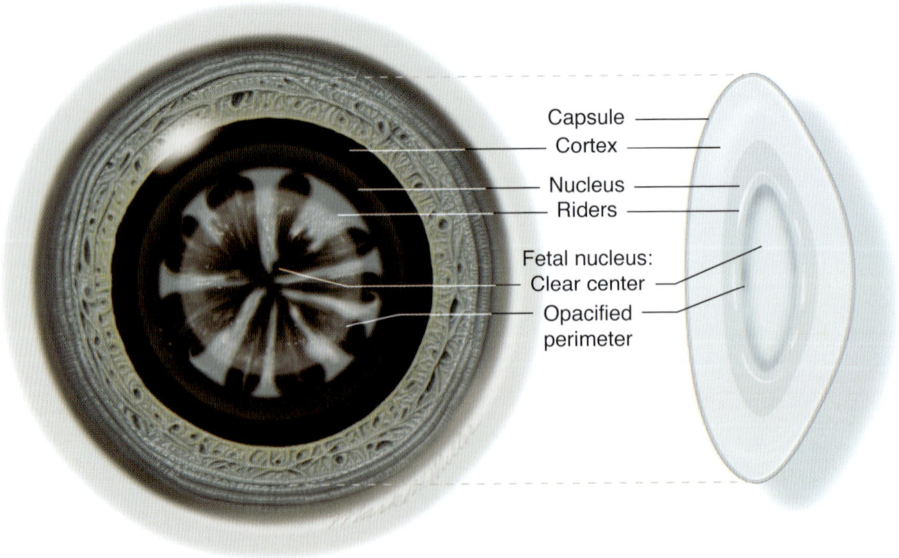

C

Figure 4-11 Lamellar cataract. **A,** Lamellar cataract, slit-lamp view. **B,** Lamellar cataract viewed by retroillumination. **C,** Schematic of lamellar cataract. *(Part C illustration by Mark Miller.)*

disc-shaped configuration. Often, additional arcuate opacities within the cortex straddle the equator of the lamellar cataract; these horseshoe-shaped opacities are called *riders.*

Polar

Polar cataracts are lens opacities that involve the subcapsular cortex and capsule of the anterior or posterior pole of the lens. *Anterior polar cataracts* are usually small, bilateral, symmetric, nonprogressive opacities that do not impair vision (Fig 4-12). Most commonly, they are congenital and sporadic, but they may be inherited in an autosomal dominant pattern. Anterior polar cataracts are sometimes seen in association with other ocular abnormalities, including microphthalmos, persistent pupillary membrane, and anterior lenticonus. They usually do not require treatment but often cause anisometropia.

Posterior polar cataracts are generally associated with more profound decrease in vision than anterior polar cataracts, because they tend to be larger and are positioned closer to the nodal point of the eye. Capsular fragility has been reported in association with these cataracts, which are usually stable but occasionally progress. They may be familial or sporadic. Familial posterior polar cataracts are usually bilateral and inherited in an autosomal dominant pattern. Sporadic posterior polar cataracts are often unilateral and may be associated with remnants of the tunica vasculosa lentis or with an abnormality of the posterior lens surface such as lenticonus or lentiglobus.

Sutural

The sutural, or stellate, cataract is an opacification of the Y-sutures of the fetal nucleus (Fig 4-13). It usually does not impair vision. These opacities often have branches or knobs projecting from them. Sutural cataracts are bilateral and symmetric and are frequently inherited in an autosomal dominant pattern.

Coronary

Coronary cataracts are so named because they consist of a group of club-shaped cortical opacities that are arranged around the equator of the lens like a crown, or corona. They cannot be seen unless the pupil is dilated, and they usually do not affect visual acuity. Coronary cataracts are often inherited in an autosomal dominant pattern.

A
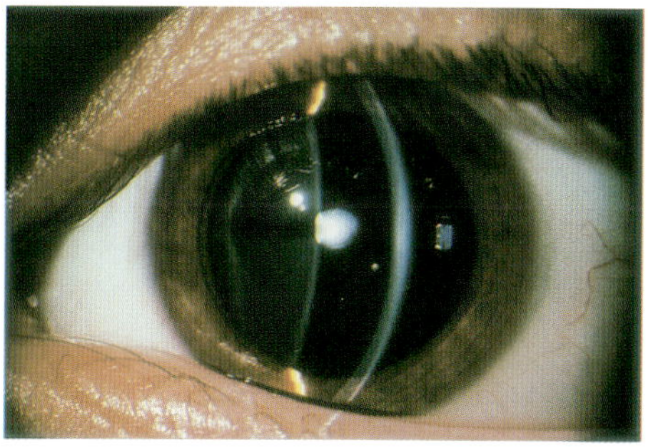
B
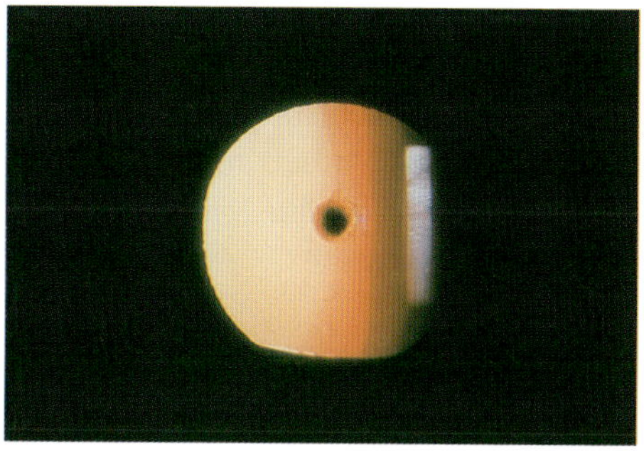

Figure 4-12 Anterior polar cataract. **A,** Anterior polar cataract, slit-lamp view. **B,** Anterior polar cataract viewed by retroillumination.

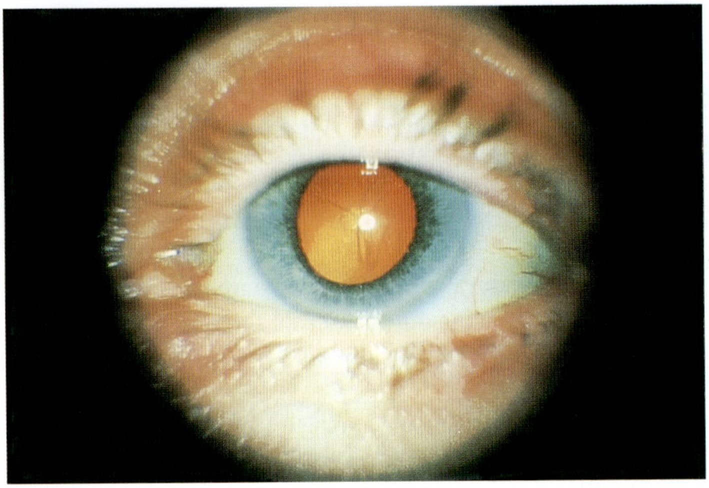

Figure 4-13 Sutural cataract.

Cerulean

Also known as *blue-dot cataracts,* cerulean cataracts are small bluish opacities located in the lens cortex (Fig 4-14). They are nonprogressive and usually do not cause visual symptoms.

Nuclear

Congenital nuclear cataracts are opacities of the embryonic nucleus alone or of both embryonic and fetal nuclei (Fig 4-15). They are usually bilateral, with a wide spectrum of severity. Lens opacification may involve the complete nucleus, or it may be limited to discrete layers within the nucleus. Eyes with congenital nuclear cataracts tend to be microphthalmic, and they are at increased risk of developing aphakic glaucoma.

Capsular

Capsular cataracts are small opacifications of the lens epithelium and anterior lens capsule that spare the cortex. They are differentiated from anterior polar cataracts by their protrusion into the anterior chamber. Capsular cataracts generally do not adversely affect vision.

Complete

In cases of complete, or total, cataract, all of the lens fibers are opacified. The red reflex is completely obscured, and the retina cannot be seen with either direct or indirect ophthalmoscopy. Some cataracts may be subtotal at birth and progress rapidly to become complete cataracts. Complete cataracts may be unilateral or bilateral, and they cause profound visual impairment.

Membranous

Membranous cataracts occur when lens proteins are resorbed from either an intact or a traumatized lens, allowing the anterior and posterior lens capsules to fuse into a dense white membrane (Fig 4-16). The resulting opacity and lens distortion generally cause significant visual disability.

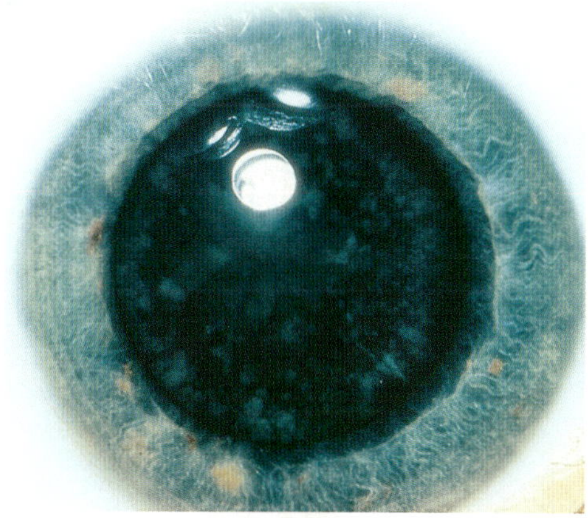

Figure 4-14 Cerulean cataract. *(Courtesy of Karla J. Johns, MD.)*

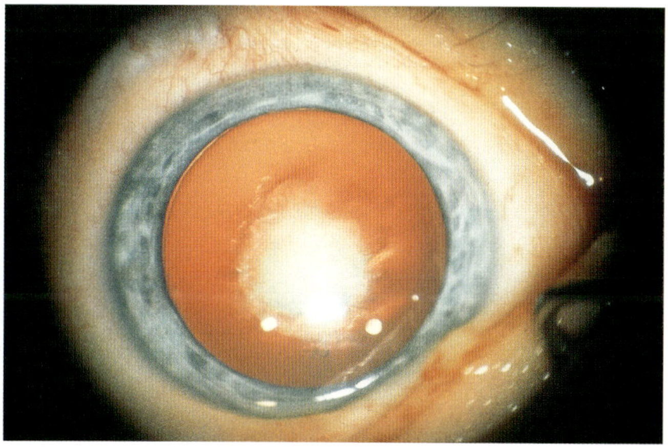

Figure 4-15 Congenital nuclear cataract. *(Reproduced from Day SH.* Understanding and Preventing Amblyopia: Slide & Script Presentation. *Eye Care Skills for the Primary Care Physician Series. American Academy of Ophthalmology; 1987.)*

Rubella

Maternal infection with the rubella virus, an RNA togavirus, can cause fetal damage, especially if the infection occurs during the first trimester of pregnancy. Cataracts resulting from *congenital rubella syndrome* are characterized by pearly white nuclear opacifications. Sometimes the entire lens is opacified (complete cataract), and the cortex may liquefy (Fig 4-17). On histologic examination, lens-fiber nuclei are retained deep within the lens substance. Live virus particles may be recovered from the lens as late as 3 years after the patient's birth. Cataract removal may be complicated by excessive postoperative inflammation caused by release of these particles. (See also BCSC Section 6, *Pediatric Ophthalmology and Strabismus.*) Other ocular manifestations of congenital rubella syndrome include diffuse pigmentary retinopathy, microphthalmos, glaucoma, and transient or permanent corneal clouding. Although congenital rubella syndrome may cause cataract or glaucoma, both conditions are usually not present simultaneously in the same eye.

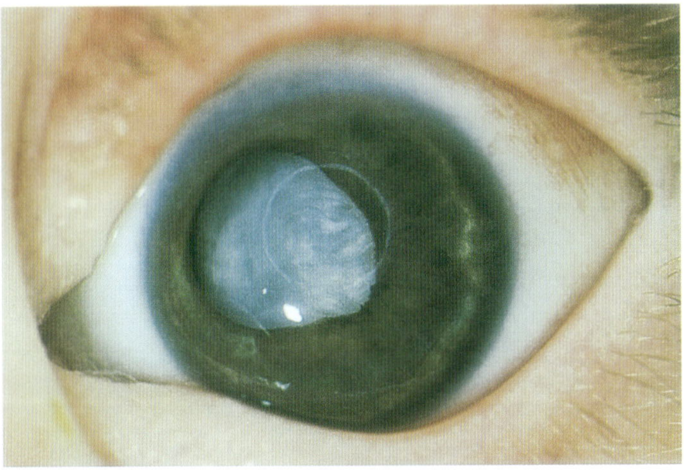

Figure 4-16 Membranous cataract.

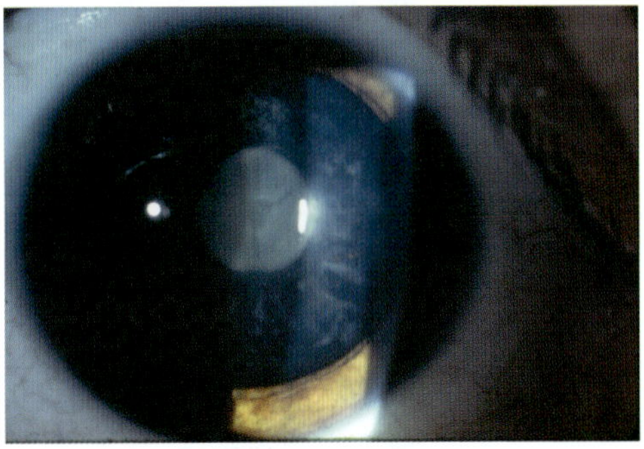

Figure 4-17 Rubella cataract. *(Courtesy of Thomas L. Steinemann, MD.)*

Developmental Defects

Ectopia Lentis

Ectopia lentis is a displacement of the lens that may be congenital, developmental, or acquired. A *subluxated* lens is partially displaced from its normal position but remains in the pupillary area. A *luxated,* or *dislocated,* lens is completely displaced from the pupil, implying separation of all zonular attachments. Findings associated with lens subluxation include decreased vision, marked astigmatism, monocular diplopia, and iridodonesis (tremulous iris). Potential complications of ectopia lentis include cataract and displacement of the lens into the anterior chamber or the vitreous space. Dislocation into the anterior chamber or pupil may cause pupillary block and angle-closure glaucoma. Dislocation of the lens posteriorly into the vitreous cavity often has no adverse sequelae aside from a profound change in refractive error.

Trauma is the most common cause of acquired lens displacement. Nontraumatic ectopia lentis is commonly associated with Marfan syndrome, homocystinuria, aniridia, and congenital glaucoma. Less frequently, it appears in association with Ehlers-Danlos syndrome, hyperlysinemia, Weill-Marchesani syndrome, and sulfite oxidase deficiency. Ectopia lentis may occur as an isolated anomaly (simple ectopia lentis), which is usually inherited as an autosomal dominant trait. Ectopia lentis can also be associated with pupillary abnormalities in the ocular syndrome ectopia lentis et pupillae (discussed later in this chapter).

Marfan syndrome

Marfan syndrome is a heritable disorder with ocular, cardiovascular, and skeletal manifestations. Though usually inherited as an autosomal dominant trait, the disorder appears in individuals with no family history in approximately 15% of cases. Marfan syndrome is caused by mutations in the fibrillin gene on chromosome 15. Affected individuals are tall, with arachnodactyly (Fig 4-18A) and chest wall deformities. Associated cardiovascular abnormalities include dilated aortic root and mitral valve prolapse.

Between 50% and 80% of patients with Marfan syndrome exhibit ectopia lentis (Fig 4-18B). The lens subluxation tends to be bilateral and symmetric (usually superior and temporal), but variations do occur. The zonular attachments commonly remain intact but become stretched and elongated. Ectopia lentis in Marfan syndrome is probably congenital in most cases. Progression of lens subluxation occurs in some patients over time, but in many patients the lens position remains stable.

Other ocular abnormalities associated with Marfan syndrome include axial myopia and an increased risk of retinal detachment. Patients with Marfan syndrome may develop pupillary block glaucoma if the lens dislocates into the pupil or anterior chamber. Open-angle glaucoma may also occur. Amblyopia may develop in children with lens subluxation if their refractive error shows significant asymmetry or remains uncorrected in early childhood. Spectacle or contact lens correction of the refractive error provides satisfactory vision in most cases. Pupillary dilation is sometimes helpful. The clinician may refract both the phakic and the aphakic portions of the pupil to determine the optimum visual acuity. A reading add is often necessary because the subluxated lens lacks sufficient accommodation.

In some cases, adequate visual acuity cannot be obtained with spectacle or contact lens correction, and removal of the lens may be indicated. Lens extraction—either extracapsular or intracapsular—in patients with Marfan syndrome is associated with a high

A

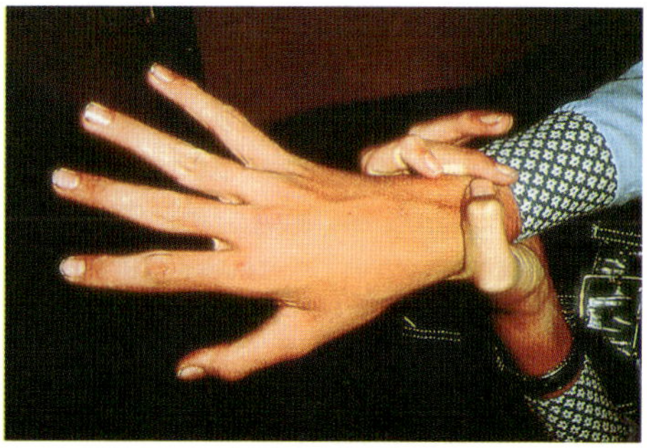

B

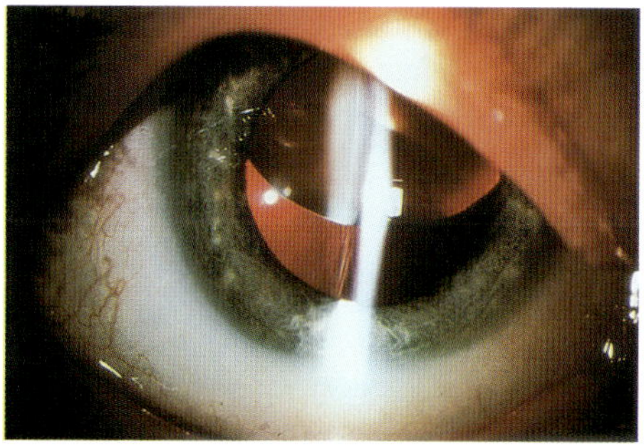

Figure 4-18 Marfan syndrome. **A,** Arachnodactyly in a patient with Marfan syndrome. **B,** Subluxated lens in Marfan syndrome. *(Part A courtesy of Karla J. Johns, MD.)*

rate of complications such as vitreous loss and complex retinal detachment. Advanced surgical techniques, including the use of capsular tension rings and capsular tension segments, are increasingly being used to improve outcomes in these cases (see Chapter 12, Preparing for Cataract Surgery in Special Situations).

Homocystinuria

Homocystinuria is an inborn error of methionine metabolism in which serum levels of homocysteine and methionine are elevated. Homocystinuria is transmitted in an autosomal recessive pattern. Affected individuals are healthy at birth; however, seizures and osteoporosis typically develop within the first year of life, and cognitive impairment soon becomes apparent. These individuals are usually tall and have light-colored hair. Persons with homocystinuria are prone to thromboembolic episodes, and surgery and general anesthesia are thought to increase the risk of thromboembolism.

Lens dislocation in individuals with homocystinuria tends to be bilateral and symmetric. The dislocation appears in infancy in approximately 30% of affected individuals, and by the age of 15 years, it appears in 80% of those affected. The lenses are usually subluxated inferiorly and nasally, but variations have been reported. Because zonular fibers of the lens are known to have a high concentration of cysteine, deficiency of cysteine is thought to disrupt normal zonular development; affected fibers tend to be brittle and easily disrupted. In studies of infants with homocystinuria treated with a low-methionine, high-cysteine diet and vitamin supplementation with the coenzyme pyridoxine (vitamin B_6), the incidence of sequelae, including ectopia lentis, was reduced in some patients who received this therapy. (See also BCSC Section 6, *Pediatric Ophthalmology and Strabismus.*)

Hyperlysinemia

Hyperlysinemia, an inborn error of metabolism of the amino acid lysine, is associated with ectopia lentis. Affected individuals also show cognitive impairment and muscular hypotony.

Genetic Contributions to Age-Related Cataracts

Studies of identical and fraternal twins and of familial associations suggest that a large proportion of the risk of age-related cataracts is inherited. It is estimated that inheritance accounts for more than 50% of the risk of cortical cataracts. Studies have identified mutations in the gene associated with congenital and age-related cortical cataracts, *EPHA2,* which has been mapped to 1p36. This is the first gene known to cause hereditary, nonsyndromic age-related cortical cataracts, although mutations at this locus account for only a small fraction of cortical opacities. Similarly, 35%–50% of the risk of nuclear cataracts can be traced to inheritance. Identification of the genes associated with increased risk of cortical and nuclear cataracts is important, because understanding the biochemical pathways in which they function may suggest ways to slow the progression or prevent the development of age-related cataracts in a large number of cases.

Jun G, Guo H, Klein BE, et al. *EPHA2* is associated with age-related cortical cataract in mice and humans. *PLoS Genet.* 2009;5(7):e1000584.

Shiels A, Bennett TM, Knopf HL, et al. The *EPHA2* gene is associated with cataracts linked to chromosome 1p. *Mol Vis.* 2008;14:2042–2055.

Ectopia Lentis et Pupillae

In the autosomal recessive disorder ectopia lentis et pupillae, the lens and the pupil are displaced in opposite directions. The pupil is irregular, usually slit shaped, and displaced from the normal position. The dislocated lens may bisect the pupil or may be completely absent from the pupillary space. This disorder is usually bilateral but not symmetric. Characteristically, the iris dilates poorly. Associated ocular anomalies include severe axial myopia, retinal detachment, enlarged corneal diameter, cataract, and abnormal iris transillumination.

Beebe DC. The lens. In: Kaufman PL, Alm A, eds. *Adler's Physiology of the Eye: Clinical Application.* 11th ed. Mosby; 2011:131–163.

Congdon NG, Chang MA, Botelho P, Stark WJ, Datiles MB III. Cataract: clinical types. In: Tasman W, Jaeger EA, eds. *Duane's Clinical Ophthalmology.* Lippincott Williams & Wilkins; 2006; vol 1, chapter 73.

Hiles DA, Kilty LA. Disorders of the lens. In: Isenberg SJ, ed. *The Eye in Infancy.* 2nd ed. Mosby; 1994:336–373.

Streeten BW. Pathology of the lens. In: Albert DM, Jakobiec FA, eds. *Principles and Practice of Ophthalmology.* 2nd ed. Saunders; 2000:3685–3749.

CHAPTER 5

Pathology

Highlights

- The lens changes color, density, and clarity in response to increasing age, trauma, and toxic exposures.
- Age-related cataract development takes several forms, causing varying degrees of visual impairment.
- Smoking, use of smokeless tobacco, and excessive alcohol consumption are modifiable risk factors for developing cataracts; no medication or nutritional supplement has been consistently correlated with decreased cataract development.

Age-Related Lens Changes

As the lens ages, it increases in mass and thickness and decreases in accommodative power. As new layers of cortical fibers form concentrically, the lens nucleus compresses and hardens (a process known as nuclear sclerosis). Chemical modification and proteolytic cleavage of crystallins (lens proteins) result in the formation of high-molecular-mass protein aggregates. These aggregates may become large enough to cause abrupt fluctuations in the local refractive index of the lens, thereby scattering light and reducing transparency. Chemical modification of lens nuclear proteins also increases opacity, so that the lens becomes increasingly yellow or brown with advancing age (Fig 5-1). Other age-related changes include decreased concentrations of glutathione and potassium and increased concentrations of sodium and calcium in the lens cell cytoplasm.

A frequent cause of visual impairment in older adults is *age-related cataract,* the pathogenesis of which is multifactorial and not completely understood. There are 3 main types of age-related cataracts: (1) nuclear, (2) cortical, and (3) posterior subcapsular. In many patients, components of more than 1 type are present. (See also BCSC Section 4, *Ophthalmic Pathology and Intraocular Tumors.*)

Nuclear Cataracts

Some degree of nuclear sclerosis and yellowing is normal in patients older than 50 years. In general, nuclear sclerosis interferes only minimally with visual function, at least until the condition becomes severe. The central opacity causes an increased amount of light scattering, which the ophthalmologist observes as a yellow-brown central lens nucleus.

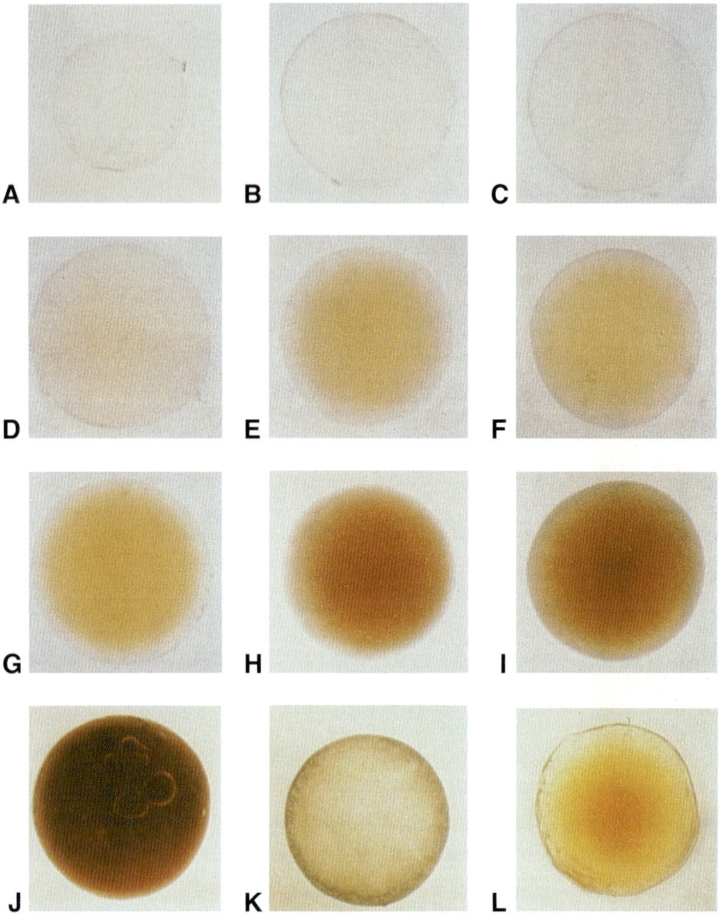

Figure 5-1 Increasing yellow-to-brown coloration of the human lens from age 6 months **(A)** to 8 years **(B)**, 12 years **(C)**, 25 years **(D)**, 47 years **(E)**, 60 years **(F)**, 70 years **(G)**, 82 years **(H)**, and 91 years **(I)**. **J,** Brown nuclear cataract in a 70-year-old patient. **K,** Cortical cataract in a 68-year-old patient. **L,** Mixed nuclear and cortical cataract in a 74-year-old patient. *(Reproduced with permission from Lerman S. Phototoxicity: clinical considerations.* Focal Points: Clinical Modules for Ophthalmologists. *American Academy of Ophthalmology; 1987, module 8.)*

A nuclear cataract (Fig 5-2) is best evaluated by using a slit-lamp biomicroscope with off-axis illumination through a dilated pupil.

Nuclear cataracts are slowly progressive. They are usually bilateral but may be asymmetric. Nuclear cataracts typically cause greater impairment of distance vision than of near vision. In the early stages of cataract development, the progressive hardening of the lens nucleus frequently causes an increase in the refractive index of the lens and a myopic shift in refraction *(lenticular myopia)*. In hyperopic or emmetropic eyes, the myopic shift enables individuals to have improved distance vision or near vision without the use of spectacles, a condition referred to as "second sight." A change in astigmatism and, in rare instances, a hyperopic shift can occur as the nucleus matures. Occasionally, the abrupt

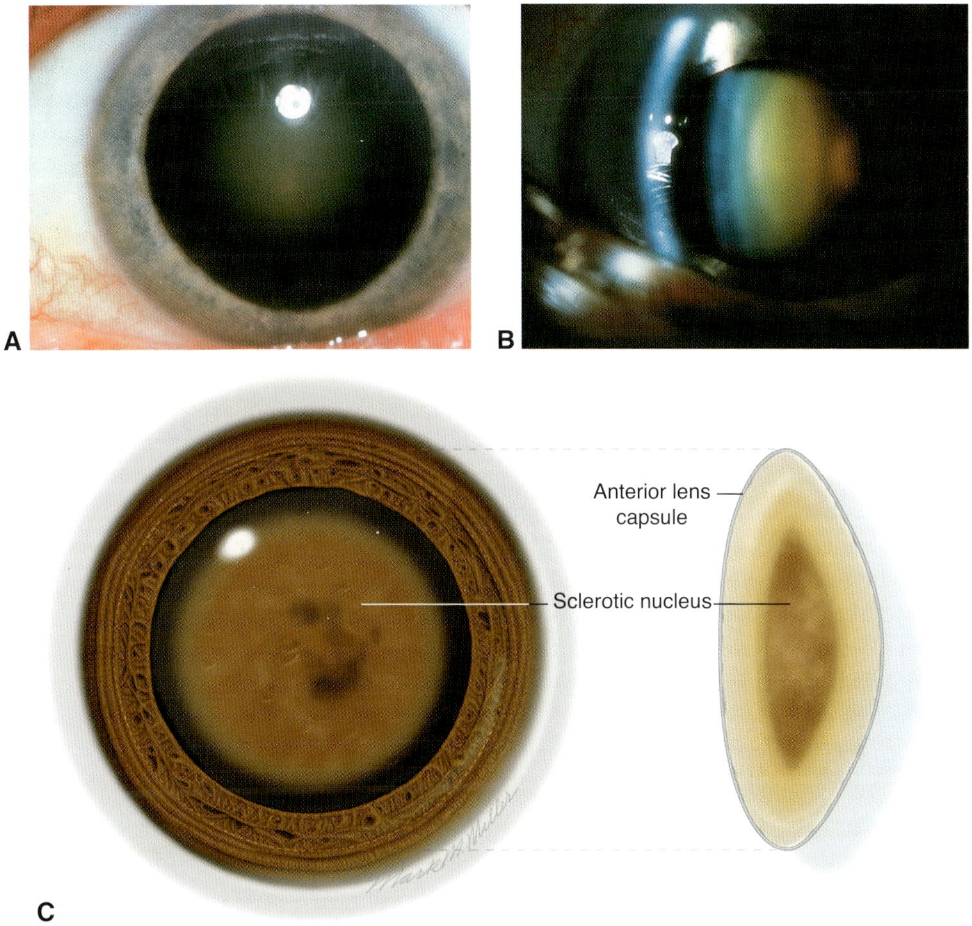

Figure 5-2 Nuclear cataract viewed with diffuse illumination **(A)** and with a slit beam **(B)**. **C,** Schematic of nuclear cataract. *(Part C illustration by Mark Miller.)*

change in refractive index between the sclerotic nucleus (or other lens opacities) and the lens cortex can cause monocular diplopia. Progressive yellowing or browning of the lens causes patients to have poor color discrimination, especially at the blue end of the visible-light spectrum. In bilateral cases, patients are frequently unaware of their altered color discrimination.

Visual dysfunction in low light often occurs with advancing nuclear cataract. In the most advanced cases, the lens nucleus becomes increasingly opaque and brown and is called a *brunescent nuclear cataract.* On histologic examination, it is difficult to distinguish the nucleus in a nuclear cataract from the nucleus of a normal, aged lens. Investigations by electron microscopy have identified an increased number of lamellar membrane whorls in some nuclear cataracts. The degree to which protein aggregates or these membrane modifications contribute to the increased light scattering of nuclear cataracts is unclear.

Cortical Cataracts

In contrast to nuclear cataracts, cortical cataracts are associated with local disruption of the structure of mature lens fiber cells. Once membrane integrity is compromised, essential metabolites are lost from the affected cells. This loss leads to extensive protein oxidation and precipitation. Like nuclear cataracts, cortical cataracts are usually bilateral but are often asymmetric. Their effect on visual function varies greatly, depending on the location of the opacity relative to the visual axis. A common symptom of cortical cataracts is glare from intense focal light sources, such as car headlights. Monocular diplopia may also result. Cortical cataracts vary greatly in their rate of progression; some cortical opacities remain unchanged for prolonged periods, while others progress rapidly.

On examination with the slit-lamp biomicroscope, the first visible signs of cortical cataract formation are vacuoles (Fig 5-3) and water clefts in the anterior or posterior cortex. The cortical lamellae may be separated by fluid. Wedge-shaped opacities (often called *cortical spokes* or *cuneiform opacities*) form near the periphery of the lens, with the pointed end of the opacities oriented toward the center (Fig 5-4). The cortical spokes appear as white opacities when viewed with the slit-lamp biomicroscope and as dark shadows when viewed by retroillumination. The wedge-shaped opacities may spread to adjacent fiber cells and along the length of affected fibers, causing the degree of opacity to increase and extend toward the visual axis. When the entire cortex, from the capsule to the nucleus, becomes white and opaque, the cataract is said to be *mature* (Fig 5-5). In mature opacities, the lens absorbs water, becoming swollen and enlarged (termed *intumescent* cortical cataract); such cataracts may lead to angle-closure glaucoma.

When degenerated cortical material leaks through the lens capsule, leaving the capsule wrinkled and shrunken, the cataract is referred to as *hypermature* (Fig 5-6). When further liquefaction of the cortex allows free movement of the nucleus within the capsular bag, the cataract is described as *morgagnian* (Fig 5-7).

On histologic examination, cortical cataracts are characterized by local swelling and disruption of the lens fiber cells. Globules of eosinophilic material (morgagnian globules)

A 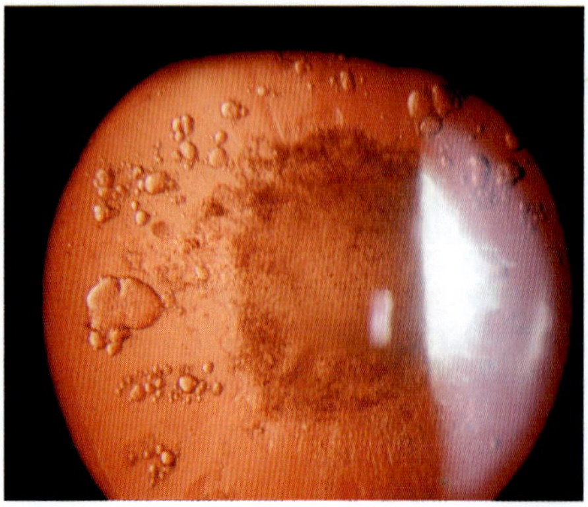

B 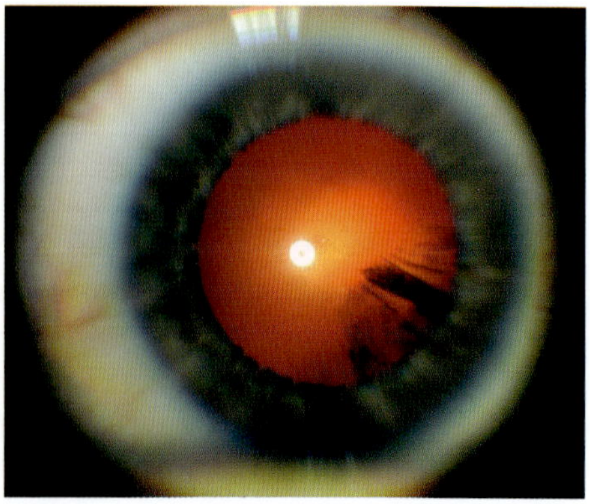

Figure 5-3 Early cortical cataract development as viewed at the slit lamp using retroillumination. **A,** Vacuoles in the periphery of a combined cataract with central PSC plaque. **B,** Typical cortical spokes. *(Courtesy of James Gilman, CRA, FOPS.)*

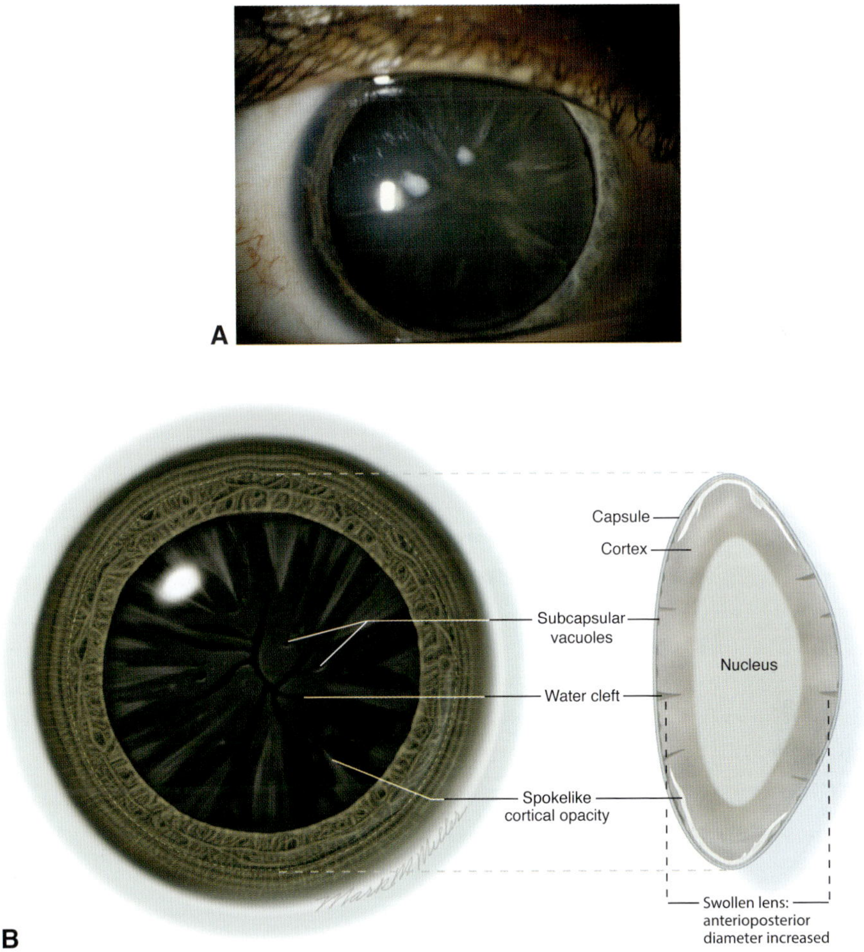

Figure 5-4 Cortical cataract. **A,** Cortical cataract viewed by oblique view at the slit lamp. **B,** Schematic of immature cortical cataract. *(Part A courtesy of James Gilman, CRA, FOPS; part B illustration by Mark Miller.)*

are observed in slitlike spaces between lens fibers (see Fig 9-11 in BCSC Section 4, *Ophthalmic Pathology and Intraocular Tumors*).

Posterior Subcapsular Cataracts

Patients who present with posterior subcapsular cataracts (PSCs) are often younger than those presenting with nuclear or cortical cataracts. PSCs are located in the posterior cortical layer and are visually significant only when they encroach on the visual axis (Fig 5-8). The first indication of PSC formation is a subtle iridescent sheen in the posterior cortical layer, which is visible with the slit lamp. At later stages, granular opacities and a plaquelike opacity of the posterior subcapsular cortex develop.

Patients with PSCs often report symptoms of glare and poor vision under bright-light conditions, because a central PSC obscures more of the pupillary aperture when miosis

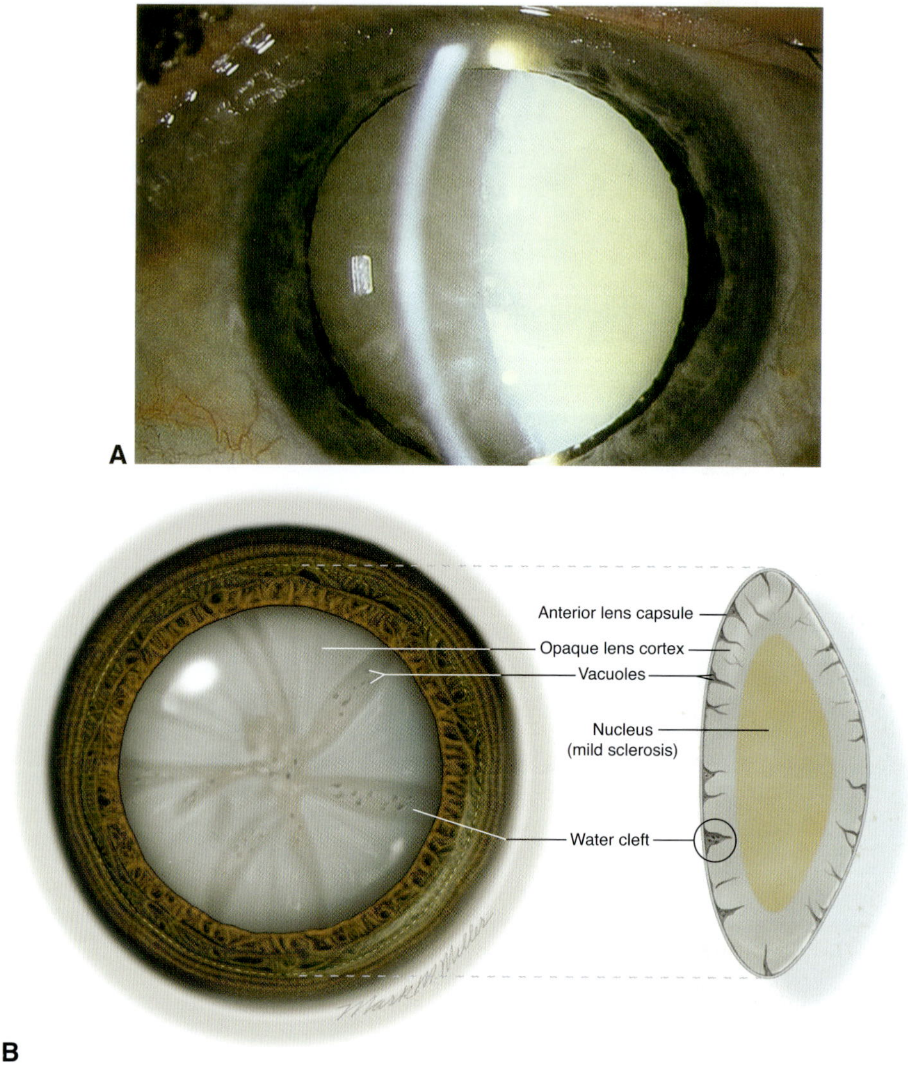

Figure 5-5 Mature cortical cataract. **A,** Mature cortical cataract viewed at the slit lamp. **B,** Schematic of mature cortical cataract. *(Part B illustration by Mark Miller.)*

is induced by bright lights, accommodation, or miotics. Near vision tends to be reduced more than distance vision in these patients. Some patients experience monocular diplopia. Slit-lamp detection of PSCs can best be accomplished through a dilated pupil. Retroillumination may also be helpful.

Although PSCs are typically related to increasing age, they can also occur after ocular trauma; systemic, topical, inhalational, or intraocular corticosteroid use; inflammation; exposure to ionizing radiation and some medications like tamoxifen; and prolonged alcohol abuse.

On histologic examination, PSCs are associated with posterior migration of the lens epithelial cells from the lens equator to the visual axis on the inner surface of the posterior

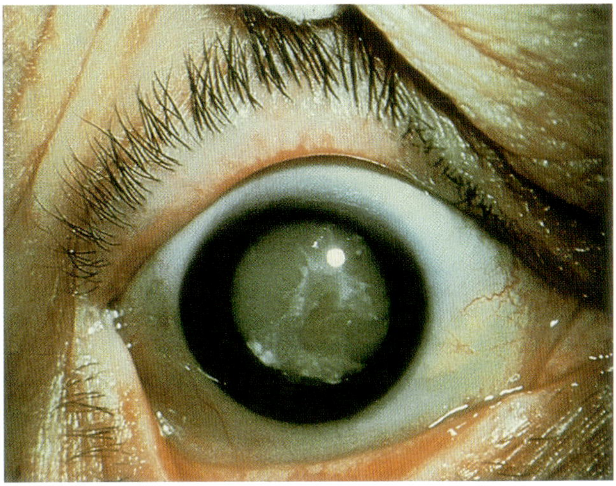

A

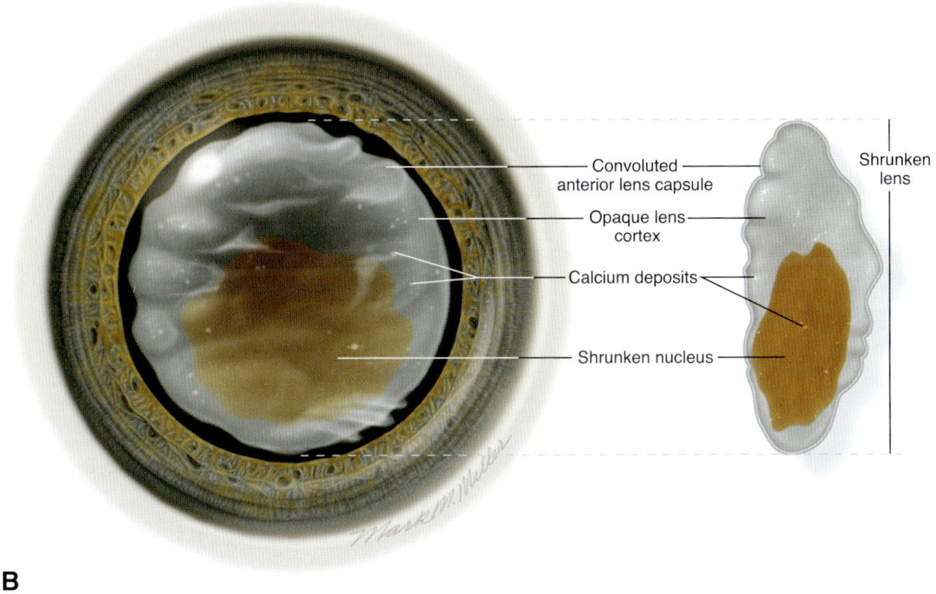

B

Figure 5-6 Hypermature cortical cataract. **A,** Clinical photo of hypermature cortical cataract. **B,** Schematic of hypermature cortical cataract. *(Part B illustration by Mark Miller.)*

capsule. During their migration to or after their arrival at the posterior axis, the cells undergo aberrant enlargement. These swollen cells are called *Wedl* (or *bladder*) cells (see Fig 9-7B in BCSC Section 4, *Ophthalmic Pathology and Intraocular Tumors*).

Keel S, He M. Risk factors for age-related cataract. *Clin Exp Ophthalmol.* 2018;46(4):327–328.

Pesudovs K, Elliott DB. Refractive error changes in cortical, nuclear, and posterior subcapsular cataracts. *Br J Ophthalmol.* 2003;87(8):964–967.

A

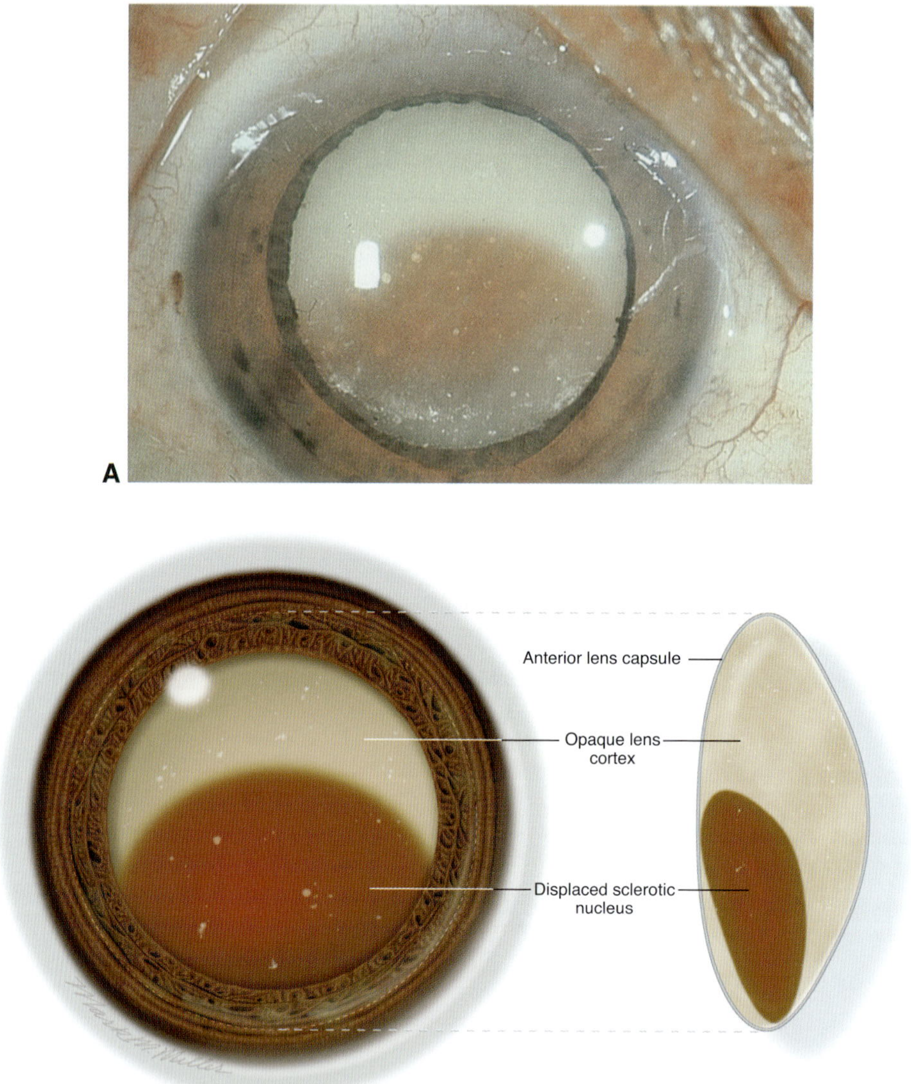

B

Figure 5-7 Morgagnian cataract. **A,** Clinical photo of morgagnian cataract. **B,** Schematic of morgagnian cataract. *(Part B illustration by Mark Miller.)*

Cataract Grading and Classification

Many systems have been proposed for grading cataract severity, using reference photographs to evaluate the color and opacity of the crystalline lens. To be clinically useful, such a grading system must be easy to learn and reproducible, and its degree of complexity should depend on the application. For instance, a grading system used in presurgical assessment may differ from one designed to quantify small changes in lens opacification over time (eg, for use in an epidemiology study or for drug development).

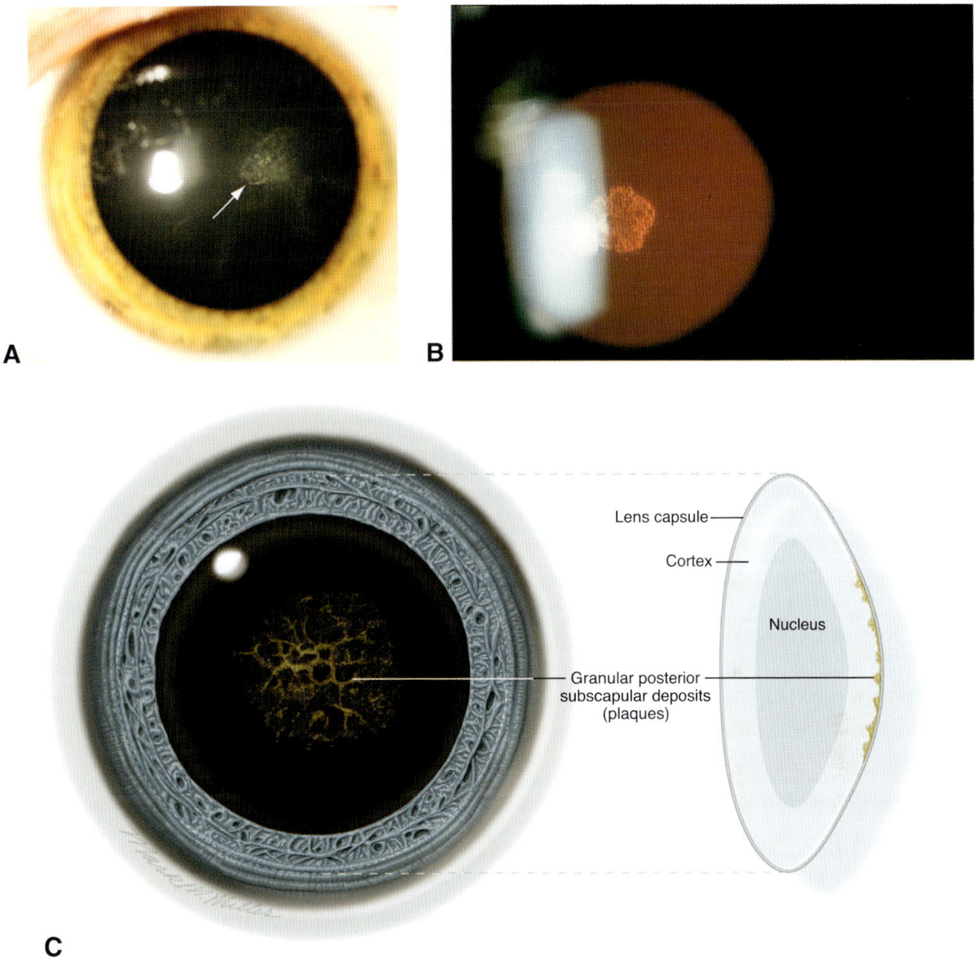

Figure 5-8 Posterior subcapsular cataract (PSC). **A,** Clinical photograph. **B,** Viewed with indirect illumination. **C,** Schematic of PSC. *(Part A courtesy of Arlene V. Drack, MD; part C illustration by Mark Miller.)*

The Lens Opacities Classification System III (LOCS III), which is widely used today, consists of a chart with 6 slit-lamp photographs used for evaluating nuclear coloration and opalescence, 5 retroillumination images used for grading cortical cataract, and 5 retroillumination photos used for evaluating PSC. A recent review suggests that although LOCS III is often used in clinical practice, it likely has little impact on the decision of when to perform cataract surgery. New systems that incorporate lens density measurements taken from anterior segment optical coherence tomography (OCT) and fundus photography and that utilize machine learning and artificial intelligence will enable researchers and clinicians to evaluate lens pathology in a standardized and objective way.

Chylack LT Jr, Wolfe JK, Singer DM, et al. The Lens Opacities Classification System III. The Longitudinal Study of Cataract Study Group. *Arch Ophthalmol.* 1993;111(6):831–836.

Gali HE, Sella R, Afshari NA. Cataract grading systems: a review of past and present. *Curr Opin Ophthalmol.* 2019;30(1):13–18.

Drug-Induced Lens Changes

Corticosteroids

Long-term use of corticosteroids has been correlated with cataract development, especially PSC formation. The development of corticosteroid-induced PSCs is related to the dose and treatment duration. Cataract formation can occur with the use of oral, topical, or inhaled corticosteroids. Treatment with intraocular steroids for retinal neovascularization and inflammation may also result in the development of PSCs, as well as ocular hypertension. The advent of slow-release steroid repositories, including subconjunctival and intravitreal implants, has not altered the risk of adverse ocular effects (eg, intraocular pressure elevation and PSC development) of these medications.

On histological and clinical examination, PSC formation that occurs subsequent to corticosteroid use cannot be distinguished from age-related PSC formation. Some corticosteroid-induced PSCs in children may resolve with cessation of the drug.

Fraunfelder FT, Fraunfelder FW, Chambers WA. *Drug-Induced Ocular Side Effects.* 7th ed. Saunders; 2015.

Jaffe GJ, Martin D, Callanan D, et al; Fluocinolone Acetonide Uveitis Study Group. Fluocinolone acetonide implant (Retisert) for noninfectious posterior uveitis: thirty-four-week results of a multicenter randomized clinical study. *Ophthalmology.* 2006;113(6):1020–1027.

Kiernan DF, Mieler WF. The use of intraocular corticosteroids. *Expert Opin Pharmacother.* 2009;10(15):2511–2525.

Phenothiazines

Phenothiazines, a group of medications used to treat mental and emotional disorders, can cause pigmented deposits in the anterior lens epithelium in an axial stellate configuration (Fig 5-9). The occurrence of these deposits appears to depend on both drug dose and treatment duration. In addition, the deposits are more likely to occur with the use of some

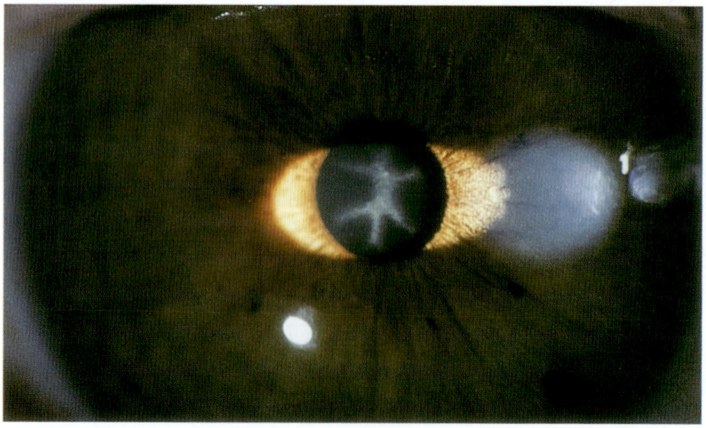

Figure 5-9 Slit-lamp image of pigmented deposits on anterior lens capsule in a patient treated with phenothiazines.

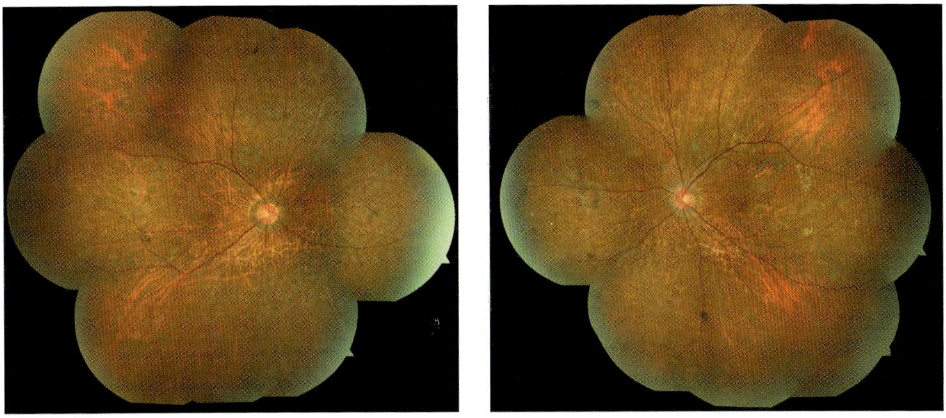

Figure 5-10 Color fundus photograph montages of right and left eyes showing thioridazine toxicity in a patient with schizophrenia. *(Courtesy of David Sarraf, MD.)*

phenothiazines, notably chlorpromazine and thioridazine, than with others. The vision changes associated with phenothiazine deposition in the lens are generally insignificant; however, the use of thioridazine may result in severe retinopathy with a deleterious effect on vision (Fig 5-10).

Miotics

Topical anticholinesterases, which have been used in the treatment of glaucoma, can cause cataract formation. However, because these medications are now used only in rare cases, this type of cataract is uncommon. The incidence of cataracts has been reported to be as high as 20% in patients after 55 months of pilocarpine use and 60% in patients after echothiophate iodide use.

Usually, this type of cataract first appears as small vacuoles within and posterior to the anterior lens capsule and epithelium. The cataract may progress to posterior cortical and nuclear lens changes. Cataract formation is more likely in patients receiving anticholinesterase therapy over a long period and in those receiving more frequent dosing.

Amiodarone

Amiodarone, an antiarrhythmic medication, has been reported to cause stellate pigment deposition in the anterior cortical axis. Only in very rare instances does this condition become visually significant. Amiodarone is also deposited in the corneal epithelium (cornea verticillata; Fig 5-11) and can cause an optic neuropathy, also only in rare instances.

Statins

Studies performed in dogs have shown that some 3-hydroxy-3-methylglutaryl coenzyme A (HMG-CoA) reductase inhibitors, known as *statins,* are associated with cataract when taken in excessive doses. Conflicting human studies have indicated that statins are both a risk factor for development of nuclear sclerotic cataracts and protective against

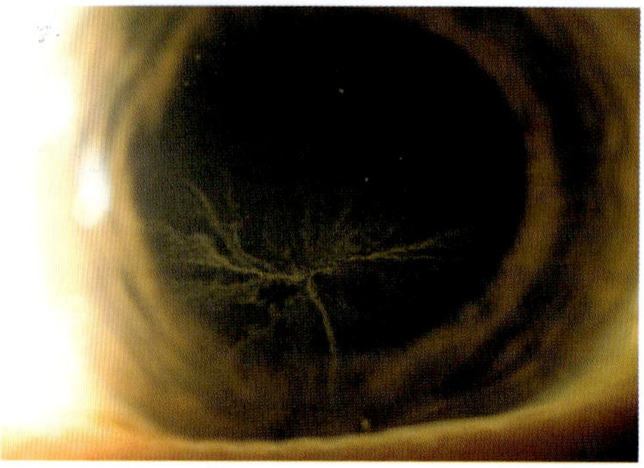

Figure 5-11 Image showing amiodarone deposits on corneal epithelium in a characteristic whorled pattern. *(Courtesy of James Gilman, CRA, FOPS.)*

them. The latest meta-analysis of human observational studies suggests an increased risk of cataract development associated with taking statins, but the magnitude of the effect is low. However, concomitant use of simvastatin and erythromycin, which increases circulating statin levels, may be associated with approximately a twofold increased risk of cataract.

Alves C, Mendes D, Batel Marques F. Statins and risk of cataracts: a systematic review and meta-analysis of observational studies. *Cardiovasc Ther.* 2018;36(6):e12480.

Leuschen J, Mortensen EM, Frei CR, Mansi EA, Panday V, Mansi I. Association of statin use with cataracts: a propensity score-matched analysis. *JAMA Ophthalmol.* 2013;131(11): 1427–1434.

Tamoxifen

Tamoxifen, an antiestrogen medication used in the prevention and adjuvant treatment of breast cancer, is thought to be related to development of cataract. Although 1 study has not substantiated this association, other studies have shown up to a fourfold increase in the risk of developing cataract, especially PSC, associated with tamoxifen use. Crystalline maculopathy has been reported in patients receiving high-dose tamoxifen therapy. Cystoid macular edema (CME) may also be present with these inner-retinal crystalline deposits and can cause significant, irreversible vision loss. See also BCSC Section 12, *Retina and Vitreous*, for discussion of tamoxifen retinopathy.

Bradbury BD, Lash TL, Kaye JA, Jick SS. Tamoxifen and cataracts: a null association. *Breast Cancer Res Treat.* 2004;87(2):189–196.

Eisner A, Luoh S-W. Breast cancer medications and vision: effects of treatments for early-stage disease. *Curr Eye Res.* 2011;36(10):867–885.

Nichols HB, DeRoo LA, Scharf DR, Sandler DP. Risk-benefit profiles of women using tamoxifen for chemoprevention. *J Natl Cancer Inst.* 2014;107(1):354.

Trauma

Traumatic lens damage may be caused by mechanical injury and by physical forces such as radiation, chemicals, and electrical current.

Contusion

Vossius ring

Blunt injury to the eye can sometimes cause a ring of pigment (known as a *Vossius ring*) from the pupillary ruff to be imprinted on the anterior surface of the lens. Although a Vossius ring is visually insignificant and gradually resolves with time, its presence indicates prior blunt trauma, and it may be associated with other ocular injuries, including damage to angle structures.

Traumatic cataract

A blunt, nonperforating injury may cause lens opacification either as an acute event or as a late sequela. A contusion cataract may involve the entire lens or only a portion of the lens. Often, the initial manifestation of a contusion cataract is a stellate or rosette-shaped opacification *(rosette cataract)*, usually axial in location, that involves the posterior lens capsule (Fig 5-12). In some cases, blunt trauma causes both dislocation and cataract formation (Fig 5-13). In rare cases, mild contusion cataracts can improve spontaneously.

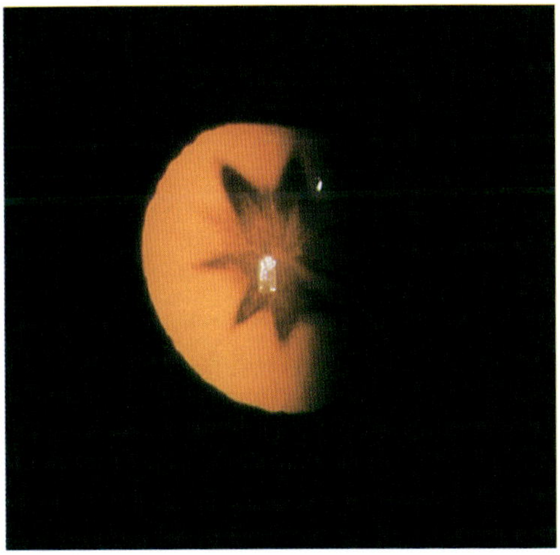

Figure 5-12 Slit-lamp retroillumination of a stellate lens opacity following contusion.

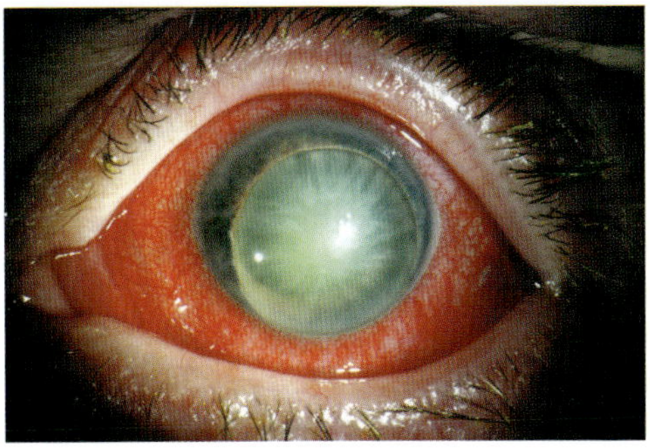

Figure 5-13 Cataractous lens has partially dislocated into anterior chamber following blunt trauma. *(Courtesy of James Gilman, CRA, FOPS.)*

Shah M, Shah S, Upadhyay P, Agrawal R. Controversies in traumatic cataract classification and management: a review. *Can J Ophthalmol.* 2013;48(4):251–258.

Smith MP, Colyer MA, Weichel ED, Stutzman RD. Traumatic cataracts secondary to combat ocular trauma. *J Cataract Refract Surg.* 2015;41(8):1693–1698.

Dislocation and subluxation

During a blunt injury to the eye, rapid expansion of the globe in an equatorial plane immediately follows compression. This rapid equatorial expansion can disrupt the zonular fibers, causing dislocation or subluxation of the lens. The lens may be dislocated in any direction, including posteriorly into the vitreous cavity or anteriorly into the anterior chamber.

Symptoms and signs of traumatic lens subluxation include fluctuation of vision, impaired accommodation, monocular diplopia, and high astigmatism. Often, iridodonesis or phacodonesis is present. Retroillumination of the lens at the slit lamp through a dilated pupil may reveal the zonular disruption.

Irvine JA, Smith RE. Lens injuries. In: Shingleton BJ, Hersh PS, Kenyon KR, eds. *Eye Trauma.* Mosby; 1991:126–135.

Perforating or Penetrating Injury

A perforating or penetrating injury of the lens often causes opacification of the cortex at the site of the rupture, which usually progresses rapidly to complete opacification (Fig 5-14). Occasionally, a small perforating injury of the lens capsule heals, resulting in a stationary focal cortical cataract (Fig 5-15).

Intraocular Procedures

Virtually any intraocular procedure may be associated with cataract formation, either shortly after surgery or following a longer period of healing. Pars plana vitrectomy, especially with gas tamponade of the retina, is strongly associated with nuclear sclerotic cataract formation. A visually significant nuclear sclerotic cataract develops in 80%–100% of phakic eyes within 2 years of undergoing vitrectomy.

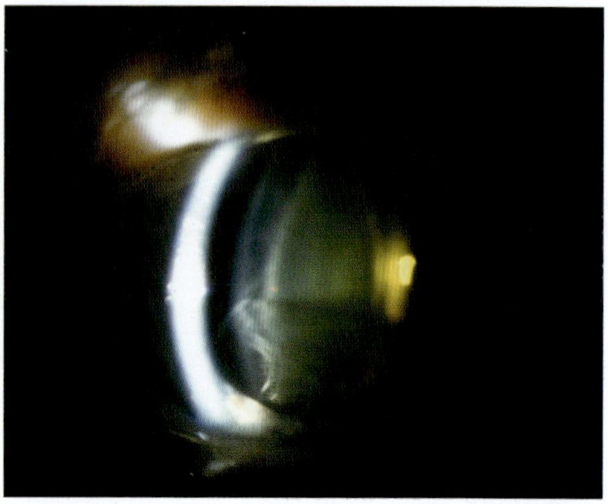

Figure 5-14 Inferior cortical opacification after capsule disruption by perforating injury. *(Courtesy of James Gilman, CRA, FOPS.)*

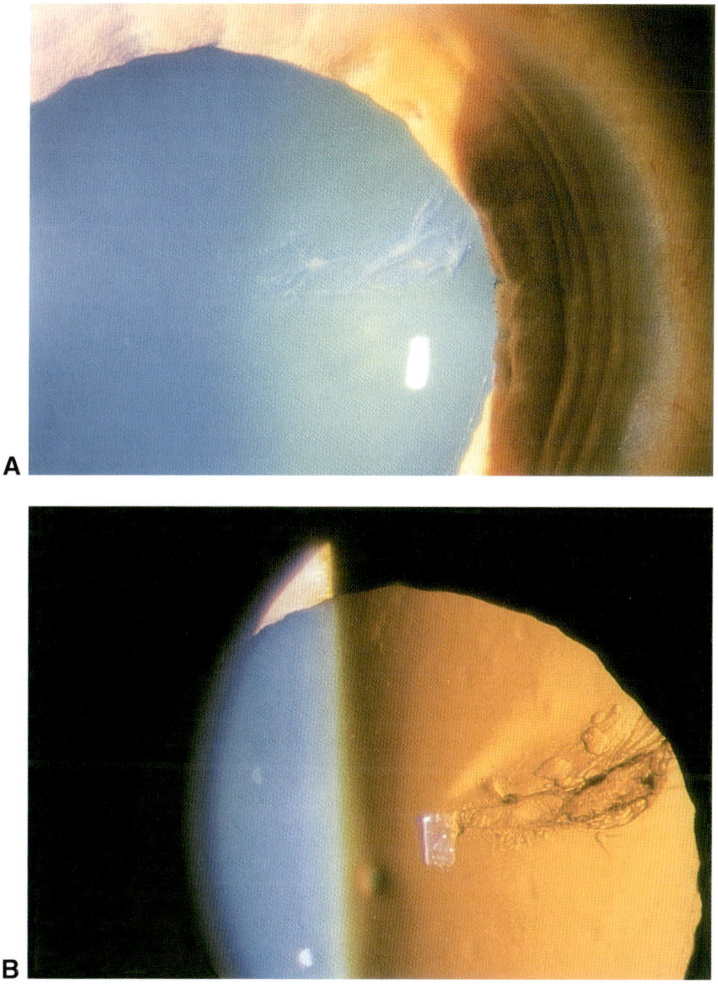

Figure 5-15 Focal cortical cataract. **A,** Focal cortical cataract from a small perforating injury to the lens capsule as viewed by direct illumination. **B,** Focal cortical cataract viewed by retroillumination.

Postvitrectomy cataracts are less common in patients younger than 50 years. The formation of nuclear cataracts after vitrectomy is associated with increases in oxygen tension in the vitreous intraoperatively and postoperatively. (See Chapter 3 for a discussion of oxygen tension in the lens.) Retinal surgery performed without vitrectomy is not associated with increased nuclear sclerosis, but any disturbance of the capsule during a vitreous procedure may precipitate a PSC.

Intravitreal injections may be associated with cataract formation either as a result of direct trauma to the lens or as an adverse effect of specific medications injected into the vitreous space.

Trabeculectomy is a known risk factor for development of visually significant cataract. The Collaborative Initial Glaucoma Treatment Study found that glaucoma patients who were initially treated with trabeculectomy were 8 times more likely to need early cataract surgery than those patients who were initially treated with medications. At 5 years following trabeculectomy, this risk decreased to 3 times more likely.

Nuclear sclerotic cataract formation also occurs at significantly higher rates in patients who have received penetrating keratoplasty or Descemet stripping endothelial keratoplasty.

Feng H, Adelman RA. Cataract formation following vitreoretinal procedures. *Clin Ophthalmol.* 2014;8:1957–1965.

Musch DC, Gillespie BW, Niziol LM, et al; Collaborative Initial Glaucoma Treatment Study Group. Cataract extraction in the Collaborative Initial Glaucoma Treatment Study: incidence, risk factors, and the effect of cataract progression and extraction on clinical and quality-of-life outcomes. *Arch Ophthalmol.* 2006;124(12):1694–1700.

Price MO, Price DA, Fairchild KM, Price FW Jr. Rate and risk factors for cataract formation and extraction after Descemet stripping endothelial keratoplasty. *Br J Ophthalmol.* 2010; 94(11):1468–1471.

Intralenticular Foreign Bodies

In rare instances, a small foreign body can perforate the cornea and the anterior lens capsule and become lodged within the lens. If the foreign body is not composed of iron or copper and the anterior lens capsule seals the perforation site, the foreign body may be retained within the lens without significant complication. Intralenticular foreign bodies may cause cataract formation in some cases but do not always lead to lens opacification.

Radiation

Ionizing radiation

The lens is extremely sensitive to ionizing radiation; however, up to 20 years may pass after exposure before a cataract becomes clinically apparent. This period of latency is related to the dose of radiation and to the patient's age; younger patients are more susceptible because they have more lens cells that are actively growing. Ionizing radiation in the x-ray range (0.001–10.0-nm wavelength) can cause cataracts in some individuals in doses as low as 2 Gy in a single fraction. (A routine chest x-ray equals 0.01-Gy exposure to the thorax.) A single computed tomography (CT) scan of the brain may expose the lens to as much as 2.5–5 cGy (100 cGy = 1 Gy).

The first clinical signs of radiation-induced cataract are often punctate opacities within the posterior capsule and feathery anterior subcapsular opacities that radiate toward the equator of the lens. These opacities may progress to complete opacification of the lens.

Infrared radiation

Exposure of the eye to infrared (IR) radiation and intense heat over time can cause the outer layers of the anterior lens capsule to peel off as a single layer. Such true exfoliation of the lens capsule, in which the exfoliated outer lamella tends to scroll up on itself, is seen today only in rare cases. Cortical cataract may be associated with this condition, in which

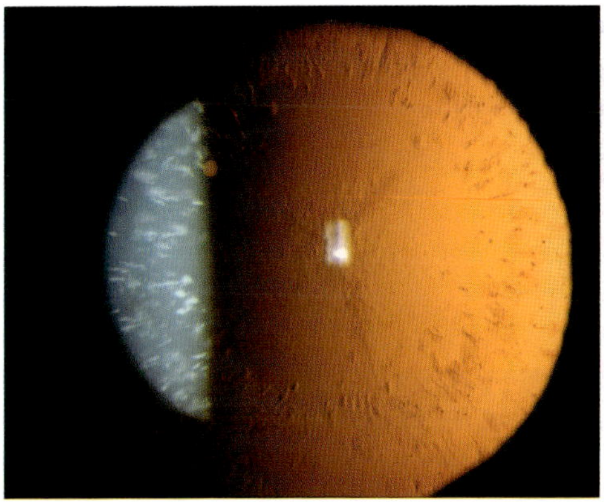

Figure 5-16 Infrared radiation may cause cortical changes, for example, this glassblower's cataract. *(Courtesy of James Gilman, CRA, FOPS.)*

case it is known as *glassblower's cataract* (Fig 5-16). (See the section Pseudoexfoliation Syndrome later in this chapter.)

Ultraviolet radiation

Experimental evidence suggests that the lens is susceptible to damage from ultraviolet (UV) radiation. Epidemiologic evidence suggests that long-term exposure to sunlight is associated with an increased risk of cortical cataracts, perhaps more frequently in men than women. Although sunlight exposure accounts for only approximately 10% of the total risk of cortical cataract in the general population in temperate climates, this risk is avoidable. Because exposure to UV radiation can lead to other morbidity, clinicians should encourage their patients to avoid excessive sunlight exposure. Lenses sold in the United States must conform to the American National Standards Institute (ANSI) requirements aimed at reducing UV transmission. Using prescription corrective lenses and nonprescription sunglasses decreases UV exposure by more than 80%, and wearing a hat with a brim decreases ocular sun exposure by 30%–50%.

Klein BE, Lee KE, Danforth LG, Schaich TM, Cruickshanks KJ, Klein R. Selected sun-sensitizing medications and incident cataract. *Arch Ophthalmol.* 2010;128(8):959–963.

Modenese A, Gobba F. Cataract frequency and subtypes involved in workers assessed for their solar radiation exposure: a systematic review. *Acta Ophthalmol.* 2018;96(8):779–788.

Metallosis

Siderosis bulbi

Intraocular iron-containing foreign bodies can cause siderosis bulbi, a condition in which iron molecules are deposited in the trabecular meshwork, lens epithelium, iris, and retina (Fig 5-17A). The epithelium and cortical fibers of the affected lens at first show a yellowish tinge, followed by a rusty brown discoloration (Fig 5-17B). Lens involvement occurs more rapidly if the retained foreign body is embedded close to the lens. Later manifestations of siderosis bulbi are complete cortical cataract formation and retinal dysfunction. See also BCSC Section 12, *Retina and Vitreous.*

A

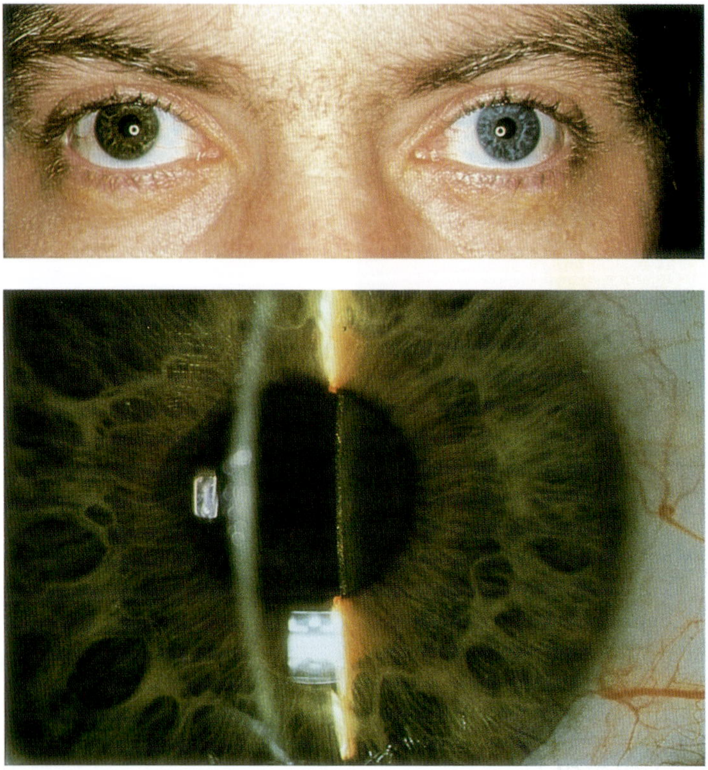

B

Figure 5-17 Siderosis bulbi. **A,** Heterochromia iridis caused by siderosis bulbi. **B,** Discoloration of the lens capsule and cortex.

Chalcosis

Chalcosis occurs when an intraocular foreign body deposits copper in Descemet membrane, anterior lens capsule, or other intraocular basement membranes. The resulting *"sunflower" cataract* is a petal-shaped deposition of yellow or brown pigment in the lens capsule that radiates from the anterior axial pole of the lens to the equator. Usually, this cataract causes no significant loss of vision. However, intraocular foreign bodies containing almost pure copper (more than 90%) can cause a severe inflammatory reaction and intraocular necrosis.

Electrical Injury

Electrical shock can cause protein coagulation and cataract formation. Lens manifestations are more likely when the transmission of current involves the patient's head. Initially, lens vacuoles appear in the anterior midperiphery of the lens, followed by linear opacities in the anterior subcapsular cortex. A cataract induced by an electrical injury may regress, remain stationary, or mature to become a complete cataract over months or years (Fig 5-18).

Portellos M, Orlin SE, Kozart DM. Electric cataracts. *Arch Ophthalmol.* 1996;114(8):1022–1023.

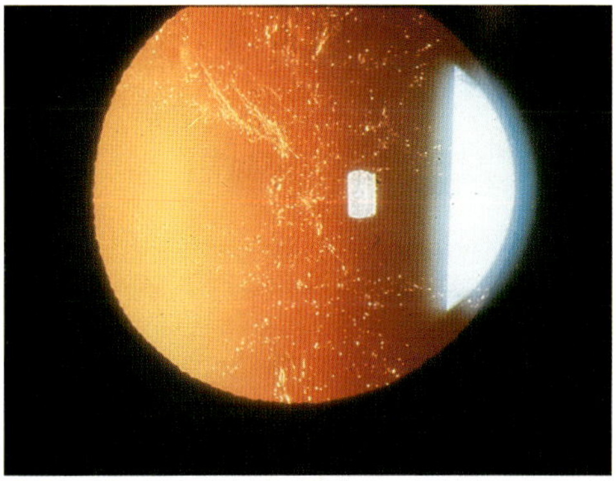

Figure 5-18 Cataract induced by electrical injury. *(Courtesy of Karla J. Johns, MD.)*

Chemical Injuries

Alkali injuries to the ocular surface often result in cataract, in addition to damaging the cornea, conjunctiva, and iris. Alkali compounds penetrate the eye readily, causing an increase in aqueous pH and a decrease in the level of aqueous glucose and ascorbate. Cortical cataract formation may occur acutely or as a delayed effect of chemical injury. Because acid tends to penetrate the eye less easily than does alkali, acid injuries are less likely to result in cataract formation.

Metabolic Cataract

Diabetes Mellitus

Diabetes mellitus can affect lens clarity as well as the refractive index and accommodative amplitude of the lens. As the blood glucose level increases, so does the glucose content in the aqueous humor (See Chapter 3 in this volume for a discussion of glucose-induced lens changes). Acute myopic shifts may indicate undiagnosed or poorly controlled diabetes mellitus. Patients with type 1 diabetes mellitus have a decreased amplitude of accommodation compared with age-matched controls, and presbyopia may present at a younger age in these patients.

Cataract is a common cause of visual impairment in patients with diabetes mellitus. Acute *diabetic cataract,* or *"snowflake" cataract,* refers to bilateral, widespread subcapsular lens changes of abrupt onset and typically occurs in young individuals with uncontrolled diabetes mellitus (Fig 5-19). Multiple gray-white subcapsular opacities that have a snowflake appearance are seen initially in the superficial anterior and posterior lens cortex. Vacuoles and clefts form in the underlying cortex. Intumescence and maturity of the cortical cataract follow shortly thereafter. Although acute diabetic cataracts are encountered in clinical practice only in rare cases today, rapidly maturing bilateral cortical cataracts in a child or young adult may indicate the presence of diabetes mellitus.

Patients with diabetes mellitus develop age-related lens changes that are indistinguishable from nondiabetic age-related cataracts, except that these lens changes tend to occur at

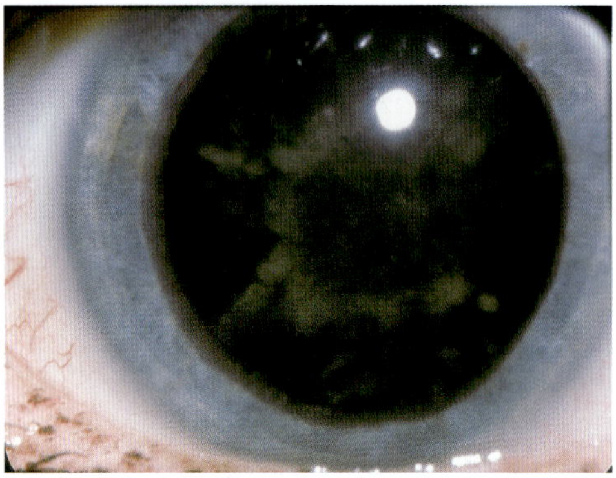

Figure 5-19 Diabetic cataract, or "snowflake" cataract, consists of gray-white subcapsular opacities. *(Courtesy of Karla J. Johns, MD.)*

a younger age than in those without the disease. The increased risk or earlier onset of age-related cataracts in diabetic patients may be a result of the accumulation of sorbitol within the lens and accompanying changes in hydration, increased nonenzymatic glycosylation of lens proteins, or greater oxidative stress from alterations in lens metabolism. These stressors may promote an increase in nuclear sclerotic cataract, cortical cataract, and PSC formation.

Cataract is the leading cause of visual impairment among children and adolescents with diabetes mellitus and may be the first sign of the disorder or may appear within 6 months of diagnosis. In various studies, the incidence of cataract among pediatric patients with diabetes was between 0.7% and 3.4% of those studied. In a study of 370 pediatric patients with diabetes mellitus, no patients were diagnosed with diabetic retinopathy, but 12 patients had cataract, and 5 of those required surgery. There is no consensus guideline for screening pediatric patients with diabetes for cataract, but some study authors have recommended an eye examination when diabetes is diagnosed and annually thereafter.

Geloneck MM, Forbes BJ, Shaffer J, Ying GS, Binenbaum G. Ocular complications in children with diabetes mellitus. *Ophthalmology.* 2015;122(12):2457–2464.

Klein BE, Klein R, Wang Q, Moss SE. Older-onset diabetes and lens opacities. The Beaver Dam Eye Study. *Ophthalmic Epidemiol.* 1995;2(1):49–55.

Li L, Wan XH, Zhao GH. Meta-analysis of the risk of cataract in type 2 diabetes. *BMC Ophthalmol.* 2014;14:94.

Šimunović M, Paradžik M, Škrabić R, Unić I, Bućan K, Škrabić V. Cataract as early ocular complication in children and adolescents with type 1 diabetes mellitus. *Int J Endocrinol.* 2018;2018:6763586.

Galactosemia

Galactosemia is an inherited autosomal recessive inability to convert galactose to glucose. As a consequence of this inability, excessive galactose accumulates in body tissues, with further metabolic conversion of galactose to galactitol (dulcitol), the sugar alcohol product of galactose. Galactosemia can result from defects in 1 of the 3 enzymes involved in the metabolism of galactose. The most common and the most severe form, known as *classic galactosemia,* is caused by a defect in galactose-1-phosphate uridyltransferase.

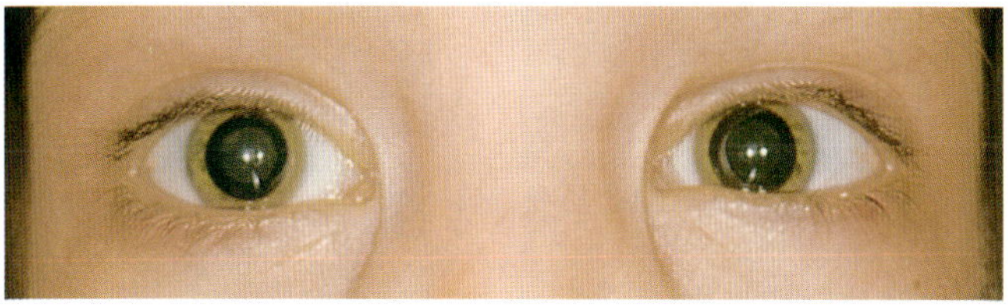

Figure 5-20 "Oil droplet" bilateral cataracts in a patient with galactosemia.

In cases of classic galactosemia, symptoms of malnutrition, hepatomegaly, jaundice, and intellectual deficiency present within the first few weeks of life. The disease is fatal if undiagnosed and untreated. The diagnosis of classic galactosemia can be confirmed by demonstration of galactose in the urine.

Typically, the nucleus and deep cortex become increasingly opacified in individuals with this condition, causing an "oil droplet" appearance on retroillumination (Fig 5-20). The cataracts can progress to total opacification.

Treatment of galactosemia includes elimination of milk and milk products from the diet. In the majority of cases, early cataract formation can be reversed by timely diagnosis and dietary intervention; other cases may require cataract surgery. The oil droplet appearance in classic galactosemia differs markedly from the similarly named oil droplet cataract of posterior lenticonus. In posterior lenticonus, it is a bulge in the posterior capsule that causes the oil droplet appearance on red reflex examination.

Karadag N, Zenciroglu A, Eminoglu FT, et al. Literature review and outcome of classic galactosemia diagnosed in the neonatal period. *Clin Lab.* 2013;59(9–10):1139–1146.

Hypocalcemia

Cataracts may develop in association with any condition that results in hypocalcemia. Hypocalcemia may be idiopathic, or it may occur as a result of unintended destruction of the parathyroid glands during thyroid surgery. Usually bilateral, hypocalcemic (tetanic) cataracts are punctate iridescent opacities in the anterior and posterior cortex. They lie beneath the lens capsule and are usually separated from it by a zone of clear lens. These discrete opacities may remain stable or may mature into complete cortical cataracts.

Wilson Disease

Wilson disease (hepatolenticular degeneration) is an inherited autosomal recessive disorder of copper metabolism. The characteristic ocular manifestation of Wilson disease is the Kayser-Fleischer ring, a golden-brown discoloration of Descemet membrane around the periphery of the cornea (Fig 5-21A). In addition, a characteristic sunflower cataract often develops. Reddish-brown pigment (cuprous oxide) is deposited in the anterior lens capsule and subcapsular cortex in a stellate shape that resembles the petals of a sunflower (Fig 5-21B). In most cases, the sunflower cataract does not cause serious visual impairment. See also BCSC Section 8, *External Disease and Cornea.*

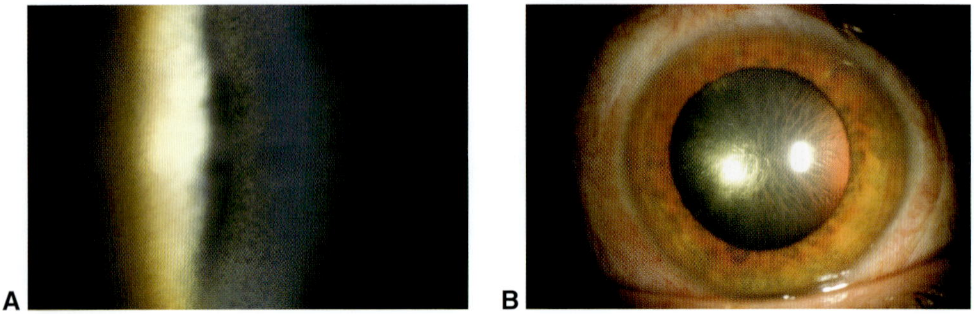

Figure 5-21 Ocular manifestations of Wilson disease. **A,** Slit-lamp image of Kayser-Fleischer ring, a golden-brown staining of Descemet membrane in corneal periphery. **B,** Clinical photo of reddish cuprous oxide deposited in the anterior lens capsule in a "sunflower" cataract. *(Courtesy of James Gilman, CRA, FOPS.)*

Myotonic Dystrophy

Myotonic dystrophy is an inherited autosomal dominant condition characterized by delayed relaxation of contracted muscles, ptosis, weakness of the facial musculature, cardiac conduction defects, and prominent frontal balding in affected male patients. Patients with this disorder typically develop polychromatic iridescent crystals in the lens cortex (Fig 5-22), with sequential PSC that progresses to complete cortical opacification. These polychromatic iridescent crystals are composed of whorls of plasmalemma from the lens fibers. Iridescent crystals that are similar in appearance are occasionally seen in the lens cortex of patients who do not have myotonic dystrophy; those crystals are thought to be caused by cholesterol deposition in the lens.

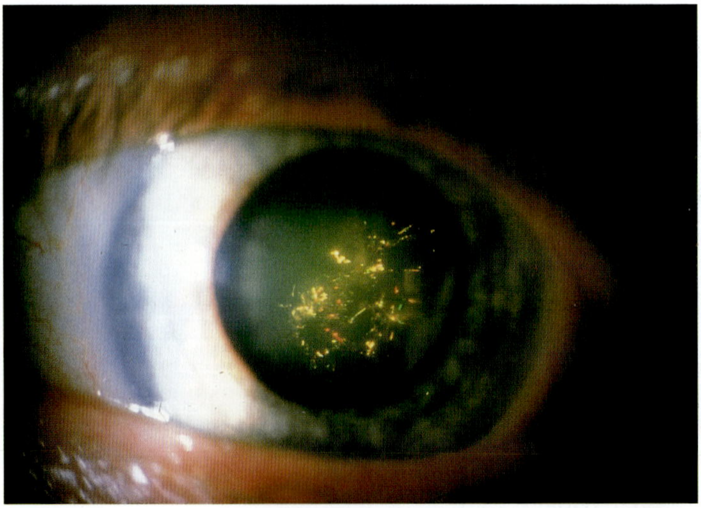

Figure 5-22 Polychromatic iridescent crystals in a patient with myotonic dystrophy. *(Courtesy of Karla J. Johns, MD.)*

Effects of Nutrition, Alcohol, and Smoking

Although nutritional deficiencies have been demonstrated to cause cataracts in animal models, this etiology has been difficult to confirm in humans. Initial population-based studies have found that increased prevalence of age-related cataracts has been associated with lower socioeconomic status, lower education level, and poorer overall nutrition. Severe episodes of dehydration caused by diarrhea may be linked to an increased risk of cataract formation. More recent studies of supplementation with vitamins, antioxidants, and estrogen have not consistently correlated these supplements with a decreased risk for cataract development.

High-dose vitamin use may pose risks. Tobacco smokers taking high doses of beta carotene appear to have an increased risk of lung cancer, death from lung cancer, and death from cardiovascular disease. In addition, women taking supplemental doses of vitamin A have an increased risk of hip fracture.

Tobacco smoking, the use of smokeless tobacco products, and excessive alcohol consumption are significant, avoidable risk factors for cataract. In numerous studies performed worldwide, these practices have consistently been associated with an increase in the frequency of nuclear opacities. Although patients may know the general health risks of smoking and excessive alcohol consumption, they may not know about the associated increased risks of ocular conditions, including macular degeneration and cataract. Ophthalmologists can inform their patients about these risks, and they are in a strong position to encourage individuals to stop smoking and reduce alcohol consumption.

Kanthan GL, Mitchell P, Burlutsky G, Wang JJ. Alcohol consumption and the long-term incidence of cataract and cataract surgery: the Blue Mountains Eye Study. *Am J Ophthalmol.* 2010; 150(3):434–440.

Raju P, George R, Ve Ramesh S, Arvind H, Baskaran M, Vijaya L. Influence of tobacco use on cataract development. *Br J Ophthalmol.* 2006;90(11):1374–1377.

Sella R, Afshari NA. Nutritional effect on age-related cataract formation and progression. *Curr Opin Ophthalmol.* 2019;30(1):63–69.

Cataract Associated With Uveitis

Lens changes may occur as a result of chronic uveitis or associated corticosteroid therapy. Typically, a PSC develops, but anterior lens opacification may also occur. The formation of posterior synechiae is common in uveitis, often with thickening of the anterior lens capsule, which may have an associated fibrous pupillary membrane. Lens changes in cataract secondary to uveitis may progress to a mature cataract. Calcium deposits may be observed on the anterior capsule or within the lens substance.

Cortical cataract formation occurs in up to 70% of cases of Fuchs heterochromic uveitis (Fig 5-23). Posterior synechiae are uncommon in this syndrome; formation of pupillary membranes is unlikely; and long-term corticosteroid therapy is not indicated. Cataract extraction in patients with Fuchs heterochromic uveitis generally has a favorable prognosis. Intraoperative anterior chamber hemorrhage at the time of cataract surgery has been reported in approximately 8%–25% of cases.

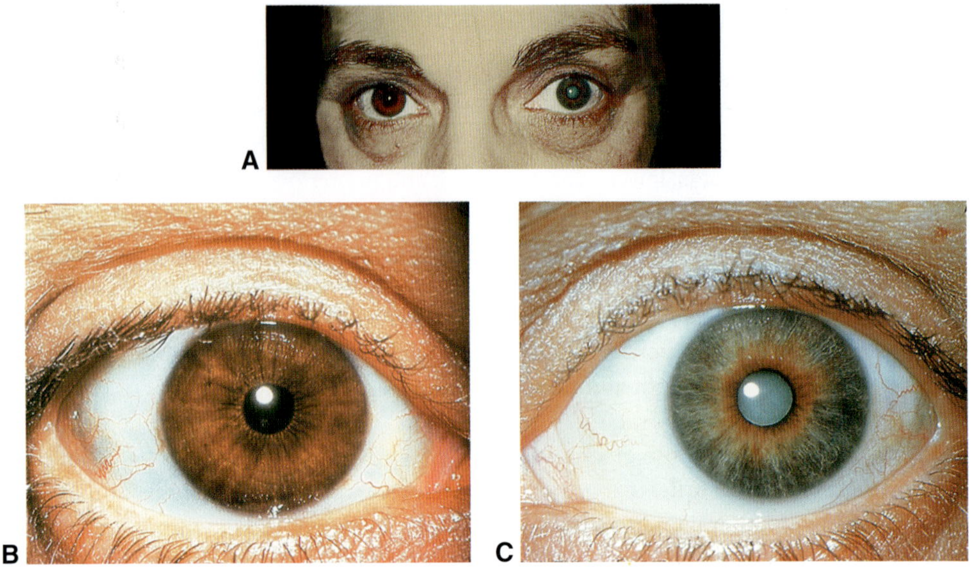

Figure 5-23 Clinical photographs from a patient with Fuchs heterochromic uveitis. **A,** The affected eye is lighter. **B,** Normal right eye. **C,** Cataract formation in the affected left eye. *(Courtesy of Karla J. Johns, MD.)*

Jones NP. Cataract surgery in Fuchs' heterochromic uveitis: past, present and future. *J Cataract Refract Surg.* 1996;22(2):261–268.

Keles S, Ondas O, Ates O, et al. Phacoemulsification and core vitrectomy in Fuchs' heterochromic uveitis. *Eurasian J Med.* 2017;49(2):97–101.

Lens Changes With Hyperbaric Oxygen Therapy

The lens may also undergo changes after hyperbaric oxygen (HBO) therapy. A myopic shift seems to occur universally during the course of treatment with HBO. This change, thought to be due to a refractive change in the crystalline lens, usually reverses after cessation of HBO treatment. However, several reports have documented the development of nuclear cataract over the course of multiple HBO treatment sessions.

Butler FK Jr, Hagan C, Murphy-Lavoie H. Hyperbaric oxygen therapy and the eye. *Undersea Hyperb Med.* 2008;35(5):333–387.

Palmquist BM, Phillipson B, Barr PO. Nuclear cataract and myopia during hyperbaric oxygen therapy. *Br J Ophthalmol.* 1984;68(2):113–117.

Pseudoexfoliation Syndrome

Pseudoexfoliation syndrome is a systemic disease in which a matrix of fibrotic material is deposited in many organs in the body. In the eye, a basement membrane–like fibrillogranular, whitish material is deposited on the cornea, iris, lens, anterior hyaloid face, ciliary processes, zonular fibers, and trabecular meshwork. These deposits, believed to

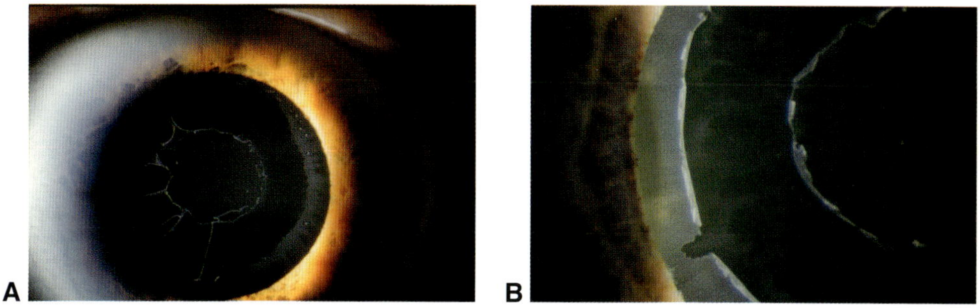

Figure 5-24 Pseudoexfoliation syndrome. **A,** Deposition of white fibrillar material in targetlike distribution on the anterior capsule. **B,** Slit-lamp photograph demonstrates atrophy of the iris margin, deposition of pigment on the anterior lens capsule, and fibrillar deposits on iris margin. *(Courtesy of James Gilman, CRA, FOPS.)*

comprise elastic microfibrils, appear as grayish-white flecks that are prominent at the pupillary margin and on the midperipheral anterior lens capsule (Fig 5-24). Associated with this condition are atrophy of the iris at the pupillary margin, deposition of pigment on the anterior surface of the iris, a poorly dilating pupil, increased pigmentation of the trabecular meshwork, capsular fragility, zonular weakness, and open-angle glaucoma. Pseudoexfoliation syndrome is a unilateral or bilateral disorder that becomes more apparent with increasing age. An association between lifetime UV-light exposure and the development of pseudoexfoliation syndrome has been documented.

Increased oxidative stress caused by abnormalities in transforming growth factor β (TGF-β) contributes to the formation of cataracts. Patients with this syndrome may also experience weakness of the zonular fibers and spontaneous lens subluxation and phacodonesis. Poor zonular integrity may affect cataract surgery technique and intraocular lens implantation. (See Chapter 12 in this volume for a discussion of cataract surgery in special situations.) The exfoliative material will continue to be produced even after the crystalline lens is removed.

Nazarali S, Damji F, Damji KF. What have we learned about exfoliation syndrome since its discovery by John Lindberg 100 years ago? *Br J Ophthalmol.* 2018;102(10):1342–1350.

Pasquale LR, Jiwani AZ, Zehavi-Dorin T, et al. Solar exposure and residential geographic history in relation to exfoliation syndrome in the United States and Israel. *JAMA Ophthalmol.* 2014;132(12):1439–1445.

Zenkel M, Lewczuk P, Jünemann A, Kruse FE, Naumann GO, Schlötzer-Schrehardt U. Proinflammatory cytokines are involved in the initiation of the abnormal matrix process in pseudoexfoliation syndrome/glaucoma. *Am J Pathol.* 2010;176(6):2868–2879.

Cataract and Atopic Dermatitis

Atopic dermatitis (AD) is a chronic, eczematous dermatitis, accompanied by itching and often seen in conjunction with increased levels of immunoglobulin E (IgE) and a history of allergic rhinitis and asthma. Cataract formation has been reported in 5%–38% of patients with atopic dermatitis. The cataracts are usually bilateral, and onset occurs most often in the second to third decade of life, although cases in young children have been

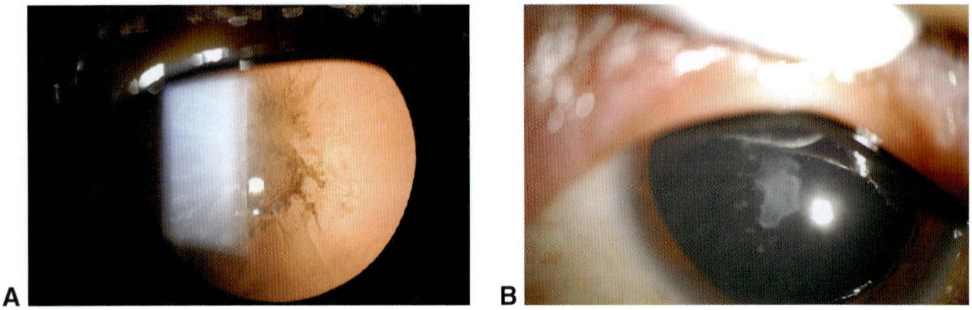

Figure 5-25 Atopic dermatitis. **A,** Characteristic subcapsular cataract. **B,** Slit-lamp retroillumination image of the same eye.

reported. Typically, these cataracts are anterior or posterior subcapsular opacities in the pupillary area that resemble shieldlike plaques (Fig 5-25). Although the pathogenesis of these cataracts is unclear, there appears to be decreased inhibition of free radical formation from decreased inducibility of superoxide dismutase in AD patients with cataracts.

Bair B, Dodd J, Heidelberg K, Krach K. Cataracts in atopic dermatitis: a case presentation and review of the literature. *Arch Dermatol.* 2011;147(5):585–588.

Mannis MJ, Macsai MS, Huntley AC, eds. *Eye and Skin Disease.* Lippincott-Raven; 1996.

Phacoantigenic Uveitis

In the normal eye, minute quantities of lens proteins leak out through the lens capsule. The eye appears to have immunologic tolerance to this limited antigenic stimulus. However, the release of a large quantity of lens proteins into the anterior chamber disrupts the immunologic tolerance and may trigger a severe inflammatory reaction. Phacoantigenic uveitis, previously termed *phacoanaphylactic endophthalmitis,* is an immune-mediated granulomatous inflammation initiated by lens proteins released through a ruptured lens capsule. This condition usually occurs following traumatic rupture of the lens capsule or after cataract surgery when cortical material is retained within the eye. Onset occurs days to weeks after the injury or surgery.

Phacoantigenic uveitis is characterized by a red, painful eye with injection, chemosis, anterior chamber cell and flare, and keratic precipitates. Occasionally, glaucoma develops due to obstruction of the trabecular meshwork and formation of synechiae. Late complications include cyclitic membrane, hypotony, and phthisis bulbi. In rare instances, phacoantigenic uveitis can give rise to an inflammatory reaction in the fellow eye. Histologic examination shows a zonal granulomatous inflammation surrounding a breach of the lens capsule. Lens extraction is the definitive therapy.

See also BCSC Section 4, *Ophthalmic Pathology and Intraocular Tumors,* and Section 9, *Uveitis and Ocular Inflammation.*

Guffey Johnson J, Margo CE. Intraocular inflammatory mass associated with lens-induced uveitis. *Surv Ophthalmol.* 2017;62(4):541–545.

Lens-Induced Glaucoma

See BCSC Section 10, *Glaucoma,* for additional discussion, including images.

Phacolytic Glaucoma

Phacolytic glaucoma is a complication of a mature or hypermature cataract. Denatured, liquefied high-molecular-weight lens proteins leak through an intact but permeable lens capsule. Macrophages ingest these lens proteins, and the trabecular meshwork becomes clogged with both the lens proteins and the engorged macrophages. The usual clinical presentation of phacolytic glaucoma consists of abrupt onset of pain and redness in a cataractous eye that has had poor vision for years. The cornea may be edematous, and significant flare reaction occurs in the anterior chamber. The lack of keratic precipitates helps distinguish phacolytic glaucoma from phacoantigenic glaucoma. White flocculent material appears in the anterior chamber and often adheres to the lens capsule as well. Intraocular pressure (IOP) is markedly elevated, and the anterior chamber angle is open, although the same material may be seen in the trabecular meshwork. Initial treatment of phacolytic glaucoma consists of controlling the IOP with IOP-lowering medications and managing the inflammation with topical corticosteroids. Surgical removal of the lens is the definitive treatment.

Lens Particle Glaucoma

Following a penetrating lens injury or surgical procedure (ie, extracapsular cataract extraction, phacoemulsification with retained cortical material, or in rare instances, Nd:YAG laser capsulotomy or vitrectomy), particles of lens cortex may migrate into the anterior chamber, where they obstruct aqueous outflow through the trabecular meshwork. In most instances, glaucoma occurs within weeks of the initial surgery or trauma, but it may occur months or years later. Gonioscopy shows that the angle is open, and cortical material can often be seen deposited along the trabecular meshwork. Medical therapy to lower IOP and to reduce intraocular inflammation is indicated. If the IOP and inflammation do not respond quickly to this treatment, the retained lens material is removed surgically.

Phacomorphic Glaucoma

As the lens thickens in the anterior–posterior dimension it can cause pupillary block and induce secondary angle-closure glaucoma, or it can physically push the iris forward and thus cause shallowing of the anterior chamber. Often, the patient presents with a red, painful eye and a history of vision changes as a result of cataract formation prior to the acute event (Fig 5-26). The cornea may be edematous, and gonioscopy reveals a closed anterior chamber angle. Initial management includes medical treatment to lower the IOP. The condition may respond to laser iridotomy, but definitive treatment consists of cataract extraction.

Glaukomflecken

Glaukomflecken are gray-white epithelial and anterior cortical lens opacities that occur following an episode of markedly elevated IOP, as in acute angle-closure glaucoma

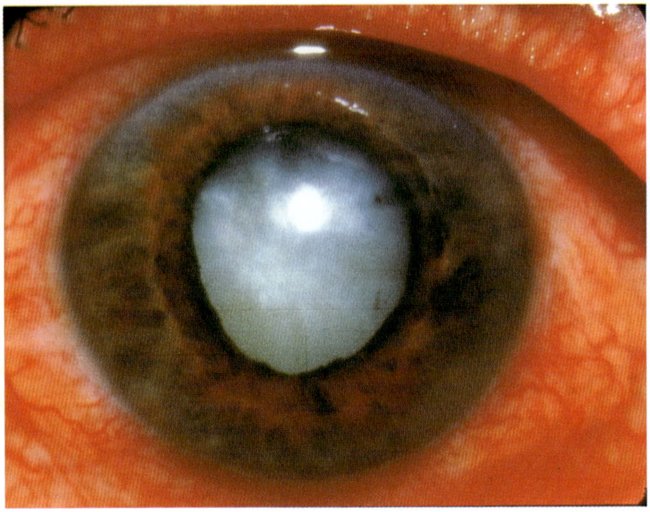

Figure 5-26 Phacomorphic glaucoma.

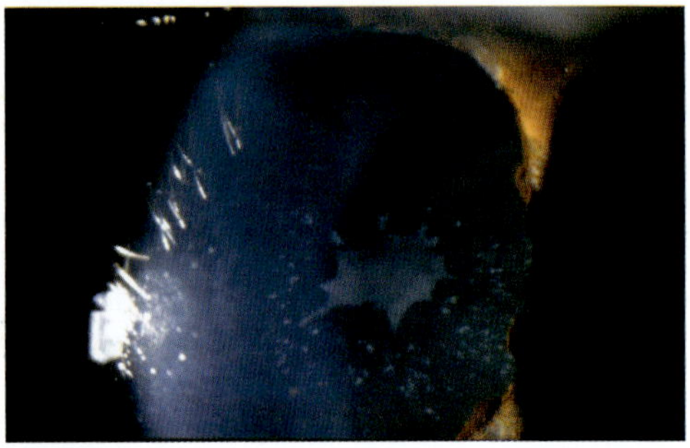

Figure 5-27 Glaukomflecken in the lens of a patient following recovery from acute angle-closure glaucoma. *(Courtesy of Thomas L. Steinemann, MD.)*

(Fig 5-27). On histologic examination, glaukomflecken are composed of necrotic lens epithelial cells and degenerated subepithelial cortex.

Ischemia

Ischemic ocular conditions, such as pulseless disease (Takayasu arteritis), thromboangiitis obliterans (Buerger disease), and anterior segment necrosis, can cause PSC. The cataract may progress rapidly to total opacification of the lens.

Cataracts Associated With Degenerative Ocular Disorders

Cataracts can occur in association with many degenerative ocular disorders, such as retinitis pigmentosa, essential iris atrophy, and chronic hypotony. These secondary cataracts usually begin as PSCs and may progress to total lens opacification. The mechanisms responsible for cataractogenesis in degenerative ocular disorders are not well understood.

CHAPTER 6

Evaluation and Management of Cataracts

Highlights

- In most cases, cataract surgery is an elective procedure. Not every cataract requires or warrants surgery.
- Preoperative evaluation is important for identifying and addressing any significant conditions that could impact the surgery or the postoperative recovery.
- Routine medical testing before routine cataract surgery has not been shown to increase the safety of the procedure.

Introduction

When evaluating a patient with cataracts, the ophthalmologist must assess the degree to which the lens opacity affects the patient's vision and determine whether surgery will improve the patient's quality of life. Considering the answers to the following questions is important in the evaluation and management of cataract:

- What is the functional impact of the cataract?
- What are the morphological characteristics of the cataract?
- Is surgery indicated either to improve the patient's quality of life or to aid in the management of other ocular conditions?
- What are the patient's expectations regarding the refractive results of surgery?
- Does the patient have ocular or systemic comorbidities that might affect the decision to proceed with surgery or alter the management plan?
- What are the possible barriers to obtaining informed consent or to ensuring good postoperative care?

In most cases, cataract surgery is an elective procedure. Thus, in addition to answering the preceding questions, it is important for the ophthalmologist to inform the patient or the patient's surrogate about the impact of the cataract, the risks and benefits of surgical management, the alternatives to surgery, and the options regarding the intraocular lens (IOL) to be used if surgery takes place. Ultimately, it is important that the patient or surrogate and physician be satisfied that surgery is the appropriate choice for improving vision.

This chapter focuses on the evaluation and management of cataracts in adults. For discussion of cataract in pediatric patients, refer to BCSC Section 6, *Pediatric Ophthalmology and Strabismus.*

Clinical History: Signs and Symptoms

Decreased Visual Acuity

Often, the clinical history of a patient with decreased vision and function due to cataract is straightforward, and the patient tells the ophthalmologist which activities have been curtailed or abandoned. Some patients, however, learn of the decline in their visual acuity only after being examined. Others deny that they are having any problems until their limitations are demonstrated or privileges are withdrawn because they are no longer visually competent.

Different types of cataract may affect vision in different ways, depending on incident light, pupil size, and refractive error (Table 6-1). The presence of even small posterior subcapsular cataracts (PSCs) can greatly disturb near vision (reading vision) without necessarily affecting distance visual acuity. Color vision disturbances may be noted by the patient, especially with unilateral or asymmetric cataract.

Glare and Altered Contrast Sensitivity

Cataract patients often report an increase in glare, which may vary from increased photosensitivity in brightly lit environments to disabling glare in the daytime or with headlights from oncoming cars. Shorter wavelengths of light cause the most scatter; the color, intensity, and direction of lighting also affect glare. This increased sensitivity is particularly prominent in eyes with PSCs and, occasionally, with anterior cortical lens changes.

Contrast sensitivity is the ability to detect subtle variations in shading. Because patients with ocular abnormalities have altered contrast sensitivity in low light, measurement of contrast sensitivity may provide a more comprehensive estimate of the visual resolution of the eye. A significant loss in contrast sensitivity may occur without a similar

Table 6-1 Characteristics and Effects of the Most Common Cataracts in Adults

Type	Growth Rate	Glare	Effect on Distance Vision	Effect on Near Vision	Induced Myopia
Cortical	Moderate	Moderate	Mild	Mild	None
Nuclear	Slow	Mild	Moderate	None	Moderate
Posterior subcapsular	Variable (rapid>slow)	Marked	Mild	Marked	None

loss in Snellen acuity. However, loss in contrast sensitivity is not a specific indicator of vision loss due to cataract.

Myopic Shift

The development of cataract may increase the dioptric power of the lens, commonly causing a mild to moderate degree of myopic shift. Hyperopic and emmetropic patients find that their need for distance or reading spectacles diminishes as they experience this "second sight." This phenomenon is encountered with nuclear sclerotic cataracts and disappears when the optical clarity of the crystalline lens further deteriorates. Less commonly, hyperopic or astigmatic refractive errors can be induced by cataractous lens changes. Asymmetric development of lens-induced myopia may produce intolerable anisometropia.

Monocular Diplopia or Polyopia

Occasionally in cataractous eyes, nuclear changes are localized to the inner layers of the lens nucleus, resulting in multiple refractile areas at the center of the lens. Such areas may best be seen as irregularities in the red reflex on retinoscopy or direct ophthalmoscopy. This type of cataract can result in monocular diplopia or polyopia, including ghost images and occasionally a true second image. Use of a pinhole occluder can eliminate the symptoms and be helpful in evaluation (for more on the pinhole test, see the section Potential Acuity Estimation later in this chapter). Monocular diplopia can also occur with abnormalities of the cornea and retina or other disorders of the eye (see BCSC Section 5, *Neuro-Ophthalmology*).

Decreased Visual Function

Assessing the overall effect of the cataract on visual function is a more appropriate way to determine visual disability than is acuity testing alone. This assessment includes asking patients whether their vision (at near, at distance, and under different lighting conditions) is adequate to allow them to perform relevant activities of daily living and participate in any hobbies. Questionnaires for measuring visual function may be useful, such as the Activities of Daily Vision Scale (ADVS), the Visual Function Index (VF-14), the National Eye Institute Visual Function Questionnaire (NEI-VFQ), and the Visual Disability Assessment (VDA).

Mangione CM, Lee PP, Gutierrez PR, Spritzer K, Berry S, Hays RD; National Eye Institute Visual Function Questionnaire Field Test Investigators. Development of the 25-item National Eye Institute Visual Function Questionnaire. *Arch Ophthalmol.* 2001;119(7):1050–1058.

Mangione CM, Phillips RS, Seddon JM, et al. Development of the 'Activities of Daily Vision Scale'. A measure of visual functional status. *Med Care.* 1992;30(12):1111–1126.

Pesudovs K, Wright TA, Gothwal VK. Visual disability assessment: valid measurement of activity limitation and mobility in cataract patients. *Br J Ophthalmol.* 2010;94(6):777–781.

Steinberg EP, Tielsch JM, Schein OD, et al. The VF-14. An index of functional impairment in patients with cataract. *Arch Ophthalmol.* 1994;112(5):630–638.

Nonsurgical Management

Nonsurgical approaches may be attempted to improve visual function in cataract patients who do not desire surgery or for whom surgical management is not feasible. Careful refraction may improve spectacle correction for distance and near vision. Use of specialized tints on spectacles may reduce glare, and brighter illumination can improve the contrast of reading material. Handheld monoculars may facilitate spotting objects at a distance; high-plus spectacles, magnifiers, closed-circuit televisions, and telescopic loupes may be used for reading and close work.

Referral to low vision services may be appropriate. The American Academy of Ophthalmology's Initiative in Vision Rehabilitation page on the ONE Network (www.aao.org/low-vision-and-vision-rehab) provides resources for low vision management, including patient handouts and information about additional vision rehabilitation opportunities beyond those provided by the ophthalmologist.

In patients with small axial cataracts, dilating the pupils either pharmacologically or by laser pupilloplasty may improve visual function by allowing more light to pass through peripheral portions of the lens. However, there is a risk of inducing additional glare with this approach.

Pharmacologic treatment of cataracts is the subject of ongoing research. No commercially available medication has been proven to delay or reverse cataract formation in humans. Aldose reductase inhibitors, which block the conversion of glucose to sorbitol, have been shown to prevent cataracts in animals with experimentally induced diabetes mellitus. However, studies of the use of these inhibitors in humans show no such effect. Antioxidants such as zinc and beta carotene and vitamins E and C had no significant effect on the development or progression of cataracts on participants in the Age-Related Eye Disease Study (AREDS); the role of vitamins in cataract prevention requires further study.

American Academy of Ophthalmology Cataract and Anterior Segment Panel, Hoskins Center for Quality Eye Care. Preferred Practice Pattern® Guidelines. *Cataract in the Adult Eye.* American Academy of Ophthalmology; 2016. www.aao.org/ppp

Indications for Surgery

Although patients with visually significant cataracts may express the desire for improved vision, the decision to operate is not based solely on a specific level of reduced acuity. Key to the decision is determining whether the patient's visual function would improve enough to warrant cataract surgery. Some governmental agencies and industries have minimum standards of visual function for their workers for tasks such as driving, flying, and operating complex equipment. A patient whose best-corrected visual acuity (BCVA; also called corrected distance visual acuity) does not meet these visual requisites may need to consider cataract surgery. The ophthalmic surgeon must determine whether cataract surgery is advisable, through discussion with the patient and/or the patient's surrogate and analysis of the results of subjective and objective testing.

Some third-party payers require that patients have a certain level of vision loss before approving reimbursement for cataract surgery; in such cases, glare testing may be useful for documenting loss of visual function beyond that measured by Snellen acuity. In some cases, patients have lens changes that cause unwanted refractive errors or symptoms but do not meet criteria for third-party reimbursement. After a careful discussion of the risks, benefits, alternatives, and costs, surgery may be offered to patients who would benefit from the procedure.

Medical indications for cataract surgery include phacolytic glaucoma, phacomorphic glaucoma, phacoantigenic uveitis, and dislocation of the lens. An additional indication for surgery is a cataract that is sufficiently opaque so as to obscure the view of the fundus and impair the diagnosis or management of other ocular diseases, such as diabetic retinopathy, macular degeneration, or glaucoma.

Cataract in elderly persons, especially those with significant deafness or early dementia, may lead to isolation. The quality of life of such patients may be greatly improved following cataract surgery, with possible spectacle independence. Cataract extraction has been shown to decrease the frequency of falls and hip fractures and to reduce morbidity and mortality.

Common indications for surgery in a patient with a monocular cataract include loss of stereopsis, diminished peripheral vision, disabling glare, and symptomatic anisometropia. The presence of cataract in 1 eye has a negative effect on driving performance and accident avoidance.

There are many possible treatment strategies for a patient with bilateral, visually significant cataracts. The strategy ultimately chosen, and the time waited before performing surgery on the second eye, is based on a combination of the surgeon's preference and the patient's needs, expectations, and visual potential. Surgery is usually performed first in the eye with the more advanced cataract, although the dominant or more ametropic eye may be addressed first in order to facilitate the patient's adaptation after surgery. In patients with active or severe systemic illness, or in those with other ocular diseases contributing to decreased vision, it may be appropriate to operate only on the eye with better visual potential.

Traditionally, before proceeding with the second surgery, the physician and the patient allow some time to confirm the success and safety of the first operation and to assess the refractive outcome. However, symptomatic anisometropia may occur as a result of the first cataract surgery, and the patient may find this disabling enough to justify prompt surgery on the second eye, even if the cataract in that eye is at a relatively early stage of development. After undergoing second-eye cataract surgery, patients have been shown to experience significant improvements not only in acuity and satisfaction with their vision but also in measures of bilateral visual function, such as stereopsis and contrast sensitivity.

Interest has increased in immediate sequential (same-day) bilateral cataract surgery (ISBCS). Indications for ISBCS might include patients with bilateral cataracts or unilateral cataract with a high refractive error that could result in significant postoperative anisometropia or patients who require general anesthesia where the risks of anesthesia outweigh the risks of surgery. ISBCS may be most useful in regions with limited surgical access or for patients with transportation issues. If same-day surgery is performed, each eye is treated as an entirely separate case by using new gloves, draping, instruments, and tubing. When proper safety techniques are used, ISBCS has a demonstrated record of safety. However, most ophthalmologists still do not use this approach due to reimbursement issues, as well as the potential for bilateral complications. The inability to incorporate information regarding refractive outcome into planning for the second eye is another concern; however, with the use of intraoperative aberrometry and improved refractive formulas, this is becoming less significant.

Brown GC, Brown MM, Menezes A, Busbee BG, Lieske HB, Lieske PA. Cataract surgery cost utility revisited in 2012. *Ophthalmology.* 2013;120(12):2367–2376.

Herinton LJ, Liu LL, Alexeeff S, Carolan J, Shorstein NH. Immediate sequential vs. delayed sequential bilateral cataract surgery. *Ophthalmology.* 2017;124(8):1126–1135.

Ishii K, Kabata T, Oshika T. The impact of cataract surgery on cognitive impairment and depressive mental status in elderly patients. *Am J Ophthalmol.* 2008;146(3):404–409.

Ivers RQ, Cumming RG, Mitchell P, Attebo K. Visual impairment and falls in older adults: the Blue Mountains Eye Study. *J Am Geriatr Soc.* 1998;46(1):58–64.

Sarikkola AU, Uusitalo RJ, Hellstedt T, Ess SL, Leivo T, Kivela T. Simultaneous bilateral versus sequential bilateral cataract surgery: Helsinki Simultaneous Bilateral Cataract Surgery Study Report 1. *J Cataract Refract Surg.* 2011;37(6):992–1002.

Preoperative Evaluation

To determine whether cataract surgery is advisable, the following information is obtained, and the suggested parameters are tailored to the individual patient.

General Health of the Patient

A complete medical history is the starting point for the preoperative evaluation. The ophthalmologist can work with the patient's primary care physician to achieve optimal management of all medical problems, especially diabetes mellitus, ischemic heart disease, chronic obstructive pulmonary disease, bleeding disorders, or adrenal suppression caused by systemic corticosteroid use. The ophthalmologist should be aware of the patient's drug sensitivities and use of medications that might alter the outcome of surgery, such as immunosuppressants and anticoagulants. Given the low risk of significant hemorrhage with scleral tunnel or clear corneal incisions, anticoagulant medications generally do not need to be discontinued prior to routine cataract surgery. Any alteration in the patient's use of these medications is ideally done in consultation with the prescribing physician.

It is important to specifically ask the patient about the use of systemic α_1-adrenergic antagonist medications (including prazosin, terazosin, doxazosin, silodosin, alfuzosin, and tamsulosin, as well as herbal supplements, such as saw palmetto) for the treatment of benign prostatic hyperplasia, urinary incontinence, urolithiasis, and hypertension. These medications are strongly associated with intraoperative floppy iris syndrome (IFIS) and fluctuations in pupil size. All α_1-blockers can bind to postsynaptic nerve endings of the iris dilator muscle for a prolonged period, causing excessive iris mobility and diffuse atrophy of the iris dilator smooth muscle. This effect may occur after only 1 dose of the medication and may persist indefinitely, even after discontinuation of the drug. Anecdotal reports document potential α_1-antagonist properties and potential associations with IFIS in other medications, including certain antipsychotic and antihypertensive medications. See Chapter 10 in this volume for further discussion of IFIS.

It is important for the ophthalmologist to inquire about and document any allergies, adverse reactions, and sensitivities to sedatives, narcotics, anesthetics, povidone-iodine, and latex. Factors limiting the patient's ability to cooperate in the operating room or to lie comfortably on the operating room table (eg, deafness, language barriers, dementia, claustrophobia, restless legs syndrome, head tremor, musculoskeletal disorders, psychiatric disorders including anxiety) will influence the choice of anesthesia and the surgical plan.

The extent of the formal medical preoperative evaluation is based on the patient's overall health and may be guided by requirements of the facility where the procedure is to take place. Screening with self-reported information gained from health questionnaires may help identify patients who are at higher risk for medical difficulties related to surgery, but this method should not be the only form of evaluation. Certainly, for all patients with risk factors related to their ability to undergo surgery, a history should be obtained, and a physical examination and relevant laboratory work should be performed. However, routine medical testing before routine cataract surgery has not been shown to increase the safety of the procedure.

See also Chapter 12 in this volume and BCSC Section 1, *Update on General Medicine,* for specific recommendations for preoperative cataract surgery planning in patients with special medical conditions.

American Academy of Ophthalmology Quality of Care Secretariat, Hoskins Center for Quality Eye Care. Routine preoperative laboratory testing for patients scheduled for cataract surgery—2014. *Clinical Statement.* American Academy of Ophthalmology; 2014. Accessed October 5, 2021. www.aao.org/clinical-statement/routine-preoperative-laboratory-testing-patients-s

Pertinent Ocular History

The ocular history helps the ophthalmologist identify conditions that could affect the surgical approach and the visual prognosis. Trauma, inflammation, amblyopia, strabismus, glaucoma, optic nerve abnormalities, or retinal disease might affect the visual outcome after cataract removal. In addition, an understanding of the patient's history of refractive error and spectacle or contact lens correction, as well as the patient's experience with monovision or progressive lenses, may aid refractive planning for cataract surgery.

Controlling active uveitis before cataract surgery is performed helps minimize the risk of complications from postoperative inflammation, such as macular edema and iris adhesion to the lens implant. Ideally, the eye is quiet without the use of topical corticosteroids for at least 3 months before surgery. This is not always possible, and surgery may be needed before the clinician is able to completely quiet the eye. Systemic immunomodulation may be necessary to achieve remission. Systemic steroids may be required perioperatively to manage ocular inflammation, even in eyes that were quiet prior to surgery. The presence of zonular abnormalities, fibrin membranes, and posterior synechiae will require the surgeon to adjust his or her surgical technique, as discussed in Chapter 12 of this volume.

A family history of retinal detachment or a history of retinal detachment in either of the patient's eyes is a risk factor for postoperative retinal detachment. Previous vitrectomy for the treatment of retinal disease or vitreous hemorrhage may cause intraoperative chamber fluctuations, which increase the risk of posterior capsule disruption and loss of nuclear fragments posteriorly.

Ideally, in patients with glaucoma, optimal control of intraocular pressure (IOP) is achieved prior to cataract surgery. If this cannot be accomplished, the surgeon may wish to consider a combined operation (cataract surgery along with an intervention to lower IOP). New techniques combining cataract surgery with minimally invasive glaucoma surgery (MIGS) may allow for the reduction of medications while maintaining a risk profile similar to that of cataract surgery alone. See Chapter 12 in this volume and BCSC Section 10, *Glaucoma.*

Past records document the patient's visual acuity before the development of cataract. If the patient has had cataract surgery in the fellow eye, it is important to obtain information about the operative and postoperative course. If problems such as IFIS, elevated IOP, vitreous loss, cystoid macular edema, endophthalmitis, hemorrhage, or a refractive surprise occurred during or after the first operation, the surgical approach and postoperative follow-up could be modified for the second eye in order to reduce the risk of similar complications.

If the patient has previously undergone refractive surgery, it is helpful to perform additional ocular measurements prior to and after the cataract surgery. See Chapters 7 and 12 for further discussion on surgical preparation.

Foster CS. Cataract surgery and uveitis. *Current Insight.* American Academy of Ophthalmology; 2006: Q3. Accessed October 5, 2021. www.aao.org/current-insight/cataract-surgery-uveitis

Social History

As discussed earlier, the decision to undertake cataract surgery is based not only on the patient's visual acuity but also on the ramifications of reduced vision on the individual's quality of life. Many factors affect postoperative recovery, including the patient's occupation, hobbies, and lifestyle. Any surrogate decision makers must be identified and included in preoperative planning.

Measurements of Visual Function

Visual Acuity Testing

It is useful to measure Snellen acuity under lighted and darkened examination conditions. Although visual acuity testing in the ophthalmologist's office is commonly performed in a darkened room, diminished Snellen acuity from a symptomatic cataract is sometimes demonstrated only in a lighted room. Distance and near visual acuity must be tested and careful refraction performed so that BCVA can be determined. Visual acuity may improve after pupillary dilation, especially in patients with a PSC.

Refraction

Careful refraction must be performed on both eyes. This assessment is useful for choosing the IOL power necessary to obtain the desired postoperative refraction, as well as for determining whether a myopic shift has occurred. If the fellow eye has a clear lens and a high refractive error that requires correction, achieving emmetropia in the surgical eye might cause problems with postoperative anisometropia. It is important to inform the patient specifically about this possibility and discuss options including refractive surgery or use of a contact lens for the noncataractous eye. Postoperative anisometropia can also be an indication to proceed with surgery on the second eye, even if there is minimal cataract present. Aiming for a similar refractive result in the fellow eye is an option, but this will ensure long-term dependence on refractive correction. A planned monovision outcome may optimize spectacle independence, but the patient either must have experience with monovision or must be tested to find out whether adapting to unequal refractive errors will be tolerated.

Rigid contact lens overrefraction is a useful technique to assess the degree to which irregular astigmatism or other corneal irregularity is contributing to a patient's visual disability.

Glare Testing

With glare testing, the clinician attempts to measure the degree of visual impairment caused by the presence of a light source located in the patient's visual field. Testing can be done with a nonprojected eye chart in ambient light conditions or with a projected eye chart and an off-axis bright light directed at the patient. Various instruments are available to standardize and facilitate this measurement. Patients with significant cataracts commonly show a decrease of 3 or more lines under these conditions, compared with results obtained when visual acuity is tested in a darkened room. It is best to perform this assessment prior to dilation. Glare testing performed after dilation must be adjusted to account for the change in visual acuity after dilation; the results may be less accurate, especially in patients with a PSC.

Wiggins MN, Irak-Dersu I, Turner SD, Thostenson JD. Glare testing in patients with cataract after dilation. *Ophthalmology.* 2009;116(7):1332–1335.

Contrast Sensitivity Testing

Patients with cataracts may experience diminished contrast sensitivity even when Snellen acuity is preserved. Various specialized charts have been developed to test contrast sensitivity in the ophthalmologist's office. Some charts are mounted on a wall; others are handheld or incorporate the use of a monitor. Certain contrast sensitivity charts feature sine wave gratings to allow evaluation of different spatial frequencies. However, no instrument is currently considered the standard for contrast sensitivity testing. Of note, contrast sensitivity may be decreased by a wide variety of ophthalmic conditions affecting the cornea, optic nerve, and retina. It is therefore essential that the ophthalmologist identify any comorbidities before attributing an irregularity in test results solely to cataract.

External Examination

The preoperative evaluation of a patient with cataract includes the body habitus and any abnormalities of the external eye and ocular adnexa. Conditions that may affect the surgical approach include extensive neck fat, kyphosis, ankylosing spondylitis, generalized obesity, or head tremor. The presence of enophthalmos or prominent brow may affect not only the surgical approach but also the chosen route of anesthesia.

Entropion, ectropion, or eyelid closure abnormalities, as well as abnormalities in the tear film, may have an impact on the ocular surface and thus adversely affect postoperative recovery if not addressed preoperatively. Severe blepharitis or acne rosacea may pose an increased risk of endophthalmitis and should likewise be treated before cataract surgery. Active nasolacrimal disease should also be treated, particularly if there is a history of inflammation, infection, or obstruction.

Motility and Ocular Dominance

Ocular motility can be determined by evaluating ocular alignment and testing the range of movement of the extraocular muscles. Cover testing helps determine any muscle deviation. Abnormal motility may suggest preexisting strabismus with amblyopia as a cause of vision loss. Patients must be made aware that they may experience diplopia after cataract surgery if they have a significant tropia resulting in disruption of fusion. Removal of a dense cataract may improve vision but make the patient aware of ocular misalignment.

The examination can also include an assessment of ocular dominance. Ocular dominance can be important if considering monovision; however, the importance of this in planning monovision is debatable.

Pupils

In addition to checking direct and consensual constriction of the pupil to light, the swinging flashlight test is performed to detect a *relative afferent pupillary defect* (*RAPD;* also known as a *Marcus Gunn pupil*), the presence of which indicates extensive retinal disease or optic nerve dysfunction. (See also BCSC Section 5, *Neuro-Ophthalmology.*) Although the vision of a patient with RAPD in the cataractous eye may improve after cataract surgery, the visual outcome may be limited by optic nerve dysfunction. The patient must be made aware of the possibility of less than complete restoration of vision.

It is important to measure the size of the pupil under different lighting conditions, because this information may affect selection of the IOL. For example, small-optic lenses may be inappropriate for a patient who has a large pupil in moderate or dim illumination. The edge of the optic can fall inside the pupil border, allowing light to pass around the optic edge, with resultant glare or dysphotopsias. Also, the function of a multifocal

IOL may be affected by a pupil that is small, atonic, or eccentric. It is helpful to assess pupil size before and after dilation, because the risk of surgical complications is higher in small pupils that do not dilate adequately (eg, in patients with diabetes mellitus, posterior synechiae, pseudoexfoliation syndrome, a history of opioid use, or a history of systemic α_1-adrenergic antagonist or long-term topical miotic use); in such cases, the surgeon may need to use expansion devices. These devices are discussed in Chapter 12.

Slit-Lamp Examination

Conjunctiva

Vascularization or scarring of the conjunctiva due to previous inflammation, injury, or ocular surgery may indicate compromised healing and limit surgical exposure. Symblepharon or shortening of the fornices may be associated with underlying systemic or ocular surface diseases. It is important that infectious processes receive appropriate treatment before cataract surgery in order to ensure optimal postoperative healing.

Cornea

Examination of the cornea includes an assessment of corneal thickness and whether corneal abnormalities, including edema, ectasia, guttae, or dystrophy, are present. Abnormalities could increase the risk of poor healing and decompensation postoperatively. Specular reflection with the slit lamp may provide an estimate of the endothelial cell count and information regarding cell morphology. Descemet membrane irregularity associated with cornea guttae, as well as any central opacity, may affect the surgeon's view of the lens during surgery and limit visual acuity after surgery. In patients with pannus due to long-term contact lens use or other conditions, the surgeon can plan to avoid making corneal incisions in areas of vascularization, if possible. Also, weakened or thinned areas in the cornea can be identified so that they can be avoided intraoperatively.

The ocular surface is the first and principal refracting interface of the eye. Tear film quantity and quality are thus critical to visual results. Diagnosis and management of keratitis sicca, blepharitis, and epithelial basement membrane dystrophy are of critical importance in cataract patients, particularly if multifocal or toric IOLs are being considered.

If areas of scarring possibly consistent with a history of herpetic eye disease are present, prophylactic antiviral medication and careful monitoring of steroid therapy in the perioperative period may be advisable to prevent reactivation.

If the patient has undergone previous corneal refractive surgery, it is important to document the type of surgery and any associated corneal findings, including haze after photorefractive keratectomy (PRK), the location of a LASIK (laser in situ keratomileusis) flap, and the placement of radial or astigmatic incisions. It is also important to note any apparent problems with healing. If the patient has undergone previous radial keratotomy (RK), the surgeon must take care to develop a surgical plan that attempts to avoid corneal splitting at the site of the RK incisions. See also Chapters 7 and 12 in this volume and BCSC Section 13, *Refractive Surgery.*

Anterior Chamber and Iris

Knowing the depth of the anterior chamber and the axial thickness of the lens aids in surgical planning. A shallow anterior chamber may indicate anatomically narrow angles, nanophthalmos, short axial length, an intumescent lens, or weak zonules.

Gonioscopy can be used preoperatively to rule out angle abnormalities, including peripheral anterior synechiae, neovascularization, or a prominent major arterial circle. Use of a 3-mirror lens helps in the evaluation of the lens zonules for traumatic or congenital dehiscence. Gonioscopy is essential if anterior chamber IOL implantation is anticipated.

The presence of iridodonesis or exfoliation at the margin of the undilated pupil may indicate weakened or absent zonular attachments and may affect the surgical plan. In addition, careful examination of the iris is important, because iris coloboma is often accompanied by lens coloboma and localized absence of zonular attachments.

Crystalline Lens

When examining the lens, the clinician notes its appearance both before and after dilation of the pupil. The impact of "oil droplet" nuclear cataracts and small PSCs is most closely correlated with visual symptoms before pupil dilation. After dilation, nuclear density can be evaluated, pseudoexfoliation syndrome can be detected, and opacities and distortion of the retinoscopic reflex can be visualized more easily.

To assess the lenticular contribution to the visual deficit, the clarity of the media in the visual axis is evaluated with the slit lamp. Dense, brunescent nuclear sclerotic cataracts may permit remarkably good vision, especially at near distances, whereas vacuolar cataracts, which may be detected by red reflex examination, can cause surprisingly severe vision loss. When dense cortical opacification is present, the intraoperative use of capsular dye to enhance visualization of the capsulorrhexis may be considered. The presence of a congenital posterior polar opacity is associated with a significant risk of capsule rupture and should be identified before surgery.

The position of the lens and the integrity of the zonular fibers are also evaluated. Lens coloboma, lens decentration, phacodonesis, or excessive distance between the lens and the pupillary margin indicates zonular disruption due to conditions such as lens subluxation as a result of previous trauma, metabolic disorders, or hypermature cataract. An indentation or flattening of the lens periphery may indicate focal loss of zonular support. For patients with these types of zonular disruption, the surgeon can alter surgical technique, including the use of capsular tension rings or other capsular or iris support devices intraoperatively (see Chapter 12).

Limitations of Slit-Lamp Examination

Some visually significant cataracts may appear minimal on slit-lamp biomicroscopy. However, examination of the lens with the retinoscope may clarify the lenticular contribution to the patient's vision changes. By examining the retinoscopic reflex, the clinician may detect posterior subcapsular opacities, refractile nuclear changes, or even diffuse cataracts. Similarly, examination using the direct ophthalmoscope through a +10.00 D lens at a distance of 2 ft will enhance the portions of the cataractous lens that are producing optical aberrations. This technique is particularly useful for identifying oil droplet cataracts.

Fundus Evaluation

Ophthalmoscopy

The ophthalmologist must perform a full fundus examination to evaluate the macula, optic nerve, vitreous, retinal vessels, and retinal periphery. Particular attention is paid to macular degeneration or other maculopathy that may limit visual outcome after an otherwise uneventful cataract extraction. The indirect ophthalmoscope is not generally useful for judging the visual significance of cataract, except in severe cases such as when the cataract is white. Although the direct ophthalmoscope, retinal contact lens, and noncontact fundus lens are more useful in judging media clarity, the ophthalmologist must keep in mind that these methods also provide light that is more intense than that available to the patient under ambient lighting conditions.

Patients with diabetes mellitus are examined carefully for the presence of macular edema, retinal ischemia, and background and proliferative retinopathy. Even in uncomplicated cataract surgery and in patients with minimal or no retinopathy, diabetic eye disease can progress postoperatively. Retinal ischemia may potentiate posterior or anterior neovascularization postoperatively, especially if the surgeon uses an intracapsular technique or ruptures the posterior capsule during extracapsular cataract extraction. Careful examination of the retinal periphery may reveal the presence of vitreoretinal traction or preexisting retinal holes and lattice degeneration that may warrant preoperative treatment.

Hong T, Mitchell P, de Loryn T, Rochtchina E, Cugati S, Wang JJ. Development and progression of diabetic retinopathy 12 months after phacoemulsification cataract surgery. *Ophthalmology.* 2009;116(8):1510–1514.

Optic Nerve

Examination of the optic nerve includes assessment of cupping and pallor, as well as any other abnormalities. Visual acuity, measurement of IOP, and the results of confrontation testing and the pupillary examination will help determine whether other adjunctive testing is warranted.

Fundus Evaluation With Opaque Media

B-scan ultrasonography of the posterior segment of the eye is useful whenever a dense cataract makes visualization of the retina impossible. Ultrasonography can elucidate whether a retinal detachment, vitreous opacity, posterior pole tumor, or staphyloma is present. Tests such as light projection, 2-point discrimination, gross color vision, photostress recovery, blue-light entoptoscopy, or the Maddox rod test may also be useful in detecting retinal pathology. Electroretinography and visually evoked response testing could also be considered when other modalities are inconclusive and the surgeon must decide whether cataract removal would provide any benefit.

See BCSC Section 12, *Retina and Vitreous,* and Section 3, *Clinical Optics and Vision Rehabilitation,* for discussion of these tests.

Special Tests

Potential Acuity Estimation

Potential acuity estimation can be helpful in assessing lenticular contribution to vision loss. The potential acuity pinhole test is a simple but accurate method of evaluation for patients who do not have other ocular pathology and whose visual acuity is better than 20/200. For this test, the patient is asked to read a brightly illuminated near card through a pinhole aperture. The Retinal Acuity Meter, or RAM (AMA Optics), functions in a similar manner.

The Potential Acuity Meter, or PAM (Mentor Graphics/Marco), is one of several instruments that project a numerical or Snellen vision chart through a small entrance pupil. The image can be projected onto the retina, around lenticular opacities, allowing for an estimate of what the BCVA would be if the media abnormality were absent.

It is important to note that these tests can be misleading in patients with certain disorders, including age-related macular degeneration, amblyopia, macular edema, glaucoma, small macular scars, and serous retinal detachment. An accurate clinical examination of the eye is often the best predictor of visual outcome.

Melki SA, Safar A, Martin J, Ivanova A, Adi M. Potential acuity pinhole: a simple method to measure potential visual acuity in patients with cataracts, comparison to potential acuity meter. *Ophthalmology.* 1999;106(7):1262–1267.

Visual Field Testing

It is important to perform confrontation field testing in all cataract patients, but formal visual field testing is not indicated for every patient with lens opacity. Visual field testing may help the ophthalmologist identify vision loss resulting from disease processes other than cataract. Patients with a history of glaucoma, optic nerve disease, or retinal abnormality may benefit from visual field evaluation to document the degree of visual field loss. Preoperative visual field loss does not preclude improvement in visual function following cataract surgery. Progressive cataracts may induce diffuse visual field depression that disappears after cataract removal.

Assessment of Corneal Endothelial Function

In patients with a history of endothelial dystrophy, previous ocular surgery, or trauma, additional corneal measurements may be useful. These data may aid the surgeon in counseling the patient regarding the possibility of postoperative corneal decompensation. In some cases, consideration of a combined surgery incorporating removal of the cataract and transplantation of corneal tissue may be in order.

Corneal pachymetry, a method employed to measure corneal thickness, is useful for indirectly assessing the function of the endothelium. Significantly increased central corneal thickness (>640 µm) in patients with endothelial dysfunction is associated with a greater risk of postoperative corneal decompensation.

Specular microscopy is used to determine corneal endothelial cell density per square millimeter and evaluate these cells' regularity. Because cataract surgery results in some loss of endothelial cells, the risk of postoperative corneal decompensation is increased if the preoperative endothelial cell count is low. Abnormal endothelial cell morphology, including enlargement (polymegathism) and irregularity (pleomorphism), may limit the cornea's ability to maintain its clarity after the stress of cataract surgery. (See also BCSC Section 8, *External Disease and Cornea.*)

Objective Tests of Macular Function

Optical coherence tomography (OCT) is increasingly performed as part of the preoperative testing regimen for cataract surgery in the United States. It may be useful in the assessment or detection of macular pathology, including neovascularization, edema, holes, and traction. Screening macular OCT to detect occult macular pathology may be of particular benefit for patients undergoing surgery with premium IOLs or when their vision is poorer than the degree of cataract would suggest.

Fluorescein angiography can be used to assess vascular and exudative abnormalities.

CHAPTER 7

Preoperative Considerations for Cataract Surgery

This chapter includes a related video. Go to www.aao.org/bcscvideo_section11 or scan the QR code in the text to access this content.

Highlights

- When choosing the power of the intraocular lens (IOL) for a cataract surgery, important considerations include axial length, anterior and posterior cornea power, and effective lens position.
- Informed consent is important; it includes the indications for surgery, the surgery's potential risks and benefits, any alternatives to the surgery, the surgical technique, and the IOL options.
- Recent studies have demonstrated that optical coherence tomography (OCT)–based IOL calculations and the Haigis-L and Barrett True-K No History formulas offer the lowest rate of error for postrefractive surgery IOL calculations. Intraoperative aberrometry has been shown to have similar accuracy.
- The Hill-RBF method for calculating IOL is unique because it uses adaptive learning to update its database and continually improve its IOL power predictions.
- Antimicrobial prophylaxis with intracameral antibiotics has been shown to reduce the rate of endophthalmitis.

Preoperative Measurements

Accurate preoperative or intraoperative measurements of the eye are essential to achieving the desired postoperative refractive result. Modern intraocular lens (IOL) power formulas incorporate the measurements for axial length (AL), cornea power, and effective lens position (ELP). The formulas have evolved over time, becoming increasingly more complex and theoretical in an effort to continually improve accuracy. The modalities used to obtain the measurements are also continually improving, providing better data to use when calculating IOL power calculations. Intraoperative aberrometry may also be used to directly determine the IOL power without needing to measure the patient's corneal power or AL. This technique may be particularly useful for children or patients who are unable to cooperate with office-based testing.

Axial Length

Ocular AL is a key component of IOL power calculations. An error as small as 1 mm in the AL measurement can lead to significant postoperative refractive error, especially in shorter eyes. AL can be measured with several techniques; no matter which is used, it is helpful to obtain data for both eyes, even if surgery is planned for only 1 eye. The difference in AL between the 2 eyes is typically no greater than 0.3 mm, unless there is a refractive difference or there are other relevant ocular findings. It is important to document and explain any significant disparity in AL.

Optical biometers are noncontact instruments that use infrared laser light (780 nm) and partial coherence interferometry to measure multiple parameters, such as AL, corneal curvature, anterior chamber depth, lens thickness, and horizontal white-to-white distance (corneal diameter). These devices require the patient to fixate on a target, which gives an AL along the visual axis. This technique is beneficial for patients with posterior staphyloma. Because the ocular media must be clear enough to allow voluntary fixation and light transmission, this technique is not ideal for taking measurements through dense or opacified media such as cornea scars, mature or posterior subcapsular cataracts, or vitreous hemorrhage. In some cases, measurements cannot be obtained with this modality, and ultrasound is required.

In *A-scan ultrasonography,* the transit time of the ultrasound pulse is measured. Using an estimated average velocity through the various ocular media (cornea, aqueous, lens, and vitreous), the biometric software calculates the AL. This value should be altered when velocities differ from the norm (see the Clinical Pearl sidebar). Measurements are obtained either via immersion (Fig 7-1) or contact applanation. With the immersion technique, a shell is placed on the eye between the eyelids to provide a watertight seal over the cornea, and an ultrasound transducer is mounted in the shell. This technique minimizes measurement errors when compared with contact applanation. With the contact applanation method, the examiner must be careful not to indent/compress the cornea, which results in an artificially shortened AL measurement, or to take the measurement through a tear meniscus, which results in an artificially lengthened AL. Both types of false measurement can result in postoperative refractive errors, particularly in short eyes.

CLINICAL PEARL

When measuring AL in a patient with silicone oil in the posterior chamber, the clinician must take into account the different velocity of sound waves in vitreous (1532 m/s) and in silicone oil (980 m/s or 1040 m/s, depending on the oil's viscosity) and thus the change in transit time, which is extended when silicone oil is present. Without adjustment, erroneously long ALs would be obtained, which could lead to an incorrect IOL selection that leads to an unexpectedly hyperopic result. In addition, the index of refraction of silicone oil is higher than that of vitreous; this must also be considered when selecting IOLs.

Bjeloš Rončević M, Bušić M, Cima I, Kuzmanović Elabjer B, Bosnar D, Miletić D. Intraobserver and interobserver repeatability of ocular components measurement in cataract eyes using a new optical low coherence reflectometer. *Graefes Arch Clin Exp Ophthalmol.* 2011;249(1):83–87.

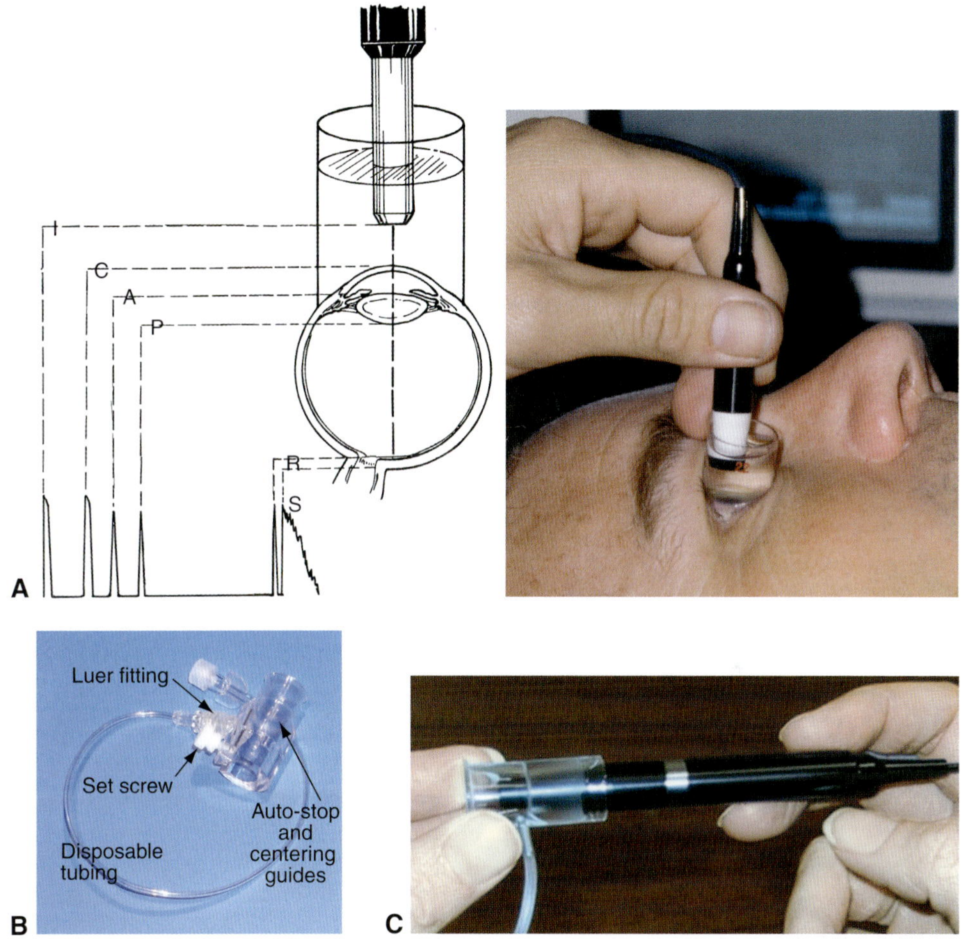

Figure 7-1 Immersion shells. Although there are other immersion shells, they are now rarely used in the United States, as visual axis alignment is more easily achieved with infusion shells than with cup shells. Infusion shells are also easier to use. **A,** In immersion ultrasonography, the probe is immersed in the solution, placing it away from the cornea. **B,** Prager shell for immersion A-scan. **C,** Ultrasound probe and Kohn shell. *(Courtesy of Kenneth J. Hoffer, MD.)*

Ianchulev T, Hoffer KJ, Yoo SH, et al. Intraoperative refractive biometry for predicting intraocular lens power calculation after prior myopic refractive surgery. *Ophthalmology.* 2014;121(1):56–60.

Roessler GF, Huth JK, Dietlein TS, et al. Accuracy and reproducibility of axial length measurement in eyes with silicone oil endotamponade. *Br J Ophthalmol.* 2009;93(11): 1492–1494.

Corneal Power

Corneal power is another major component of IOL power calculations. A 1.00-diopter (D) error in the calculation of corneal power causes a similar degree of error in the postoperative refraction. It is important to optimize the cornea prior to obtaining measurements;

this includes adequately treating any ocular surface disease, as well as minimizing warpage from contact lens wear. Preferences vary, but most surgeons require the eyes to be several weeks free from rigid gas permeable (RGP) lenses, and less time for soft contact lenses. Calculating corneal power in eyes that have undergone refractive surgery can be problematic, because traditional measures assume a particular relationship between anterior and posterior curvature. Laser refractive surgery modifies this relationship by altering the anterior curvature. In addition, accounting for posterior corneal astigmatism is increasingly recognized as an important factor in avoiding postsurgical refractive surprises, especially in patients who will be receiving toric IOLs.

Corneal power may be estimated or measured via several techniques, including manual keratometry, corneal topography, and corneal tomography:

- In *manual keratometry,* a small central portion of the cornea (3.2 mm) is measured, and the radius of curvature is calculated based on the size of a reflected image. This technique, which requires a skilled operator, allows direct visualization of tear film irregularity and can reveal cornea irregularities. It measures only the anterior surface of the cornea and extrapolates the corneal power by assuming a fixed relationship to the posterior surface.
- *In corneal topography,* a map of the corneal contour is created. Various map-creation methods exist. Placido disk–based topography, which measures the anterior surface and can provide additional information about the cornea surface, is particularly helpful in analyzing irregular astigmatism or detecting early keratoconus.
- In *corneal tomography* (ie, Scheimpflug imaging or optical coherence tomography [OCT]), the anterior and posterior curvature and cornea thickness can be measured. Scheimpflug imaging is incorporated into platforms to assist in IOL selection. OCT, which has higher axial resolution, can be useful in the presence of cornea opacities. Tomography may be particularly useful in patients who have previously undergone keratorefractive surgery, desire a toric or presbyopic IOL, or might benefit from astigmatism-correcting corneal incisions.

Effective Lens Position

ELP (sometimes called *estimated lens position*) is an estimate of the distance behind the cornea at which the intraocular lens will be located. This factor was previously called the anterior chamber depth (ACD). In older formulas, ACD was a constant value and was incorporated into the "*A* constant" value for a lens. The *A* constant was specified by the lens manufacturer and was a theoretical value that related the lens power to AL and keratometry. Formulas have become more advanced, however, and the complexity of estimating the ELP has increased. The estimate is now generally based on the relationship between the AL and central corneal power *(K)* readings. In patients with prior myopic keratorefractive surgery, the flatter anterior cornea surface can lead to errors in ELP, causing hyperopic refractive surprises.

The intended anatomic location of the lens within the eye also has an impact on the lens power selected. As the lens moves forward from in-the-bag placement to sulcus placement to anterior chamber placement, the distance from the retina increases, and the

Table 7-1 IOL Power Adjustment for Sulcus Placement

IOL Power Calculated for In-the-Bag Placement	Power Adjustment for Sulcus Placement
+28.50 D to +30.00 D	Subtract 1.50 D
+17.50 D to +28.00 D	Subtract 1.00 D
+9.50 D to +17.00 D	Subtract 0.50 D
+5.00 D to +9.00 D	No change

power required for the implant decreases. In general, an anterior chamber IOL (ACIOL) will be about 3.00 D lower in power than a planned in-the-bag posterior chamber IOL (PCIOL). This measurement will be different for eyes at the extremes of AL (ie, those with high myopia or high hyperopia). When shifting a PCIOL from the capsular bag to the sulcus, an adjustment can be made relative to the AL and projected in-the-bag IOL power (Table 7-1). If the lens is placed in the sulcus and optic capture is performed, no adjustment needs to be made, because the optic is then effectively in the capsular bag.

Koch DD, Jenkins RB, Weikert MP, Yeu E, Wang L. Correcting astigmatism with toric intraocular lenses: effect of posterior corneal astigmatism. *J Cataract Refract Surg.* 2013; 39(12):1803–1809.

IOL Power Determination

Classic Regression Formula

Although it is no longer regularly used for IOL calculation, the SRK formula developed by Sanders, Retzlaff, and Kraff in the 1980s helps illustrate the relative impact of AL and keratometric power in attaining the proper implant power. A small error in AL can have a much larger impact than a small error in keratometry.

$$P = A - (2.5L) - 0.9K$$

where

P = lens implant power for emmetropia (diopters)
L = axial length (mm)
K = average keratometric reading (diopters)
A = constant specific to implant to be used

IOL Calculation

Prior to surgery, the ophthalmologist discusses the refractive goals with the patient and determines the desired refractive result. This information with the IOL power calculation formulas can then be used to determine the power of the IOL to be implanted. It is important to make sure that the patient realizes that the formulas are not perfect. Despite extensive research to determine the optimal IOL calculation formulas, large case series show that significant percentages of postoperative results miss the refractive target by up to 0.50 D, while smaller percentages miss by over 1.00 D. The dependability of the calculations varies among

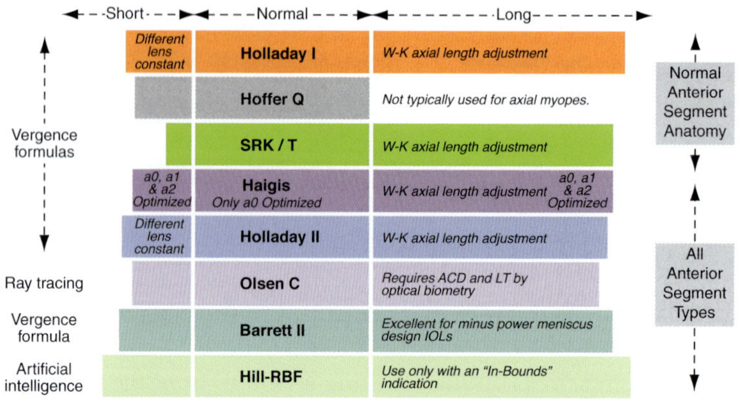

Figure 7-2 Accuracy range of commonly used intraocular lens (IOL) calculation formulas by axial length. *(Courtesy of Warren Hill, MD.)*

subgroups of patients; the greatest challenges occur in postrefractive patients or patients with axial myopia or axial hyperopia. The Hoffer Q formula has been shown to be more reliable for eyes with a short AL, while the SRK/T and Haigis formulas have shown to be more reliable in eyes with a long AL. Fourth-generation formulas (eg, Holladay 2, Haigis, Barrett True-K, and Olsen) refine refractive results by using additional variables such as preoperative refraction and age, preoperative anterior chamber depth, and lens thickness to further improve ELP accuracy. The Hill-RBF (radial base function) method is unique in that its database is continually updated, helping its adaptive learning improve its accuracy. Version 2.0 has a database of over 12,000 eyes and has been optimized for IOLs from +30.00 D to –5.00 D (Fig 7-2).

Acknowledging that no single formula is perfect, many surgeons use multiple IOL calculations to narrow in on the best choice. The American Society of Cataract and Refractive Surgery (ASCRS) hosts a website (http://iolcalc.ascrs.org/) that allows surgeons to run several calculations simultaneously.

Melles, RB, Holladay JT, Chang WJ. Accuracy of intraocular lens calculation formulas. *Ophthalmology.* 2018;125(2):169–178.

Narváez J, Zimmerman G, Stulting RD, Chang DH. Accuracy of intraocular lens power prediction using the Hoffer Q, Holladay 1, Holladay 2, and SRK/T formulas. *J Cataract Refract Surg.* 2006;32(12):2050–2053.

IOL calculations following refractive surgery

Calculating the IOL power for eyes that have undergone refractive surgery can present problems for both patients and surgeons. These patients were initially motivated to have refractive surgery because they did not want to be dependent on glasses, and they may have higher expectations regarding postoperative refractive results. It is important to inform patients who have undergone previous corneal refractive surgery about potential problems with IOL selection, as well as the potential for refractive surprise due to overcorrection or undercorrection. Refractive correction with glasses, contact lenses, refractive surgery, or IOL exchange may be required following the surgery. Documenting the discussion with the patient is extremely important.

As previously mentioned, determining the central keratometric power, a key element in lens power calculations, is complicated in eyes that have undergone previous refractive surgery because of the corneal change resulting from the original refractive procedure. In eyes in which radial keratotomy (RK) has been performed, a greater flattening of the posterior cornea relative to the anterior cornea can lead to an overestimation of corneal power, with hyperopic results. After myopic laser vision correction (LVC), conventional keratometry overestimates corneal power, with subsequent hyperopic results if adjustments are not made. The converse is true for patients with prior hyperopic LVC; in addition, the ELP (as calculated in many IOL power calculation formulas) may be incorrectly estimated.

The main challenge in calculating IOL power after refractive surgery is estimating or measuring the true posterior cornea refractive power. The challenge is compounded by the cornea change's impact on ELP estimations. As previously discussed in the section Corneal Power, traditional calculation methods assume that the relationship between anterior and posterior curvatures is fixed. However, newer corneal topography/tomography systems measure both anterior and posterior corneal curvatures, thereby improving the accuracy of IOL power calculations. Intraoperative aberrometry, which relies not on keratometric power but rather on the total refractive error of the eye, is a good option for determining IOL power in post-LVC eyes.

A variety of methods have also been developed to better estimate central corneal power in eyes that have undergone refractive surgery. Initially, many of these methods used historical data (pre–laser in situ keratomileusis [LASIK]/photorefractive keratectomy [PRK] *K*-values and the surgically induced change in manifest reaction [ΔMR]). After the discovery that these historical data models were not highly accurate, their use declined; they are no longer routinely used and are no longer incorporated into web-based calculators. Recent studies have demonstrated that OCT-based IOL calculations and the Haigis-L and Barrett True-K No History formulas give the lowest rate of error, and that averaging results can further reduce error. Intraoperative aberrometry has been shown to have similar accuracy. However, the ideal method has not yet been determined. Because each method has advantages and disadvantages, the ophthalmic surgeon may wish to consider using more than 1 method or an average value to calculate corneal power. Selecting the highest IOL power from a tightly clustered group of estimations may help avoid an undercorrection result. The IOL calculator on the ASCRS website allows users to select IOL power for eyes that have previously undergone refractive surgery (http://iolcalc.ascrs.org). The Barrett True-K No History formula is available from the Asia-Pacific Association of Cataract & Refractive Surgeons (www.apacrs.org). See also BCSC Section 13, *Refractive Surgery.*

Fram NR, Masket S, Wang L. Comparison of intraoperative aberrometry, OCT-based IOL formula, Haigis-L, and Masket formulae for IOL power calculation after laser vision correction. *Ophthalmology.* 2015;122(6):1096–1101.

Wang L, Booth MA, Koch DD. Comparison of intraocular lens power calculation methods in eyes that have undergone LASIK. *Ophthalmology.* 2004;111(10):1825–1831.

Wang L, Tang M, Huang D, Weikert MP, Koch DD. Comparison of newer intraocular lens power calculation methods for eyes after corneal refractive surgery. *Ophthalmology.* 2015;122(12):2443–2449.

Preventing Errors in IOL Calculation, Selection, and Insertion

The A-scan transducer is typically calibrated before use each day. Several scans are performed on each patient, and the measurements should cluster around a value, with a variance no greater than 0.2 mm. Both eyes are typically checked, especially if the first eye measures longer or shorter than anticipated. The difference in axial length between the eyes is usually no greater than 0.3 mm, unless there is a refractive or other anatomical reason. The patient name and K-readings, as well as AL and white-to-white measurements, are confirmed and documented. The lens power and the manufacturer's model number are also specified. Lenses and their powers for placement in the capsular bag, sulcus, or anterior chamber angle are selected.

All this information, including the IOL calculations, should be double-checked by the surgeon on the day of surgery, and the implants located, verified, and set aside preoperatively. In the operating room, a "time-out" is performed with the entire surgical team before the procedure begins to confirm the patient's identity, the operative eye, the procedure, and the IOL to be implanted.

Improving Outcomes

Refractive surgical outcomes may be tracked and evaluated by collecting information such as the following:

- whether there are overcorrections or undercorrections, and whether they occur more often with longer eyes or shorter eyes or roughly equally in both
- whether the incision routinely induces cylinder
- whether toric lenses are correcting as calculated
- whether limbal relaxing incisions have been effective for the correction of astigmatism

Commercially available programs may be useful for tracking outcomes. After the surgeon has analyzed these factors, he or she may make adjustments to improve refractive outcomes, such as including a "surgeon factor" (a modification of the parameters used that reflects the surgeon's experience) in some lens power calculations, changing the calculation software, or using immersion or optical biometry. Improving outcomes is important for increasing not only patient satisfaction but also surgeon confidence.

Patient Preparation and Informed Consent

When planning cataract surgery, the surgeon must evaluate the patient's ability to adhere to the postoperative care regimen. The surgeon should inform the patient (and caregivers, if appropriate) of the importance of using prescribed medication, maintaining proper ocular hygiene, and keeping required appointments. It is helpful to provide written instructions, along with appropriate illustrations or video presentations, and include a family member or friend in preoperative discussions in order to reinforce the patient's memory. It is important to inform the patient about any activity restrictions during the immediate postoperative period, although the advent of small-incision surgery has significantly minimized these limitations. The surgeon should also assess the patient's ability to function with only the fellow eye in the event that vision rehabilitation of the surgical eye is prolonged.

The surgeon must obtain informed consent preoperatively. Before deciding to proceed with cataract surgery, it is important to make sure that the patient has a clear understanding of the indications for surgery, the risks and benefits, the alternatives to surgery, the surgical technique, and IOL options. It is also important that the patient understands the anesthesia plan, as discussed in the following section. The surgeon should identify any risk factors for decreased visual outcome, including any preexisting ocular conditions that could adversely impact the result. In addition, the surgeon and patient should discuss the anticipated postoperative refractive status, the limitations of pseudophakic correction, and the proposed date for providing the final optical correction.

It is important that any costs associated with the surgery (eg, those related to medications or the use of premium IOL implants) are clearly outlined preoperatively. In addition, if comanagement with an optometrist or another ophthalmologist is planned, the patient must be explicitly notified and must give consent in writing.

American Academy of Ophthalmology Cataract/Anterior Segment Panel, Hoskins Center for Quality Eye Care. Preferred Practice Pattern® Guidelines. *Cataract in the Adult Eye—2016.* American Academy of Ophthalmology; 2016. www.aao.org/ppp

American Academy of Ophthalmology. Comprehensive guidelines for the co-management of ophthalmic postoperative care. American Academy of Ophthalmology website. Published 2016. Accessed October 5, 2021. www.aao.org/ethics-detail/guidelines-comanagement-postoperative-care

Anesthesia for Cataract Surgery

Consideration of the options for anesthesia is an important part of preoperative planning. A general review of the advantages and risks of the different types of anesthesia is part of the informed consent process. A discussion of what the patient will experience in the operating room increases the likelihood of comfort and cooperation on the day of surgery. (See also BCSC Section 1, *Update on General Medicine,* for a discussion of perioperative management in ocular surgery.)

Retrobulbar anesthesia for cataract surgery provides excellent ocular akinesia and anesthesia and reduces sensitivity to the microscope light. The basic technique of retrobulbar injection (Fig 7-3), first described in 1945 by Walter Atkinson, involves administration of lidocaine into the muscle cone via a 25-gauge, 1.5-inch (38-mm) blunt retrobulbar needle. Many surgeons now use a 27-gauge, 1.25-inch sharp needle and supplement the lidocaine with vitrase and bupivacaine, and sometimes bicarbonate. These modifications can enhance the patient's comfort, speed of onset, and duration of the retrobulbar block. Complications resulting from retrobulbar anesthesia are uncommon but include retrobulbar hemorrhage; globe penetration; optic nerve trauma; extraocular muscle toxicity; inadvertent intravenous injection associated with cardiac arrhythmia; and inadvertent intradural injection with associated seizures, respiratory arrest, and brainstem anesthesia. Any preexisting diplopia or ocular misalignment should be documented.

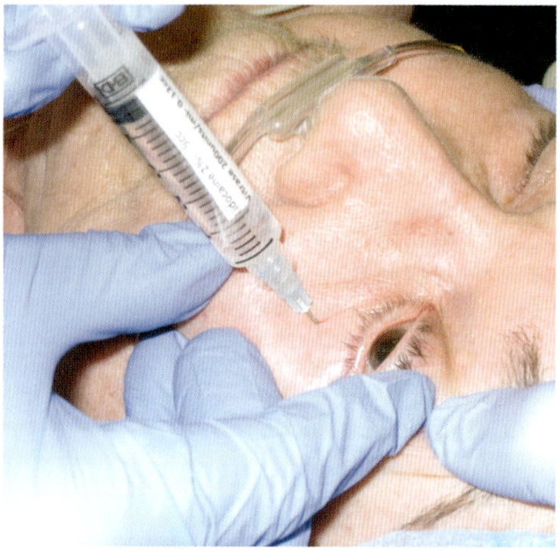

Figure 7-3 Retrobulbar injection. *(Courtesy of Michael N. Wiggins, MD.)*

Peribulbar anesthesia theoretically eliminates the risk of complications such as optic nerve injury and intradural injection. However, it is slightly less effective than the retrobulbar method for providing akinesia and anesthesia and is more likely to give conjunctival chemosis. In this technique, a shorter (1-inch) 25-gauge or 27-gauge needle is used to introduce anesthetic solution external to the muscle cone, underneath the Tenon capsule.

Sub-Tenon infusion of lidocaine has become a popular method of anesthesia during surgery. The risk of muscle injury or toxicity associated with this method is lower. A small, posterior incision is made through anesthetized conjunctiva and the Tenon capsule, and a small cannula is used to administer the anesthetic (Video 7-1; Fig 7-4).

VIDEO 7-1 Sub-Tenon injection.
Courtesy of Charles Cole, MD.
Go to www.aao.org/bcscvideo_section11 to access all videos in Section 11.

The use of *topical and intracameral anesthesia* has increased. With topical anesthesia, the risk of ocular perforation, extraocular muscle injury, and central nervous system depression is eliminated, and visual recovery is accelerated. Topical anesthesia is administered via proparacaine or tetracaine drops, cellulose pledgets soaked in anesthetic, or lidocaine jelly. Intracameral preservative-free lidocaine (which often includes a mydriatic agent) can supplement or even replace topical anesthesia. Lidocaine/phenylephrine (Shugarcaine) has the added advantage of increasing pupil dilation and reducing the effects of intraoperative floppy iris syndrome (IFIS). Only nonpreserved 1% or 2% lidocaine should be used for anterior chamber instillation, because of the toxic effect of some preservative agents on intraocular structures. Disadvantages of topical anesthesia include blepharospasm, lack of akinesia, and potential patient discomfort, which can interfere with the surgeon's ability to perform delicate maneuvers. Topical and intracameral anesthesia is typically reserved for short cataract surgeries, generally under 30 minutes in length, with cooperative patients who are well dilated and can tolerate the microscope

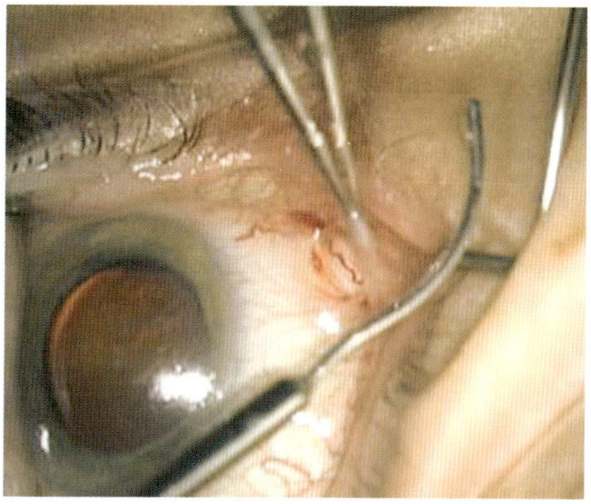

Figure 7-4 Sub-Tenon injection. *(Courtesy of Pramanik S, Doan A.* Retrobulbar Block, Peribulbar Block, and Common Nerve Blocks Used by Ophthalmologists. *February 27, 2005. Available from https://eyerounds.org/tutorials/retrobulbar-nerve-blocks.htm)*

light. Topical and intracameral anesthesia can be supplemented with oral or intravenous sedation to help reduce patient anxiety.

A *facial nerve block,* common in the era of large-incision intracapsular cataract extraction (ICCE) and extracapsular cataract extraction (ECCE), is not generally necessary with small-incision surgery. However, patients with essential or reactive blepharospasm may benefit from a facial nerve block to control squeezing during surgery. Types of facial nerve blocks include the O'Brien block, directed proximally and peripherally at the nerve trunk; the van Lint block, directed proximally and peripherally at the terminal branches; and the Atkinson block, directed between these two regions (Fig 7-5).

General anesthesia can be considered for pediatric patients and for adult patients who have any condition that would prevent their cooperation and ability to lie flat during surgery, including dementia, head tremor, deafness, language barrier, musculoskeletal disorder, restless legs syndrome, claustrophobia, or psychiatric disorder (including anxiety).

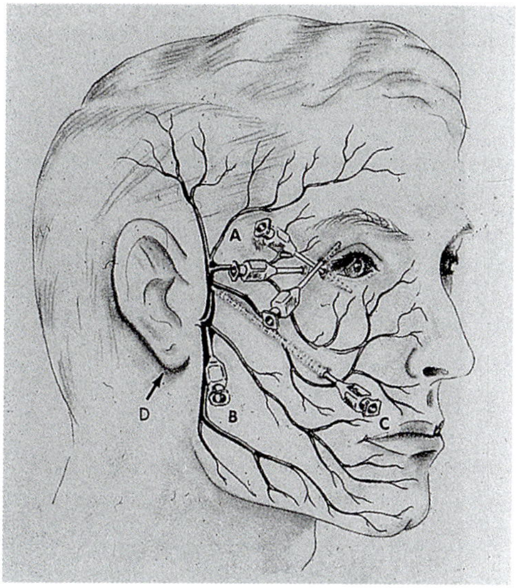

Figure 7-5 Akinesia of orbicularis oculi. **A,** Van Lint akinesia. **B,** O'Brien akinesia. **C,** Atkinson akinesia. **D,** Nadbath-Ellis akinesia. *(Reproduced with permission from Jaffe NS, Jaffe MS, Jaffe GF.* Cataract Surgery and Its Complications. *5th ed. Mosby; 1990.)*

Patient preference can also be considered as an indication. General anesthesia may require clearance from the patient's primary care physician or an anesthesiologist.

Schimek F, Fahle M. Techniques of facial nerve block. *Br J Ophthalmol.* 1995;79(2):166–173.

Zhao LQ, Zhu H, Zhao PQ, Wu QR, Hu YQ. Topical anesthesia versus regional anesthesia for cataract surgery: a meta-analysis of randomized controlled trials. *Ophthalmology.* 2012;119(4): 659–667.

Antimicrobial Therapy

Endophthalmitis remains one of the most serious complications of cataract surgery (see Chapter 11 in this volume). Therefore, a major objective of preoperative preparation and intraoperative management of the patient is to reduce the introduction of pathogenic organisms into the anterior chamber.

Before Surgery

Before the day of surgery, the surgeon should identify and reduce infectious risk factors as much as possible through preoperative treatment of coexisting eyelid disorders such as conjunctivitis, blepharitis, hordeolum, and chalazion. Systemic infections should also be identified and treated.

Cataract surgery is not considered to be an invasive procedure that induces transient bacteremia; thus, systemic antibiotic prophylaxis is not required. If questions arise about whether antibiotic prophylaxis is advisable in the perioperative period, the surgeon may wish to consult with the physicians involved in the patient's systemic care.

Although no studies have convincingly demonstrated the efficacy of topical antibiotics in reducing the risk of endophthalmitis in routine cataract surgery, there is some evidence supporting an association between the use of preoperative topical antibiotics and a reduction in ocular surface bacterial counts, as well as a lower incidence of positive aqueous cultures after surgery. Many cataract surgeons prescribe preoperative topical antibiotics.

For patients with a history of herpetic eye disease, a prescription of prophylactic antiviral medications can be considered. This topic is further discussed in Chapter 12.

Sykakis E, Karim R, Parmar DN. Management of patients with herpes simplex virus eye disease having cataract surgery in the United Kingdom. *J Cataract Refract Surg.* 2013;39(8): 1254–1259.

Yoshida J, Kim A, Pratzer KA, Stark WJ. Aqueous penetration of moxifloxacin 0.5% ophthalmic solution and besifloxacin 0.6% ophthalmic suspension in cataract surgery patients. *J Cataract Refract Surg.* 2010;36(9):1499–1502.

In Surgery

In the operating room, sterilization of the fornix is important. A 5% povidone-iodine solution (not scrub or soap) placed in the conjunctival fornix prior to surgery has been associated with a reduction in bacterial colony counts in cultures from the ocular surface at the time of surgery and a decreased risk of culture-proven endophthalmitis. In addition,

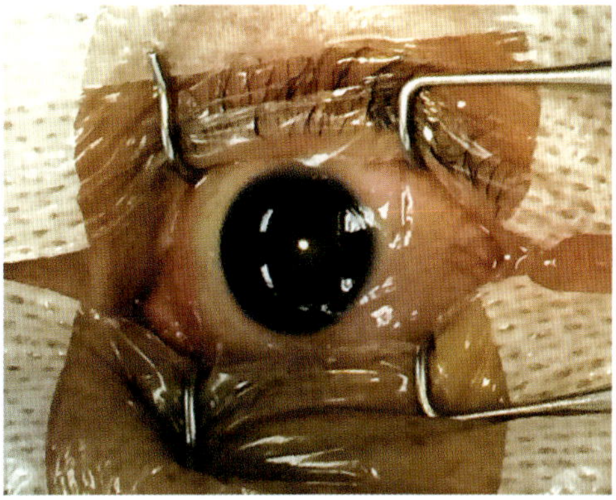

Figure 7-6 Sterile draping of the eye for surgery. *(Courtesy of Lisa Park, MD.)*

preparation of the skin around the eye with a 10% povidone-iodine solution can reduce bacterial counts on the eyelid margins. Because eyelid margins may harbor pathogens, it is important to drape the eyelashes out of the operative field (Fig 7-6).

It is important not only to limit the number of times that instruments are introduced into the eye but also to check for signs of lint, cilia, and other debris on the tips of all instruments inserted. Meticulous wound closure is imperative. Despite surgeons' best efforts, however, 7%–35% of cataract surgeries result in bacterial inoculation of the anterior chamber. The low incidence of endophthalmitis is a testament to the ability of the anterior chamber to clear itself of a potentially pathologic inoculum. The risk of endophthalmitis increases with a torn posterior lens capsule, vitreous loss, and prolonged surgery.

Some surgeons add antibiotics to the irrigating solution or inject them into the anterior chamber at the conclusion of the operation. The Endophthalmitis Study Group reported a significant reduction in endophthalmitis with the use of intracameral cefuroxime, which has not been universally adopted in the United States because of the lack of commercial antibiotic preparations for intracameral use. Intracameral vancomycin is a popular alternative; however, this antibiotic has been associated with a rare hypersensivity reaction that causes a hemorrhagic vasculitis. Intracameral moxifloxacin has become more popular; to date, it has been predominantly safe and cost-effective. There have been reported cases of pigmentary dispersion and diffuse iris depigmentation after intracameral use as well as systemic use of moxifloxacin.

Subconjunctival corticosteroids can be used in conjunction with intracameral antibiotics. Another option is the injection of a bolus of antibiotic and corticosteroid medications at the conclusion of surgery via transzonular or intravitreal injection, so that the medications are able to act over time postoperatively. "Dropless" cataract surgery can refer to any of these methods in which medications are instilled at the time of surgery and reduce or eliminate the need for postoperative drops.

Whether the risk of endophthalmitis is increased after cataract surgery performed using a sutureless clear corneal wound is controversial. After tracking the flow of fluorescein into the anterior chamber, some have suggested that inflow of bacteria from the ocular surface may be possible via a sutureless incision. For this reason, hydrating the corneal stroma to reapproximate the anterior and posterior aspects of the wound may reduce the risk of wound separation. Any possibility of leakage can be addressed with wound closure by suture or tissue adhesive.

Bowen RC, Zhou AX, Bondalapati S, et al. Comparative analysis of the safety and efficacy of intracameral cefuroxime, moxifloxacin, and vancomycin at the end of cataract surgery: a meta-analysis. *Br J Ophthalmol.* 2018;102(9):1268–1276.

Chang DF, Braga-Mele R, Henderson BA, Mamalis N, Vasavada A; ASCRS Cataract Clinical Committee. Antibiotic prophylaxis of postoperative endophthalmitis after cataract surgery: results of the 2014 ASCRS member survey. *J Cataract Refract Surg.* 2015;41(6):1300–1305.

Endophthalmitis Study Group, European Society of Cataract & Refractive Surgeons (ESCRS). Prophylaxis of postoperative endophthalmitis following cataract surgery: results of the ESCRS multicenter study and identification of risk factors. *J Cataract Refract Surg.* 2007;33(6):978–988.

Gower EW, Keay LJ, Stare DE, et al. Characteristics of endophthalmitis after cataract surgery in the United States Medicare population. *Ophthalmology.* 2015;122(8):1625–1632.

Nentwich MM, Ta CN, Kreutzer TC, et al. Incidence of postoperative endophthalmitis from 1990 to 2009 using povidone-iodine but no intracameral antibiotics at a single academic institution. *J Cataract Refract Surg.* 2015;41(1):58–66.

Witkin AJ, Chang DF, Jumper JM, et al. Vancomycin-associated hemorrhagic occlusive retinal vasculitis: clinical characteristics of 36 eyes. *Ophthalmology.* 2017;124(5):583–595.

After Surgery

After routine cataract surgery, use of antibiotic eyedrops is commonly continued or instituted. Although reduced bacterial counts have been documented with the administration of topical antibiotics, there is no definitive evidence that their use reduces the incidence of endophthalmitis.

Behndig A, Cochener B, Güell JL, et al. Endophthalmitis prophylaxis in cataract surgery: overview of current practice patterns in 9 European countries. *J Cataract Refract Surg.* 2013;39(9):1421–1431.

Ophthalmic Viscosurgical Devices

Ophthalmic viscosurgical devices (OVDs), also referred to as *viscoelastic agents,* have been employed in anterior segment surgery since 1979. They play an important role in maintaining the anterior chamber and protecting the corneal endothelium during surgery, and their use has had a profound influence on the evolution of extracapsular and phacoemulsification surgery.

OVDs contain 1 or more of the following substances in varying concentrations:

- *Sodium hyaluronate*, a biopolymer that occurs in many connective tissues throughout the body, such as synovial (joint) fluid and vitreous. It was originally isolated from human umbilical cord and rooster combs. Sodium hyaluronate has a half-life of approximately 1 day in aqueous and 3 days in vitreous.

- *Chondroitin sulfate,* a sulfated glycosaminoglycan, which is an important component of cartilage.
- *Hydroxypropyl methylcellulose (HPMC),* which does not occur naturally in animal tissues; however, cellulose is widely distributed in plant fibers such as cotton and wood. The commercial product is a cellulose polymer modified by the addition of hydroxypropyl and methyl groups to increase the hydrophilic property of the material. Methylcellulose is a nonphysiologic compound that does not appear to be metabolized intraocularly. It is eventually eliminated in the aqueous but can easily be irrigated from the eye.

Physical Properties

The physical properties of OVDs are not necessarily due to their specific biopolymer composition; rather, they are the result of chain length and molecular interactions both within chains and between chains and ocular tissue. OVDs have 4 general physical properties:

1. *Viscosity* describes resistance to flow and can be thought of as the "thickness" or "thinness" of a fluid. It is determined primarily by molecular weight and concentration, so that substances with high molecular weight and high concentration have the highest viscosity. The higher the viscosity, the better the OVD is at displacing tissue and staying in place.
2. *Elasticity* refers to the ability of a material to return to its original shape after being stressed. It describes the OVD's ability to re-form after an external force is applied to the anterior chamber and then removed. A highly elastic substance is excellent for maintaining space.
3. *Pseudoplasticity* refers to the ease with which a material can change from being highly viscous at rest to being watery at increasing rates of shear stress. This property is found in certain everyday substances such as toothpaste; when squeezed out of a tube, toothpaste flows easily, but it retains its shape when it is at rest on the toothbrush. In clinical terms, at zero shear force an OVD is a lubricant and coats tissues well, but when forced through a small-gauge cannula it functions like a liquid.
4. *Surface tension* describes how the surface of a fluid tends to stick to another surface. This property is also referred to as coatability, which is inversely proportional to surface tension. Thus, an OVD with low surface tension is better at coating tissue but is harder to remove from the eye.

Given the different combinations of all of these properties, OVDs can be classified into 2 general categories:

1. *Cohesive OVDs* are long-chain, high-molecular-weight, high-viscosity substances. These agents maintain space well at no or low shear rates, whereas at high shear rates they are easily displaced. Cohesive OVDs are easier to remove from the eye because they stick together and are aspirated as long pieces (similar to spaghetti). However, they have minimal coating ability and therefore afford less tissue protection during surgery.

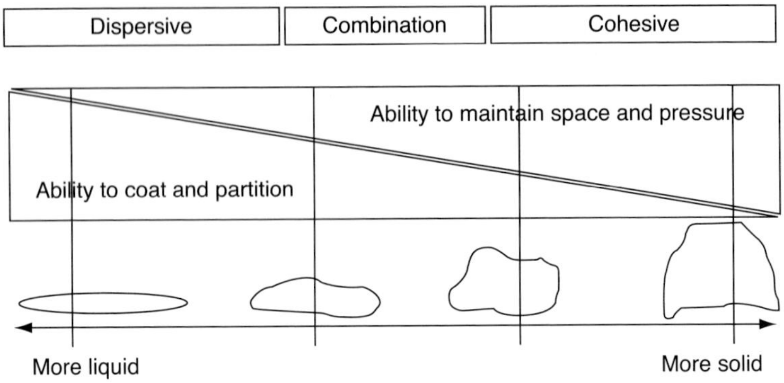

Figure 7-7 Behavior of ophthalmic viscosurgical devices (OVDs).

2. *Dispersive OVDs* are short-chain, low-molecular-weight, low-viscosity substances with low surface tension. These agents provide excellent coating and protection at high shear rates; however, they are more difficult to remove from the eye because they do not stick together and are aspirated in short fragments (similar to macaroni). They are more likely to be retained in the eye after cataract surgery, increasing the likelihood of angle obstruction with reduced outflow and subsequent IOP elevation.

Cohesive agents include Healon, Healon GV (J&J Surgical); Amvisc, Amvisc Plus (Bausch + Lomb); and Provisc (Alcon). Dispersive agents include OcuCoat (Bausch + Lomb), Viscoat (Alcon), and Healon Endocoat (J&J Surgical). Discovisc (Alcon) combines qualities of dispersive and cohesive agents. Figure 7-7 shows the full spectrum of OVDs.

Some additional OVDs, such as the viscoadaptive agent Healon5 (J&J Surgical), may need separate classification. Healon5 is a long, fragile chain with high molecular weight that changes its behavior at different flow rates. The lower the flow rate, the more viscous and cohesive the OVD is, and the higher the flow rate, the more the chains fracture. As a result, this OVD acts as a pseudodispersive agent. However, it must be carefully removed at the end of surgery because it can cause extremely elevated IOP if left in the eye.

Uses of Ophthalmic Viscosurgical Devices

The space maintenance ability of OVDs keeps the anterior chamber formed despite the presence of 1 or more corneal incisions. With expansion of the chamber, manipulations can be made away from the corneal endothelium and posterior lens capsule. A cohesive OVD can be used to enlarge a marginally dilated pupil (viscomydriasis). It can also be used to keep the plane of the anterior capsule flat to assist a controlled continuous curvilinear capsulorrhexis. Lens implantation is less traumatic to the zonular fibers and the posterior capsule when the capsular bag is inflated with an OVD.

The coatability of OVDs can be used to protect the corneal endothelium from phacoemulsification energy, particularly in dense cataracts or during long operations. The surgeon must take care to remove dispersive OVDs completely to reduce the risk of an ocular hypertensive period caused by angle outflow obstruction. In the presence of an open posterior lens capsule, a dispersive OVD can be injected over the tear to provide a vitreous tamponade and prevent prolapse of vitreous anteriorly.

The optical clarity of OVDs has prompted some surgeons to use a layer of OVD on the surface of the cornea. When slightly moistened with balanced salt solution, the agent coats the epithelium. This maneuver prevents drying and eliminates the need to irrigate the corneal surface. It also provides a slightly magnified view of anterior segment structures.

Ultimately, the choice of OVD varies depending on the clinical scenario and surgeon preference. A survey showed that 97% of surgeons vary their choice of OVD in complicated cases. For example, in pediatric cataracts or cases with a low endothelial cell count, shallow anterior chamber, or IFIS, the choice of OVD can play a critical role in management. The preferred OVD for each surgical situation is a personal decision for each surgeon, guided by experience and product availability.

Riedel PJ. Ophthalmic viscosurgical devices. *Focal Points: Clinical Modules for Ophthalmologists.* American Academy of Ophthalmology; 2012, module 7.

Surgical Checklist

Some surgeons and surgical centers employ checklists as part of the preoperative planning. A checklist enables a systematic review of the patient's general medical health, ocular concerns, and surgical planning to ensure that the correct IOL is ordered and that any special supplies needed are available. Checklist specifics will vary by location or surgeon.

CHAPTER 8

Phacoemulsification for Cataract Extraction

This chapter includes related videos. Go to www.aao.org/bcscvideo_section11 or scan the QR codes in the text to access this content.

Highlights

- Two main types of aspiration pumps are used in phacoemulsification machines: flow pumps (eg, a peristaltic pump) and vacuum pumps (eg, a Venturi pump). Flow pumps allow the surgeon to directly control aspiration flow rate and set a vacuum limit. Vacuum pumps allow direct control of the vacuum level only.
- Phacoemulsification uses ultrasound energy to emulsify a lens. Modes such as pulse and burst allow for intermittent rather than continuous delivery of phacoemulsification power, thereby decreasing the total amount of energy required for cataract extraction.
- Femtosecond laser platforms provide an alternative technology to assist in cataract extraction.
- Studies demonstrate that more than 90% of eyes achieved a postoperative spherical equivalent within 1.00 diopters (D) of that predicted by preoperative biometry.

Introduction

The modern era of cataract surgery began in 1967, when Charles Kelman invented phacoemulsification. In this procedure, an ultrasonically driven tip is used to emulsify the lens nucleus and remove the fragments with an automated aspiration system. This paradigm shift allowed cataract surgery to be performed via smaller corneal incisions, resulting in a lower incidence of wound-related and vitreous-related complications and more rapid rehabilitation of vision. Although phacoemulsification was initially met with strong resistance, the procedure gained popularity by the 1990s, coinciding with the invention of ophthalmic viscosurgical devices, the evolution of intraocular lens design, and a change to performance of cataract surgery on an outpatient basis. Today, phacoemulsification is the most commonly performed method of cataract extraction in developed areas.

In developing areas, however, the high cost of phacoemulsification technology and its associated disposable equipment have limited its adoption. Instead, extracapsular cataract extraction (ECCE) and manual small-incision cataract surgery (MSICS) remain the most common procedures. The use of historical techniques such as intracapsular cataract extraction (ICCE) and couching are rare. See the Appendix in this volume for further discussion of these techniques.

Instrumentation

Phacoemulsification (often referred to as *phaco*) makes use of ultrasound technology as well as *vacuum* (defined in the Glossary of Fluidics and Phacodynamics Terminology at the end of this chapter). Although there are several types of phaco machines, their major components are essentially the same: a handpiece, foot pedal, irrigation system, and aspiration pump.

The phaco handpiece (Fig 8-1) has been likened to a combination of a jackhammer, vacuum, and garden hose. The surgeon uses the handpiece to simultaneously emulsify and aspirate the crystalline lens while keeping the tip cool and maintaining anterior chamber depth. The mechanical energy of phacoemulsification is produced by the to-and-fro oscillation generated by *piezoelectric crystals* in the phaco handpiece. The amplitude of the movement, or *stroke length,* is variable and increases when the power is raised. As the phaco tip moves forward, compression of gas atoms in solution occurs; as the tip moves backward, expansion of gas atoms occurs, and bubbles of gas form (known as *cavitation*; see the Glossary of Ultrasonic Technology Terminology at the end of this chapter). The bubbles are subject to the same compression and expansion. When the bubbles implode, they release heat and shock waves, which disassemble the nucleus at the phaco tip. Nonaxial vibrations generated by a torsional or elliptical motion of the tip can augment the primary oscillation and aid the mechanical breakdown of nuclear material. These mechanisms are specific to the type of phaco machine used.

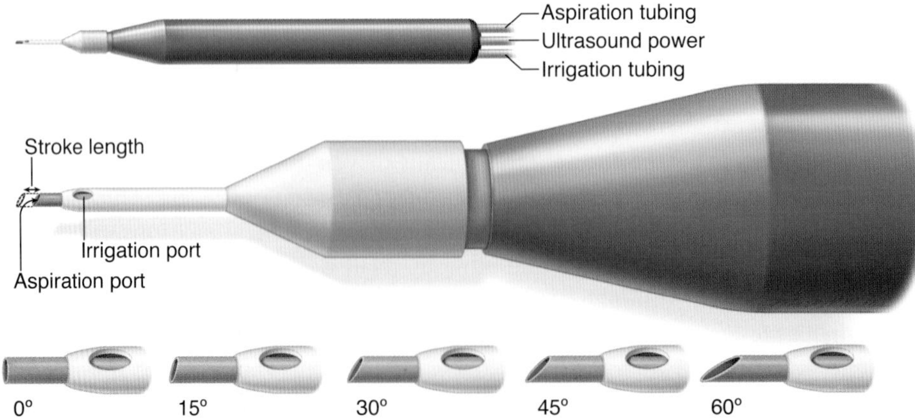

Figure 8-1 Illustration of the parts of a phaco handpiece. The smaller drawings depict the different tip bevels available. *(Illustration courtesy of Mark Miller.)*

Mastering use of the phaco foot pedal is critical to successful phacoemulsification technique. All current phaco machines have foot pedal controls with at least 3 positions. Position 1 activates irrigation, with the infusion pressure determined by irrigation bottle height or its equivalent. Position 2 engages the aspiration or vacuum mode at a fixed or variable rate. Position 3 adds ultrasound power at a fixed or variable level. In the fixed power mode, the level may be set from 0% to 100%, and the chosen power level is delivered immediately when the foot pedal is depressed into position 3. With variable ultrasound, the surgeon controls the amount of phaco power delivered by varying the depth of depression of the foot pedal while it is in position 3.

Key Concepts and Advances in Phaco Power Delivery

The delivery of phaco power can have both favorable and unfavorable consequences. Cavitation, shock waves, shear forces, and heat buildup at the tip may facilitate disassembly of the lens nucleus. However, more power is not necessarily better; the longitudinal stroke of the phaco tip tends to push nuclear fragments away even as the aspiration attracts them, resulting in *chatter.* In addition, heat buildup from the delivery of phaco power may cause thermal injuries such as wound burns or damage to the corneal endothelium.

Many parameters can be adjusted to deliver phaco power more efficiently and safely. The size and angle of the phaco tip can be altered to increase cutting efficiency. Intermittent rather than continuous phacoemulsification modes, such as pulse and burst, can also be used. Various mechanical strategies, including torsional and elliptical movement of the phaco tip (rather than only longitudinal movement), may also minimize heat generation.

Phaco Tip

Phaco tips vary by angle and size of the lumen. Phaco tips are available with bevels of 0°, 15°, 30°, 45°, and 60° (see Fig 8-1). The surgeon generally chooses the bevel angle of the phaco tip according to personal preference. A tip with a steeper bevel has an oval port with a larger surface area, which can generate more holding force (Fig 8-2) and greater cutting efficiency. The disadvantage of steeper bevels is that the larger opening may be more difficult to occlude to achieve full vacuum. End configurations can be round, ellipsoid, bent, or flared.

Pulse and Burst Modes

To reduce the total energy delivered into the eye, the surgeon can use an intermittent rather than a continuous mode of phacoemulsification (Fig 8-3). The delivery of phaco power for only a portion of the cycle also reduces repulsion of material by the vibrating tip (ie, reduces chatter) and improves followability. This method of breaking up the delivery of ultrasonic power into smaller packets of pulses and bursts is called *phaco power modulation.*

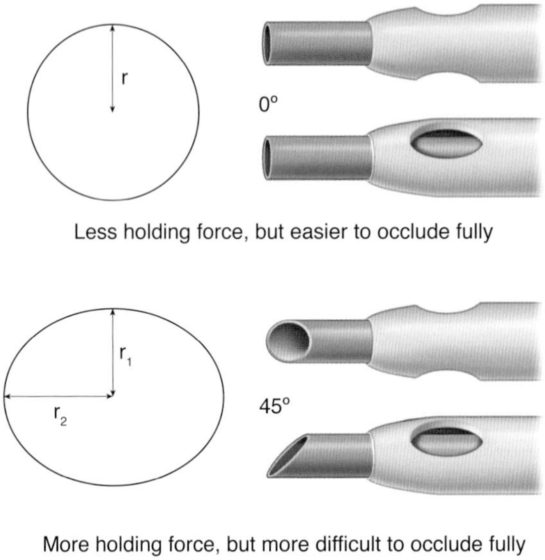

Figure 8-2 Illustration demonstrating the relationship between the phaco tip bevel and holding force. *r*=radius of the tip. *(Modified with permission from Seibel BS.* Phacodynamics: Mastering the Tools and Techniques of Phacoemulsification Surgery. *3rd ed. Slack; 1999. Illustration by Mark Miller.)*

Pulse-mode phacoemulsification involves setting the number of pulses per second (ie, the number of intervals during which phaco power is turned on) while the foot pedal is in position 3. These intervals alternate with "rest" intervals during which phaco power is off. The phaco power of each pulse increases as the foot pedal is depressed farther in position 3. When the foot pedal is fully depressed in position 3, each pulse will have the preset maximum power.

Burst-mode phacoemulsification involves delivery of preset power (0%–100%) in single bursts that are separated by decreasing intervals as the foot pedal is depressed through position 3. When the foot pedal is fully depressed in position 3, the power is no longer delivered in bursts but is continuous. Burst mode allows the tip of the phaco needle to be buried into the lens, an essential step for chopping techniques.

The ratio of "power on" time to total time is referred to as the *duty cycle*. The traditional pulse mode has a default duty cycle of 50%, with the phaco energy on and then off for equal periods (50:50). Modern pulse modes allow detailed control of the duty cycle and the number of pulses per second. As mentioned previously, during burst-mode phacoemulsification, foot pedal position 3 allows linear control between minimum and maximum set duty cycles, with the maximum usually being continuous.

Torsional and Elliptical Phacoemulsification

Other advances in phacoemulsification technology can also reduce chatter and the total amount of phaco energy used. For example, in torsional phacoemulsification, the piezoelectric crystals of the phaco handpiece produce an oscillatory (torsional) movement, which is amplified by use of a bent phaco tip (eg, a Kelman-style phaco tip).

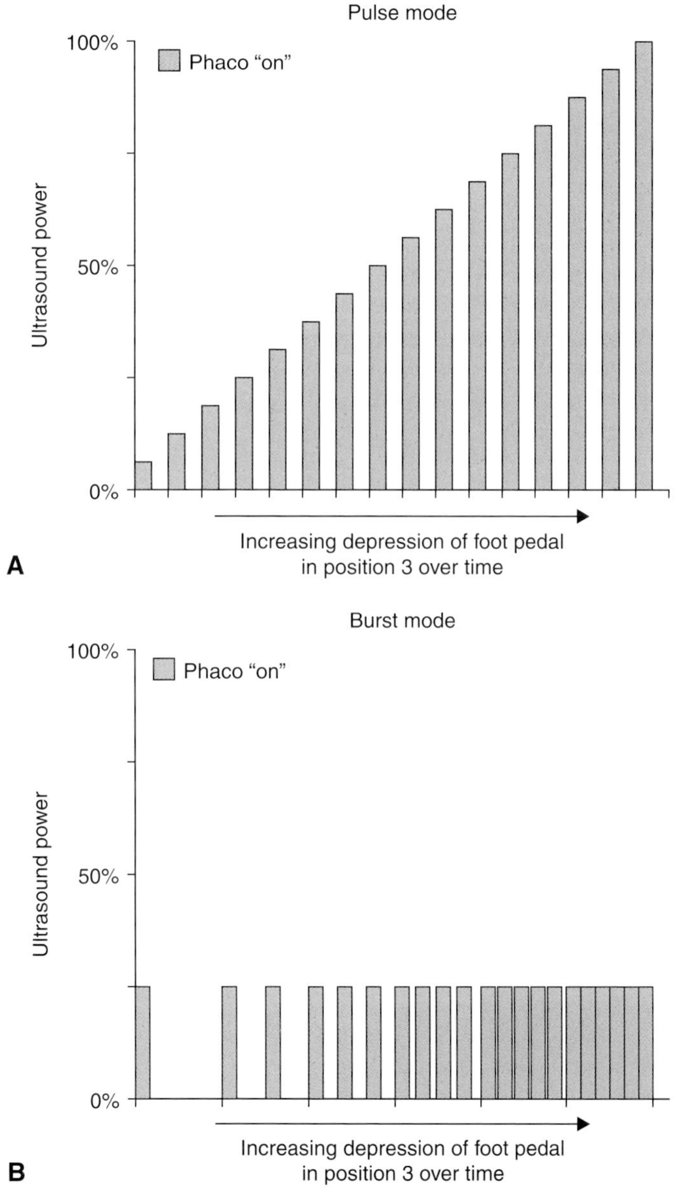

Figure 8-3 Pulse- versus burst-mode phacoemulsification. **A,** In pulse mode, foot pedal excursion provides linear control of ultrasound power, with a fixed duty cycle (50% in this case) and number of pulses per second. **B,** In burst mode, foot pedal excursion provides linear control of number of bursts per second, with a fixed ultrasound power (25% in this case) and burst duration. *(Data modified from Seibel BS.* Phacodynamics: Mastering the Tools and Techniques of Phacoemulsification Surgery; *4th ed. Slack; 2005:121, Fig 1-55.)*

The greater side-to-side movement at the tip may allow for greater shearing forces to assist in nucleus disassembly. Another system utilizes a combination of transverse and longitudinal modalities; the resulting elliptical cutting pattern may enhance nucleus emulsification.

Irrigation

The fluid dynamics of phacoemulsification require constant irrigation through the sleeve around the ultrasound tip with minimal egress of fluid through the incisions. Coaxial irrigation with balanced salt solution cools the phaco tip, preventing heat buildup and consequent damage to adjacent tissue.

Another important purpose of irrigation is maintenance of a stable anterior chamber during surgery. The surgeon can adjust intraocular pressure and anterior chamber depth by changing the infusion pressure. In some phaco machines, infusion pressure is controlled by the height of the irrigation bottle, with gravity providing the force necessary to increase the level of irrigation. Air infusion can also be used to pressurize the irrigation bottle. In other phaco machines, infusion pressure is controlled by a collapsible saline bag that is compressed by pressure plates that provide continuous feedback to maintain a stable anterior chamber.

Some surgeons put additives in the irrigation bottle to maintain pupillary dilation. Others add antibiotics to the bottle as prophylaxis against endophthalmitis (see the section Antimicrobial Therapy in Chapter 7).

Donnenfeld ED, Whitaker JS, Jackson MA, Wittpenn J. Intracameral ketorolac and phenylephrine effect on intraoperative pupil diameter and postoperative pain in cataract surgery. *J Cataract Refract Surg*. 2017;43(5):597–605.

Aspiration Pumps

The aspiration system of the phaco machine is a critical element in the performance of various maneuvers. Thus, an understanding of this system can greatly improve the efficiency of the surgeon's phacoemulsification technique. Ideally, the surgeon is able to utilize fluidics to maximize phacoemulsification efficiency and to grasp nuclear fragments without inadvertently damaging the iris, capsule, or other intraocular tissues. For example, adjusting the aspiration flow rate can help attract nuclear or cortical material into the aspiration port of the phaco tip or irrigation/aspiration handpiece. Adjusting the vacuum determines how tightly particulate material that has occluded the aspiration port is grasped.

Two main types of aspiration pumps are used in phaco machines: *flow pumps* (of which peristaltic pumps are the most common example) and *vacuum pumps* (of which Venturi pumps are the most common example) (Table 8-1). In general, both peristaltic and Venturi pumps are effective, although the vacuum rise time varies between the different pump designs. The latest generation of machines feature continuous feedback sensors that measure flow and vacuum and make immediate adjustments.

Table 8-1 Flow Pump Versus Vacuum Pump: Machine Parameter Effects With and Without Aspiration Port Occlusion

Type of Aspiration Pump	Machine Parameter (Controlled by Surgeon)	Aspiration Port Status	Clinical Effect
Flow pump (eg, peristaltic pump)	Aspiration flow rate (cc/min)	No occlusion	Attracts material to aspiration port
		Occlusion	Controls rise time
	Vacuum limit (mm Hg)	No occlusion	No effect
		Occlusion	Provides gripping force
Vacuum pump (eg, Venturi pump)	Vacuum (mm Hg)	No occlusion	Controls aspiration flow rate, attracting material to aspiration port
		Occlusion	Provides gripping force

Data from Seibel BS. *Phacodynamics: Mastering the Tools and Techniques of Phacoemulsification Surgery;* 4th ed. Slack; 2005:169, Fig 2-7A.

Peristaltic (or Flow) Pumps

A *peristaltic pump* (Fig 8-4) directly creates flow by moving a set of rollers along flexible tubing, pushing fluid through it. The pressure differential between the lower-pressure aspiration tubing and the higher-pressure anterior chamber creates a relative vacuum at the aspiration port of the phaco tip. Direct linear control of the aspiration flow rate can be achieved by depressing the foot pedal farther down into position 2, thereby increasing the speed of the pump rollers. Higher aspiration flow rates will cause the nuclear fragments to more quickly approach the phaco tip. If the anterior chamber collapses while there is steady flow, the irrigation bottle height can be increased, or the aspiration flow rate can be decreased.

Although a *vacuum limit* is set on the machine, a peristaltic pump does not directly produce this level of vacuum. Rather, the peristaltic pump directly controls the aspiration flow rate, which indirectly controls the vacuum level produced. The vacuum level depends on the resistance in the fluidic circuit. Vacuum (grip) builds upon occlusion of the aspiration port. When the aspiration port is not occluded, a higher aspiration flow rate will attract material to the aspiration port more quickly. With complete occlusion, the vacuum level will build up to (but not exceed) the preset vacuum limit and will determine how tightly a nuclear fragment is held onto the aspiration port. The vacuum *rise time* (the amount of time required

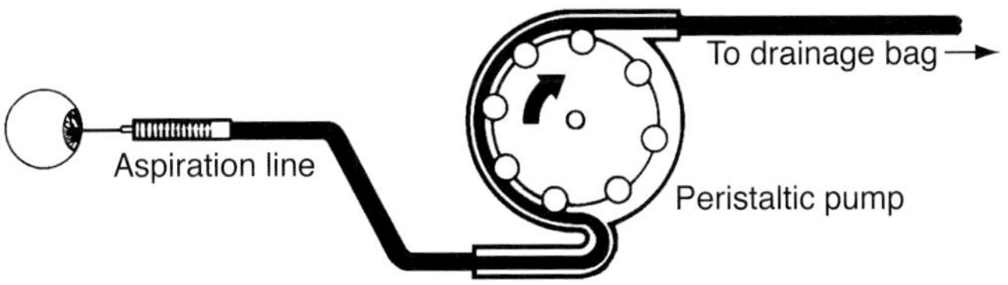

Figure 8-4 Illustration of the peristaltic pump. *(Redrawn with permission from* Practical Phacoemulsification: Proceedings of the Third Annual Workshop. *Medicopea International; 1991:43–48.)*

to reach a given level of vacuum) is related to the aspiration flow rate: during occlusion, a higher aspiration flow rate will cause a faster vacuum rise time.

During complete occlusion, modern peristaltic phaco machines *do* allow for linear control of the vacuum because there is no flow. For example, if the vacuum limit has been reached during full occlusion, lifting the foot pedal up while still remaining in position 2 will decrease the amount of applied vacuum (by a slight reversal of the pump rollers), even though the aspiration port is still completely occluded.

Venturi (or Vacuum) Pumps

Vacuum pumps directly control only the level of vacuum in the aspiration tubing (indirectly controlling the aspiration flow rate). A *Venturi pump* (Fig 8-5) directly creates vacuum based on the Venturi effect: a flow of gas across a port creates vacuum proportional to the rate of flow of the gas. This direct control of the vacuum level in the pump cassette then indirectly produces flow (while the aspiration port is not occluded) by "pulling" on the fluid in the aspiration tubing. The actual aspiration flow rate that is produced depends on the resistance in the fluidic circuit. In the absence of significant occlusion, higher vacuum levels will produce a faster aspiration flow rate, attracting material to the aspiration port more quickly.

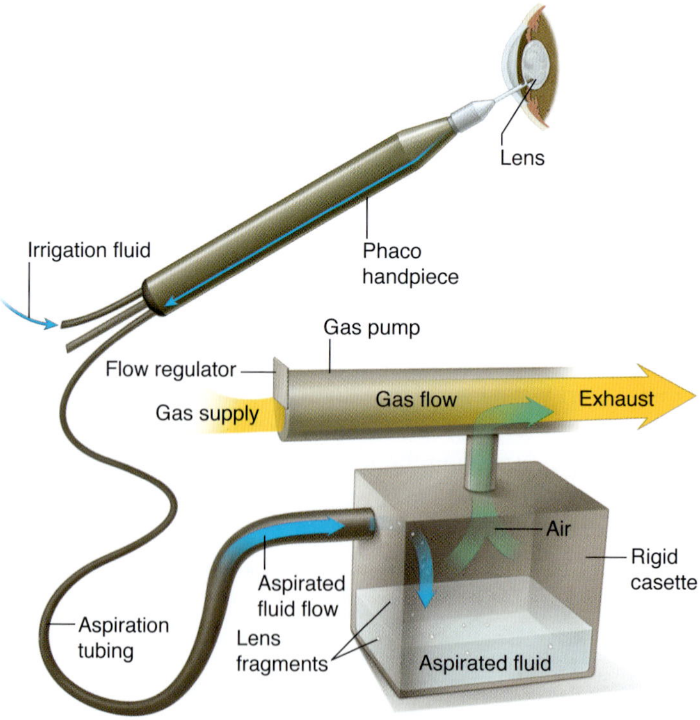

Figure 8-5 Illustration of the Venturi pump. The volume of gas flowing through the pump dictates the amount of air pulled from the rigid cassette, which in turn creates a vacuum that pulls fluid through the aspiration tubing. *(Illustration courtesy of Mark Miller.)*

With occlusion, the surgeon can attenuate the inherently rapid rise time of a vacuum pump via a programmed time delay or by controlling the speed at which the foot pedal is depressed through position 2. That is, direct linear control of vacuum is achieved by varying the foot pedal's excursion through position 2. During complete occlusion, the effect produced by a Venturi pump's linear control of vacuum is clinically equivalent to that produced by a modern peristaltic pump's linear control.

Seibel BS. *Phacodynamics: Mastering the Tools and Techniques of Phacoemulsification Surgery.* 4th ed. Slack; 2005.

Outline of the Phacoemulsification Procedure

Eye Marking and Time-Out

Before surgery, a designated member of the surgical team, typically the surgeon, uses marking pens or stickers to identify the operative eye to prevent errors in surgical site (eg, wrong eye). Depending on the surgical drape being used, the mark may be placed on the cheek or under the eyebrow, rather than on the forehead. In this way, the surgeon can see the identifying mark immediately before placing the surgical drape.

A "time-out" is an opportunity for the surgeon and the rest of the operating room team, including the anesthesiologist and nursing staff, to ensure that they are prepared for the correct surgical procedure on the correct eye with the correct implant. Information typically reviewed during the time-out includes patient name, patient date of birth, procedure, operative eye, and type and power of the intraocular lens (IOL). When 2 patients share the same name, use of 2 patient identifiers (eg, name and date of birth) helps prevent errors.

Exposure of the Globe

After the anesthesia has been administered and the eye has been prepared and draped in sterile fashion (see the section Antimicrobial Therapy in Chapter 7 and Fig 7-6), the eyelids are held apart with an eyelid speculum. When selecting the speculum, it is important to ensure that it will accommodate the phaco handpiece and other instruments (Fig 8-6).

The surgeon may choose to be seated superiorly or temporally. This preference may be dictated by the prominence of the patient's brow, the presence of a large pterygium or filtering bleb, or patient history of ocular surgery. Another factor to consider is the axis of astigmatism, with mild flattening induced at the site of a clear corneal wound.

Paracentesis

The paracentesis incision is used for multiple purposes, including insertion of a second instrument, introduction of intracameral additives, and placement of iris hooks. A small sharp blade, such as a 15° blade or microvitreoretinal (MVR) blade, is used to create 1 or 2 paracentesis incisions approximately 2 or 3 clock-hours away from the site where an incision will be made for the phaco handpiece. A straight entry plane is made parallel

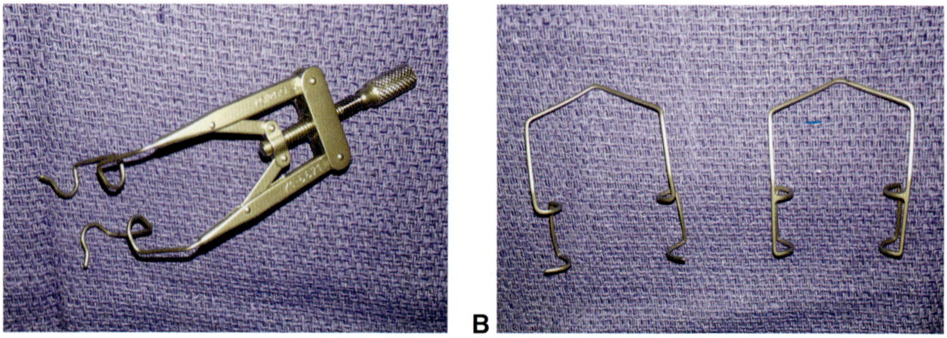

A B

Figure 8-6 Eyelid specula. **A,** Lieberman speculum. **B,** Open-loop speculum *(left)* and closed-loop wire speculum *(right)*. *(Courtesy of Lisa Park, MD.)*

to the iris or at a slight downward angle. Alternatively, these incisions may be made by femtosecond laser (see the section Alternative Technologies for Cataract Extraction later in this chapter). Once the paracentesis is complete, an ophthalmic viscosurgical device (OVD; also referred to as a viscoelastic agent; see Chapter 7) is often instilled to protect intraocular structures and to give the surgeon more control during creation of the phaco incision.

CLINICAL PEARL

The operating microscope's light reflecting off the paracentesis blade can be used to ensure that the blade is parallel to the iris plane.

Clear Corneal Incision

During phacoemulsification, most surgeons use a clear corneal approach for the main incision (Fig 8-7). These small incisions are typically 2.2–3.2 mm wide, just large enough to accommodate the phaco handpiece and allow insertion of the IOL. Globe stabilization is important in clear corneal incisions, especially when the procedure is performed with topical anesthesia. Fixation rings, 0.12-mm toothed forceps, or instruments supplying counterpressure can be used to stabilize the globe as the incisions are made.

Various types of corneal phacoemulsification incisions have been described, including biplanar and multiplanar incisions. Regardless of which type of clear corneal incision is used, an important objective is to create a stable, watertight incision to minimize the risk of wound leak and endophthalmitis. In the multiplanar technique, a diamond or metal blade is used to create a 0.3-mm-deep groove perpendicular to the corneal surface. Another blade is inserted into the groove, and its tip is then directed tangentially to the corneal surface, creating a tunnel through clear cornea into the anterior chamber.

Another approach is the beveled, self-sealing biplanar incision. A beveled blade is flattened against the eye, and the tip is used to enter the cornea just anterior to the vascular arcade. The blade is advanced tangentially to the corneal surface until the shoulders of the

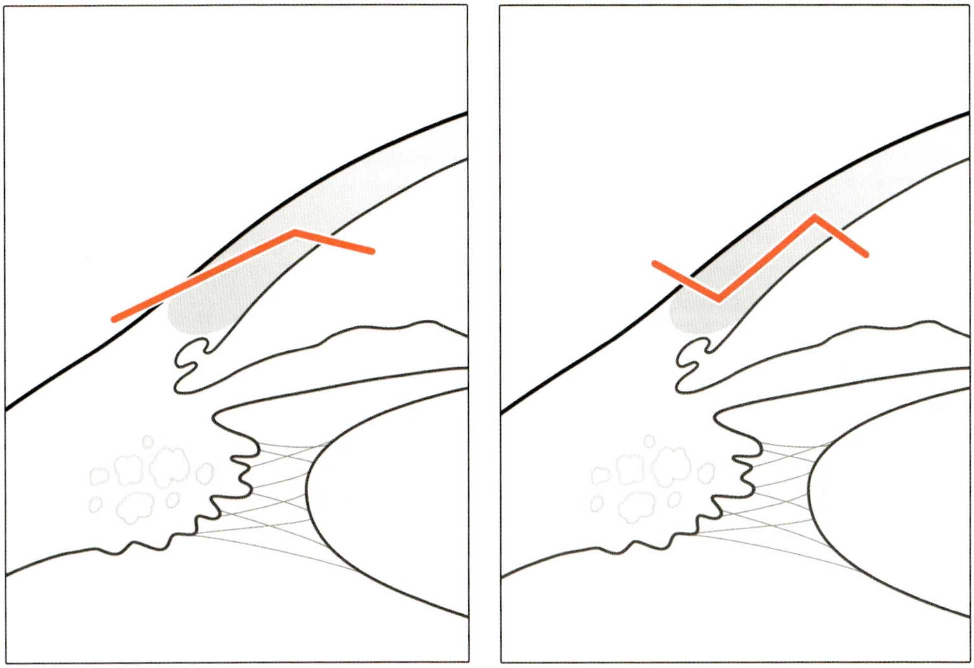

Figure 8-7 Illustration of the architecture of clear corneal incisions: biplanar *(left)* and triplanar *(right)*. *(Illustration developed by Lisa Park, MD, and rendered by Christine Gralapp.)*

blade are fully buried in the stroma. The point of the blade is then redirected posteriorly so that the point and the rest of the blade enter the anterior chamber parallel to the iris.

Self-sealing clear corneal incisions can be created with beveled, trapezoidal diamond blades. Such blades can be advanced in one motion and in one plane, from the clear cornea into the anterior chamber. The blade is oriented parallel to the iris, and the tip is placed at the start of the clear cornea, just anterior to the vascular arcade. The blade is tilted up and the heel down so that the blade is angled 10° from the iris plane; it is then advanced into the anterior chamber in one smooth, continuous motion.

Another type of incision uses the "near-clear" approach, in which the incision begins within the vascular arcade. Proponents of this approach cite better wound closure and a reduced incidence of induced astigmatism. However, there may be slight bleeding during surgery, and conjunctival ballooning may occur. In addition, a subconjunctival hemorrhage may be present postoperatively.

Clear corneal incisions may also be made using a femtosecond laser; see the section Alternative Technologies for Cataract Extraction for further discussion.

Regardless of which type of clear corneal incision is used, the length of the wound should permit optimal visualization and instrument manipulation during phacoemulsification. If the corneal incision is too long, the surgeon may have problems manipulating the phaco tip within the anterior chamber and corneal striae may reduce visibility as the surgeon manipulates the handpiece. If the tunnel is too short, the incision may not seal postoperatively. The phaco tip may also abrade the iris, causing atrophy and possible pupil distortion.

Scleral Tunnel Incision

An alternative to the clear corneal incision is a scleral tunnel incision (Fig 8-8). One advantage of this incision is that it may reduce the incidence of both early and late surgically induced astigmatism. Another advantage may be more-controlled conversion to ECCE when this becomes necessary.

For this incision, a limited conjunctival peritomy is created over the intended incision site. The surgeon then clears the overlying Tenon capsule from the sclera and may apply light bipolar cautery to achieve hemostasis. Excessive cautery should be avoided because it can cause scleral shrinkage and postoperative astigmatism.

The scleral incision is usually linear, but it may be either curvilinear (smile shaped, following the limbus, or frown shaped, following the curve opposite the limbus) or chevron shaped. After making the incision, the surgeon uses a blade to enter the scleral groove at a depth of half the scleral thickness, dissecting anteriorly into clear cornea just anterior to the vascular arcade, creating a partial-thickness scleral tunnel. If the scleral groove is entered too deeply, the scleral flap will be very thick, and the blade may penetrate the anterior chamber earlier than anticipated, closer to the vascular iris root. If the scleral groove is entered too superficially, the scleral flap will be very thin and prone to tears or buttonholes.

To enter the anterior chamber from beneath the scleral flap, the surgeon uses a keratome sized to match the width of the phaco tip. The keratome is inserted into the corneal stroma until the tip reaches the clear cornea beyond the vascular arcade. The heel of the keratome is elevated, and the tip of the keratome is pointed posteriorly, aiming toward the center of the lens and creating a dimple in the peripheral cornea. The keratome is then slowly advanced in this posterior direction, creating an internal corneal lip as it enters the anterior chamber.

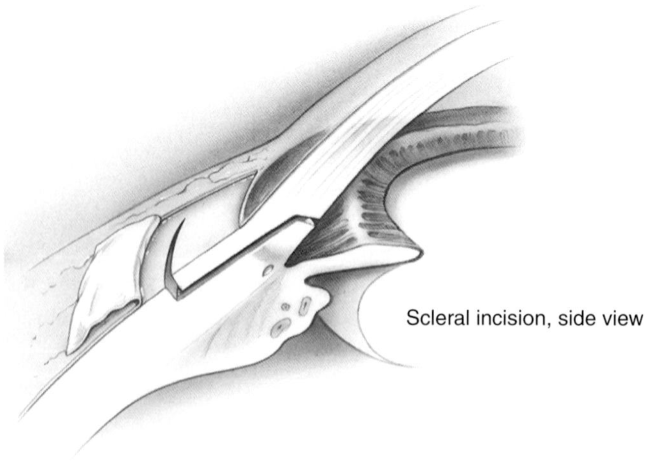

Figure 8-8 Illustration showing scleral tunnel incision, side view: The initial groove is one-third to one-half of the scleral depth. The incision is traditionally 2–3 mm posterior to the limbus. The tunnel is traditionally dissected past the vascular arcade. A short third plane is made by changing the angle of the blade before entering the anterior chamber. *(Reproduced with permission from Johnson SH. Phacoemulsification.* Focal Points: Clinical Modules for Ophthalmologists. *American Academy of Ophthalmology; 1994, module 6. Illustration by Christine Gralapp.)*

Continuous Curvilinear Capsulorrhexis

After the main incision has been made, the next step is to open the lens capsule. Opening the capsule with a continuous curvilinear capsulorrhexis (CCC) offers a number of advantages:

- allows the surgeon to choose from a wide range of phacoemulsification techniques (Fig 8-9)
- resists radial anterior capsule tears that could extend around and open the posterior capsule
- stabilizes the lens nucleus, allowing maneuvers to disassemble it within the capsular bag (thereby reducing trauma to the corneal endothelium)
- transfers haptic forces circumferentially and helps stabilize and center the lens implant

In addition, a CCC sized just smaller than the IOL optic may allow for tighter contact between the posterior surface of the posterior chamber IOL (PCIOL) and the posterior capsule, possibly reducing the incidence of posterior capsule opacification.

The surgeon begins a CCC with a central, radial cut in the anterior capsule using a cystotome needle or capsulorrhexis forceps with special tips for grasping and tearing. At the end of the radial cut, the needle is either pushed or pulled in the direction of the desired tear, allowing the anterior capsule to fold over on itself. The surgeon then engages the free edge with either forceps or the cystotome needle, and the flap is carried around in a circular manner (Video 8-1). For maximum control of the size of the CCC, frequent regrasping of the flap near the tear is helpful. An OVD may be added to keep the lens surface flat and reduce the likelihood of peripheral extension.

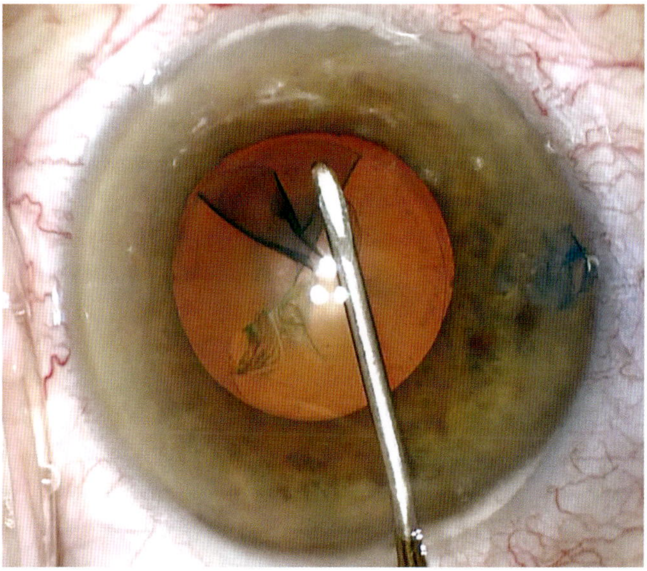

Figure 8-9 A capsulorrhexis is initiated with a puncture into the anterior capsule, which is then extended radially, and a flap turned over. A cystotome or forceps is then used to grasp this flap and tear circumferentially. *(Courtesy of Lisa Park, MD.)*

VIDEO 8-1 Continuous curvilinear capsulorrhexis.
Courtesy of Lisa Park, MD.
Go to www.aao.org/bcscvideo_section11 to access all videos in Section 11.

If the capsulorrhexis tear is allowed to turn too far inward, it can result in a central opening that is too small. If the tear turns too far outward, it can result in an opening that is too large or to extension of the tear to the posterior capsule. An opening that is too small complicates most nucleus disassembly techniques and may contract postoperatively (capsular phimosis). A capsulorrhexis that is too large may allow the IOL optic or haptic to become decentered or dislocate anteriorly. For these reasons, many surgeons advocate a size that just allows the capsular rim to cover the optic edge for 360°. This technique has become increasingly important with the use of premium IOLs, which require a stable position within the eye for optimal refractive results.

If a CCC cannot be completed, conversion to a can-opener capsulotomy is an acceptable strategy (see the Appendix, Fig A-3). A can-opener capsulotomy is performed by using a cystotome or bent 27-gauge needle to create multiple small tears or punctures in the anterior capsule. These are circumferential to the equator and pulled centrally in a clockwise or counterclockwise direction to create a complete opening. However, this type of anterior capsulotomy makes hydrodissection, hydrodelineation, and endocapsular phacoemulsification more challenging because of the increased likelihood of an anterior capsule tear extending around to the posterior capsule.

Alternatively, a circular capsulotomy may be made by a handheld electronic capsulotomy device or by a femtosecond laser (see the section Alternative Technologies for Cataract Extraction later in this chapter).

Little BC, Smith JH, Packer M. Little capsulorhexis tear-out rescue. *J Cataract Refract Surg.* 2006;32(9):1420–1422.

Hydrodissection

Hydrodissection is performed to separate the peripheral and posterior cortex from the underlying posterior lens capsule. In addition to loosening the lens–cortex complex, this procedure facilitates nucleus rotation during phacoemulsification and hydrates the peripheral cortex, making it easier to aspirate after nucleus removal.

In this procedure, the surgeon places a bent, blunt-tipped 25- to 30-gauge cannula or flattened hydrodissection cannula attached to a 3- to 5-mL syringe under the anterior capsule flap. While carefully lifting the capsular flap, the surgeon injects balanced salt solution in a radial direction. Exerting gentle posterior pressure on the nucleus will express posterior fluid and prevent fluid pressure from rupturing the posterior capsule. Gentle irrigation continues until the surgeon sees a wave of fluid moving under the nucleus and across the red reflex (Video 8-2). In mature cataracts or in cases without a red reflex, careful hydrodissection continues until nucleus rotation can be performed. Irrigation in the subincisional area may require a right-angled or J-shaped hydrodissection cannula.

VIDEO 8-2 Hydrodissection.
Courtesy of Linda M. Tsai, MD.

If the nucleus is displaced into the anterior chamber, it can be reposited into the posterior chamber with injection of OVD and application of slight posterior pressure. Alternatively, a supracapsular phacoemulsification technique may be selected in this situation. Hydrodissection is riskier after a can-opener capsulotomy has been performed, with weakened zonular fibers, or with a posterior polar cataract (see Chapter 12 for further discussion of posterior polar cataracts).

Hydrodelineation

After hydrodissection, some surgeons also inject balanced salt solution into the substance of the nucleus for *hydrodelineation,* or separation, of the various layers of the nucleus. This separates the harder endonucleus from the softer epinucleus, which can be left to cushion the underlying posterior capsule. In less brunescent cataracts, a fluid wave can be seen separating the endonucleus from the epinucleus and producing the "golden ring" sign. In cataracts with a white or densely brunescent nucleus, the epinucleus layer may not be present, making hydrodelineation ineffective.

Nucleus Rotation

If hydrodissection has succeeded in breaking the attachments between the peripheral and posterior cortex and the posterior capsule, the surgeon should be able to rotate the nucleus within the capsular bag. Phacoemulsification techniques are easier to perform when the lens rotates freely. Difficulty in rotation may suggest inadequate hydrodissection, loose zonular fibers, or posterior capsule rupture. Attempting to rotate the nucleus in patients with loose zonular fibers can weaken the stability of the capsular bag.

Nucleus Disassembly and Removal

Most methods of nucleus disassembly and removal consist of several distinct steps: sculpting, cracking, chopping, grasping, and emulsifying. With modern phaco machines, all parameters (power levels and intervals of delivery, aspiration flow rate, and vacuum) can be adjusted for each step of the procedure as well as for the density of the cataract, giving the surgeon maximum control of the process.

> **CLINICAL PEARL**
>
> Immediately before initiating phacoemulsification, the surgeon can use the phaco handpiece to aspirate some of the dispersive OVD above the anterior lens surface to create a "working space," thereby decreasing the risk of thermal wound burn (see Chapter 10 for a discussion of intraoperative thermal injury to the cornea).

Two main modes or settings are used during phacoemulsification: (1) sculpt (if using a "divide and conquer" technique) or chop (if using a chopping technique; see the section Techniques of Nucleus Disassembly) and (2) segment removal. Although exact settings will depend on the machine and can be optimized for a surgeon's technique, preliminary relative settings for the major steps of nucleus removal are shown in Table 8-2.

With the *sculpt* setting, the central nucleus is debulked. This process involves a shaving maneuver in which the phaco tip is never fully occluded in order to generate minimal vacuum. Thus, the portion of the phaco needle that is in contact with the lens passes through it without grabbing, and the lens material can be emulsified and aspirated in a controlled fashion. Because of the scaphoid shape of the posterior lens, the sculpted groove should be deeper centrally and shallower peripherally to avoid sculpting through the peripheral posterior capsule. Sculpting is usually performed with low vacuum, low aspiration flow rate, and linear continuous or pulsed ultrasound mode (with high duty cycle and high pulses per second) with a relatively high maximum power setting.

The *chop* setting is used to impale and hold the nucleus with the fully occluded phaco tip, allowing for mechanical chopping of the nucleus with a second instrument. This can be effectively performed with burst-mode longitudinal phacoemulsification, high vacuum, and a 0° to 30° bevel phaco tip (which is easier to occlude to achieve full vacuum than is a 45° or 60° bevel phaco tip).

The *segment removal* setting is employed once the nucleus has been divided (using one of the techniques described later in this chapter); the resulting fragments are grasped using moderately high vacuum and pulled centrally for emulsification. Full occlusion of the phaco tip is required for vacuum to build to the desired level. Once this level has been reached, ultrasound power may be applied. After the nucleus has been emulsified, the epinuclear material may be removed with a lower aspiration flow rate setting with either the phaco handpiece or the irrigation/aspiration (I/A) instrument (discussed in the section Irrigation and Aspiration later in this chapter).

Alternatively, nonphaco mechanisms for nuclear disassembly include fracturing the lens mechanically with a nitinol loop or prechopper or segmenting and softening the nucleus by femtosecond laser (see the section Alternative Technologies for Cataract Extraction later in this chapter).

Table 8-2 Preliminary Relative Settings for the Steps of Nucleus Removal

	Vacuum Limit	Aspiration Flow Rate	Ultrasound Mode
Sculpting	Low	Low	Continuous mode, or pulse mode (with high duty cycle and high pulses per second)
Chopping	High	Low/moderate	Burst mode (with longitudinal ultrasound)
Segment Removal	Moderate/high	Moderate/high	Pulse mode

Location of Emulsification

The nucleus may be emulsified at various locations within the eye, including the posterior chamber, iris plane, and anterior chamber. The location determines which techniques are used to emulsify the nucleus.

Posterior chamber

The posterior chamber is a common location for nucleus disassembly and emulsification. Removal of the nucleus at this location is facilitated by hydrodissection and nucleus rotation. The advantages of posterior chamber phacoemulsification include a reduced risk of corneal endothelial trauma and the ability to minimize the size of the capsulorrhexis opening, which is helpful with suboptimal pupil dilation. Disadvantages include increased risk of complications because emulsification takes place closer to the posterior capsule, greater stress placed on the capsule and zonular fibers when the nucleus is being manipulated, and the need for sophisticated methods of nucleus splitting.

Iris plane

When phacoemulsification is performed at the iris plane, one piece (or pole) of the nucleus is prolapsed anteriorly. Once prolapsed, the nucleus can be manipulated with less stress on the posterior capsule and zonular fibers. Emulsification occurs between the corneal endothelium and the posterior capsule, thereby reducing the risk of damage to either structure.

This location is often suitable for the beginning phacoemulsification surgeon and advantageous in patients who have compromised capsular or zonular integrity. In patients with small pupils, this technique permits good visualization and enables safe emulsification. The disadvantages of working at the iris plane include difficulty prolapsing the nucleus and risk of damage to the corneal endothelium if the surgeon emulsifies the nucleus too close to the cornea.

Anterior chamber

This supracapsular approach involves prolapsing the nucleus through the capsulorrhexis during hydrodissection, which requires a medium to large capsulorrhexis and a relatively soft nucleus. This technique theoretically reduces the stress on the zonular fibers during manipulation of the nucleus. The risks include a greater chance of aspirating the iris in the phaco tip, as well as damaging the corneal endothelium. Nevertheless, phacoemulsification in a supracapsular location is useful in situations such as the presence of posterior capsule rupture. Using an OVD to protect the endothelium and minimizing phaco energy are recommended.

Techniques of Nucleus Disassembly

Phaco fracture "divide and conquer" technique

The most widely used 2-handed technique, referred to as "divide and conquer nucleofractis," can be effectively applied to all but very soft cataracts.

After adequate hydrodissection (and hydrodelineation if desired), continuous ultrasound is used to sculpt a deep central linear groove or trough in the nucleus that is 1 to 1½ times the width of the phaco tip. Signs of adequate groove depth include smoothing of the striations in the groove, brightening of the red reflex in the groove, and sculpting to a central depth of 2 or 3 phaco tip diameters (Fig 8-10).

CLINICAL PEARL

Because of the scaphoid shape of the posterior lens, the sculpted groove should be deeper centrally and progressively shallower toward the periphery of the nucleus to avoid sculpting through the peripheral posterior capsule.

At this point, the surgeon can either separate the nucleus into 2 pieces (nucleus cracking) or rotate the nucleus 90° and sculpt a perpendicular groove (Video 8-3). The phaco tip and second instrument are then inserted into each groove and spread apart, thereby achieving complete separation/cracking of the pieces (Fig 8-11).

VIDEO 8-3 Nucleus cracking.
Courtesy of Lisa Park, MD.

The surgeon can then engage a quadrant using the phaco tip and a segment removal setting. After adequate vacuum has been attained, the nuclear quadrant is pulled toward

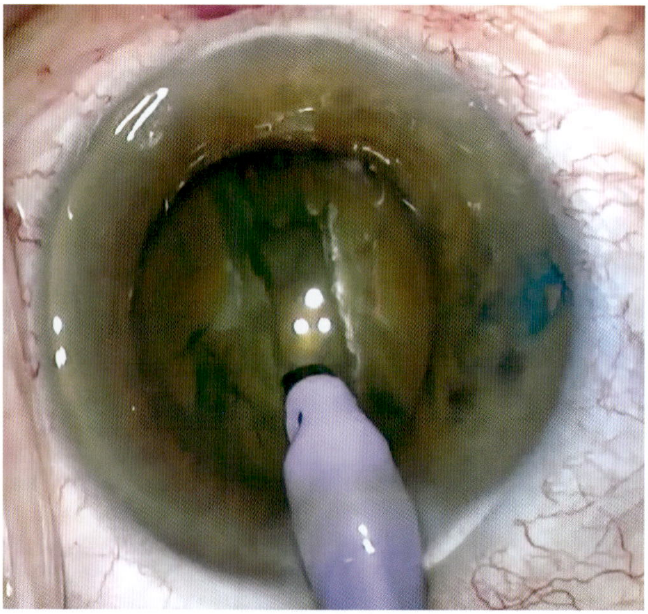

Figure 8-10 A central groove is sculpted under conditions of low vacuum. The ideal groove is deeper centrally than peripherally to allow for effective cracking of the lens. *(Courtesy of Lisa Park, MD.)*

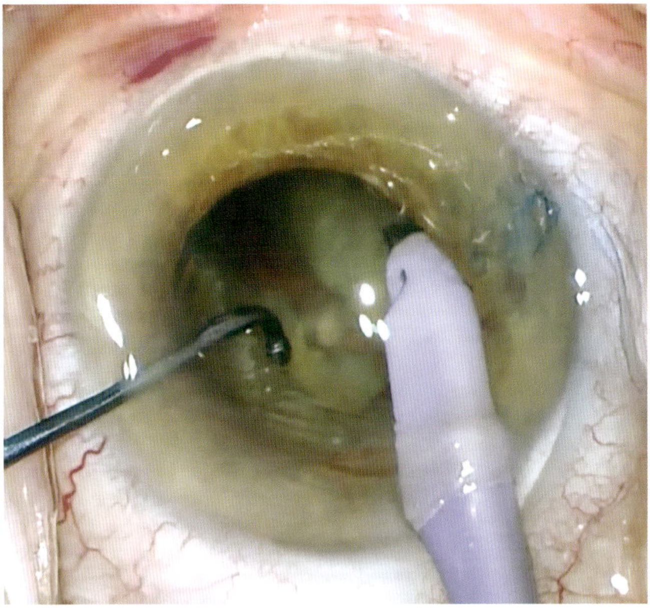

Figure 8-11 Photograph showing 2 instruments used to crack the crystalline lens. These may include the phaco tip and a second instrument introduced through a side port, as shown here. A nucleus cracker or 2 spatulas may also be used to separate the 2 hemispheres. *(Courtesy of Lisa Park, MD.)*

the center of the capsular bag and emulsified. Each quadrant is sequentially removed in the same manner.

Chopping techniques

The *horizontal phaco chop* technique does not entail creation of a central groove but instead uses the natural fault lines in the lens nucleus to create a fracture plane. After burying the phaco tip in the center of the nucleus while using high vacuum, the surgeon inserts a chopping instrument under the anterior capsule flap (Fig 8-12), deeply engages the endonucleus in the periphery, and draws it toward the phaco tip, thereby cracking the nucleus into 2 pieces (Video 8-4). This technique requires the surgeon to place the chopper under the capsular rim and around the equatorial nucleus. The phaco tip is then buried in 1 of the nuclear halves, and the surgeon uses the chopping instrument in the same fashion to create multiple small wedges of nucleus for emulsification.

VIDEO 8-4 Horizontal phaco chop technique.
Courtesy of Lisa Park, MD.

A modification of this procedure entails sculpting a central groove and then cracking the nucleus into 2 pieces. The resulting heminuclei are then chopped into smaller pieces. This technique, known as *stop and chop,* affords the surgeon more room to manipulate the nuclear pieces in the capsular bag.

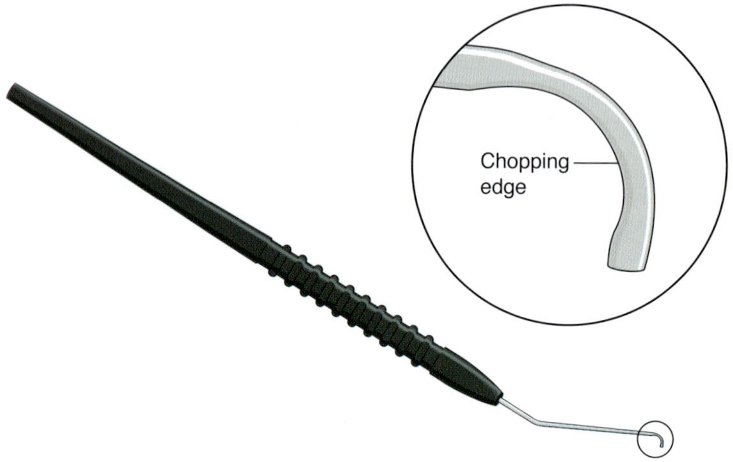

Figure 8-12 An example of a horizontal chopper. *(Illustration courtesy of Mark Miller.)*

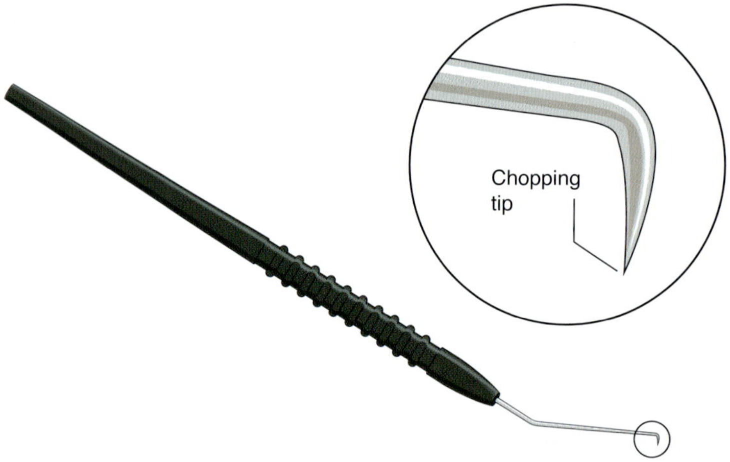

Figure 8-13 An example of a vertical chopper. *(Illustration courtesy of Mark Miller.)*

Vertical chopping techniques have also been described. After the center of the nucleus is impaled with the phaco tip using high vacuum, the surgeon buries a chopper with a sharp tip within the nucleus, just adjacent to the phaco tip (Fig 8-13). The phaco tip lifts while the chopper depresses, and the surgeon separates the instruments to complete the chop, which occurs along natural fault lines in the nucleus (Video 8-5).

VIDEO 8-5 Vertical phaco chop technique.
Courtesy of Lisa Park, MD.

In practice, either the vertical or the horizontal chopping technique can be used with almost any other strategy for disassembly of the nucleus. Chopping may be difficult in soft nuclei, for example, as with pure posterior subcapsular cataracts. Other techniques, such as hydrodelineation and aspiration with minimal phaco power, may be more appropriate in these cases.

Chang DF. *Phaco Chop and Advanced Phaco Techniques: Strategies for Complicated Cataracts.* 2nd ed. Slack; 2013.

Steinert RF, ed. *Cataract Surgery.* 3rd ed. Saunders; 2010.

Irrigation and Aspiration

Once phacoemulsification of the nucleus has been completed, a plate of soft epinucleus or transitional cortex may rest on the posterior capsule. The surgeon can use the phaco needle to accomplish irrigation and aspiration (I/A) without ultrasound; reduced vacuum and flow settings can be employed to aspirate this material from the capsular fornix or posterior capsule.

The coaxial or bimanual I/A technique can also be used to remove peripheral cortical material. With coaxial cortical removal, the port is rotated toward the equator of the lens capsule, and the cortical material is engaged under low vacuum and stripped to the center of the inflated capsular bag. The surgeon rotates the port so that it is fully visible, and the cortex can be aspirated under greater vacuum. This procedure is repeated until all of the cortex is removed. If the surgeon finds it difficult to reach the subincisional cortex, a 45°, right-angled (90°), or U-shaped (180°) aspiration cannula may be useful.

The I/A functions may also be separated using a bimanual technique in which the aspiration port is introduced through the paracentesis incision while irrigation through a second paracentesis maintains the anterior chamber. The instruments may be interchanged as needed (Video 8-6). An advantage of this technique is that it allows the surgeon to more easily reach the subincisional cortex. A disadvantage is that the anterior chamber may become unstable if the flow rate through the aspiration handpiece outpaces the influx of fluid through the separate irrigation handpiece. This issue can be resolved by either decreasing the aspiration flow rate or increasing the infusion pressure.

VIDEO 8-6 Bimanual irrigation and aspiration of cortex.
Courtesy of Lisa Park, MD.

Cortex resistant to aspiration can be separated from the capsular bag with OVD (ie, viscodissection) to allow easier access with the I/A handpiece. Another strategy is to postpone removal of residual cortex until after IOL implantation. The implant can be rotated within the capsular bag so the haptics further loosen the cortex. The surgeon must weigh the benefits of attempting to remove small amounts of residual cortex against the risk of damaging the posterior capsule. Very small amounts of retained fine cortical strands may easily be resorbed postoperatively.

The surgeon may then polish the posterior and/or anterior capsule surface to remove residual lens epithelial cells, which contribute to development of postoperative capsular opacification and capsular phimosis. Polishing can be accomplished either with a mechanical polishing instrument or with gentle aspiration using an I/A tip. The surgeon must take care to avoid posterior capsule rupture during this maneuver.

Insertion of the Intraocular Lens

For discussion of the history of IOL design and development, see the Appendix. IOLs are also discussed in BCSC Section 3, *Clinical Optics and Vision Rehabilitation*, and Section 13, *Refractive Surgery*. For a more detailed discussion of currently available IOLs, see Chapter 9.

In uncomplicated cataract surgery, the surgeon's goal is generally to place an IOL into the capsular bag. The surgeon must determine whether the support structures within the eye are adequate to maintain IOL centration and stability. With posterior capsule rupture, sufficient anterior capsule support may allow a 3-piece PCIOL to be safely placed in the ciliary sulcus. Complete lack of capsular support warrants placement of an anterior chamber lens (ACIOL) or a scleral- or iris-fixated posterior chamber lens.

In all cases, an OVD is used to fill the capsular bag or expand the ciliary sulcus, stabilize the anterior chamber during IOL insertion, and protect the corneal endothelium from contact with the IOL. The phacoemulsification incision must be large enough to accommodate the IOL and inserter; if necessary, the incision may be enlarged after removal of the cataract.

Foldable single-piece IOLs

Foldable single-piece and 3-piece IOLs are the most commonly used IOL styles. A foldable single-piece IOL (Fig 8-14) is loaded into an injector cartridge that has been prefilled with OVD. The cartridge is then inserted into a handpiece, which is operated using a manual plunger or screw mechanism. Preloaded IOL injector systems and automated inserters are also available. The tip of the injector is then introduced into the corneal wound and the IOL inserted, with the first haptic placed carefully into the capsular bag under direct visualization. The trailing haptic is flexed and placed into position, or "dialed in," by rotating it clockwise with slight posterior pressure utilizing either the tip of the injector or a second instrument, such as a hook, so that the second haptic slides under the anterior

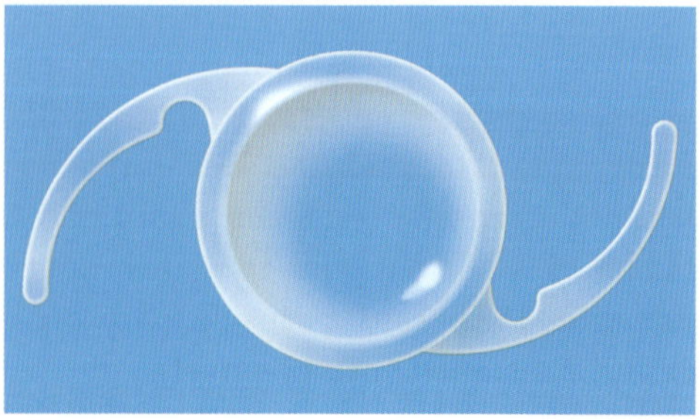

Figure 8-14 An illustration of a modern foldable single-piece posterior chamber intraocular lens (IOL). *(Illustration courtesy of Mark Miller.)*

capsule (Video 8-7). A foldable single-piece IOL should never be placed in the ciliary sulcus or anterior chamber because of the risk of iris chafing and uveitis-glaucoma-hyphema (UGH) syndrome (see Chapter 11).

VIDEO 8-7 Injection of a single-piece intraocular lens.
Courtesy of Lisa Park, MD.

Foldable 3-piece IOLs

Foldable 3-piece IOLs are generally made of either an acrylic or a silicone optic with polypropylene haptics (Fig 8-15). These lenses can be placed into either the capsular bag or the ciliary sulcus using an injector, or they can be folded in half and placed through the incision using implant forceps. The optic and trailing haptic are positioned using forceps or by dialing in the lens, as described in the preceding section.

Polymethyl methacrylate IOLs

Polymethyl methacrylate (PMMA) IOLs are not foldable and may be safely inserted with standard, fine-tip, smooth forceps. The phacoemulsification incision must be widened to accommodate the size of the lens, and the IOL is advanced by first placing the leading haptic into position and then rotating the optic and trailing haptic into place.

Scleral- or iris-fixated posterior chamber IOLs

Several techniques have been described for securing a PCIOL behind the iris when capsular support is inadequate. If the lens is to be sutured to the sclera, polypropylene sutures or Gore-Tex sutures (W. L. Gore & Associates) are typically used instead of nylon sutures, because nylon degrades over time and lens dislocation may result. Transscleral polypropylene or Gore-Tex sutures may be used to secure the IOL haptics in the ciliary sulcus, or the haptics may be sutured to the overlying iris with polypropylene sutures. Note that the Gore-Tex suture packaging explicitly states that the product is not for ophthalmic use. Alternative techniques have been described whereby the PCIOL haptics are secured via a scleral tunnel, with or without the use of surgical glue.

A scleral-fixated PCIOL is a valuable alternative to an ACIOL in situations when an angle-supported lens may be problematic, such as when peripheral anterior synechiae are

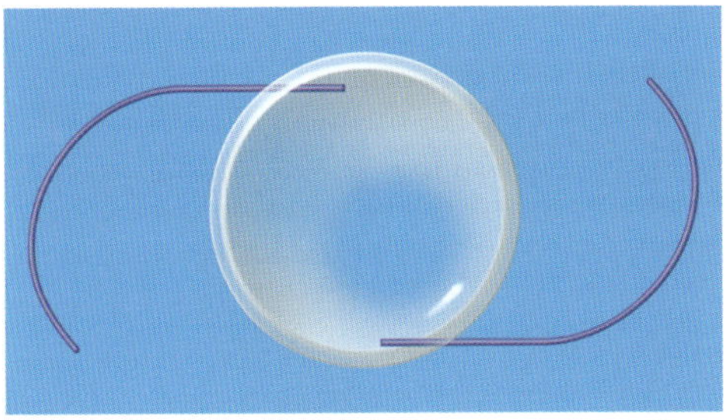

Figure 8-15 An illustration of a modern foldable 3-piece posterior chamber IOL. *(Illustration courtesy of Mark Miller.)*

present or there is significant corneal endothelial compromise. Scleral-fixation techniques are more difficult than those used in standard implantation and are associated with a greater risk of complications such as vitreous hemorrhage, lens dislocation, lens tilt, or late endophthalmitis (see Chapters 10 and 11).

Agarwal A, Jacob S, Kumar DA, Agarwal A, Narasimhan S, Agarwal A. Handshake technique for glued intrascleral haptic fixation of a posterior chamber intraocular lens. *J Cataract Refract Surg.* 2013;39(3):317–322.

Yamane S, Sato S, Maruyama-Inoue M, Kadonosono K. Flanged intrascleral intraocular lens fixation with double-needle technique. *Ophthalmology.* 2017;124(8):1136–1142.

Anterior chamber IOLs

Modern, flexible, open-loop ACIOLs with 4-point fixation are supported by the anterior chamber angle and considered acceptable for use when implantation in the posterior chamber is not feasible (Fig 8-16). The appropriate length of the ACIOL is commonly determined using 1 mm plus the horizontal diameter of the limbus, as measured externally with a caliper ("white to white").

If an ACIOL is being implanted during the initial phacoemulsification procedure, it is generally advisable that the primary clear corneal phacoemulsification incision be sutured and abandoned in favor of a wider scleral tunnel incision at a secondary site. Otherwise, the corneal phacoemulsification incision will have to be enlarged with the keratome or with corneal scissors to enable insertion of an ACIOL, and this could lead to inadequate wound integrity. The pupil is generally constricted pharmacologically before IOL implantation, and any vitreous is removed from the anterior chamber. At least one peripheral iridectomy is performed to avoid pupillary block. The anterior chamber depth is stabilized, and the corneal endothelium is protected with an OVD. A lens glide may be inserted across the anterior chamber into the distal angle to isolate the iris from the advancing IOL haptic. The IOL is then inserted, with its leading haptic placed into the angle while the iris is observed for any indication of distortion. If a glide has been used, it is removed as the IOL is stabilized with forceps. The posterior lip of the incision is gently retracted to allow placement of the trailing haptic in the angle (Video 8-8).

VIDEO 8-8 Placement of an anterior chamber intraocular lens.
Courtesy of Lisa Park, MD.

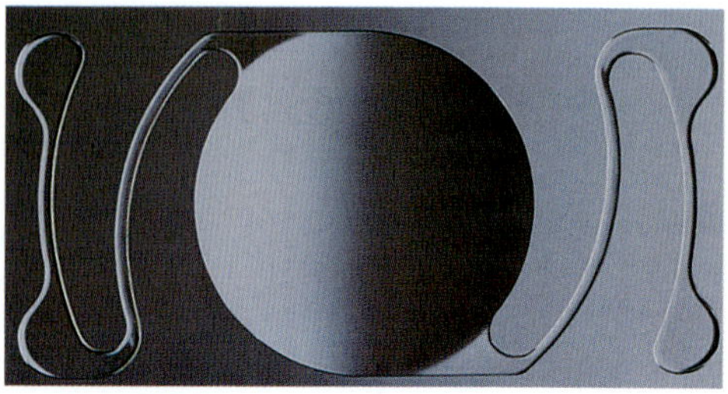

Figure 8-16 Kelman-style open-loop anterior chamber IOL with flexible 4-point fixation. *(Courtesy of Robert C. Drews, MD.)*

Careful inspection confirms the proper insertion. The pupil will peak toward any area of iris "tuck," in which case the IOL can be repositioned until the pupil is round and the optic is centered. The surgeon can adjust the position of the ACIOL by using a hook to flex the optic toward either angle.

Donaldson KE, Gorscak JJ, Budenz DL, Feuer WJ, Benz MS, Forster RK. Anterior chamber and sutured posterior chamber intraocular lenses in eyes with poor capsular support. *J Cataract Refract Surg.* 2005;31(5):903–909.

After IOL Insertion

After removing the cataract and inserting the IOL, the surgeon removes the OVD from the anterior segment to minimize the risk of increased postoperative IOP. In an uncomplicated case with the IOL in the capsular bag, the OVD may be removed by inserting the I/A tip behind the optic or pushing the optic posteriorly to prolapse the OVD and allow its aspiration from the anterior chamber. In the setting of capsular rupture or sulcus IOL placement, removal of the OVD is performed with minimal manipulation of the IOL to avoid destabilization.

To reproduce physiologic IOP, balanced salt solution is instilled via the paracentesis incision to reform the anterior chamber. The main incision is then examined for adequate closure. If the incision leaks, both sides and/or the roof of the corneal tunnel incision can be hydrated with balanced salt solution injected via a syringe with a blunt 25- to 30-gauge irrigating tip. Hydration of the corneal incision causes temporary stromal swelling and increases the wound apposition between the roof and the floor of the tunnel. This anterior–posterior reapproximation, rather than apposition of the external corneal edges, is the critical anatomical feature that determines good wound closure.

With the continuing evolution of techniques for self-sealing incisions and the use of foldable IOLs, many surgeons elect not to suture the incision at the conclusion of a routine case. Long-term results have shown that the small incisions used in modern cataract surgery heal quickly, are relatively stable, and induce minimal astigmatism.

When there is wound leakage, however, the surgeon must be ready to use additional means of closure, such as placement of a 10-0 nylon suture that can be removed postoperatively at the slit lamp. Incisions may also be closed with corneal sealants.

Dewey S, Beiko G, Braga-Mele R, Nixon DR, Raviv T, Rosenthal K; ASCRS Cataract Clinical Committee, Instrumentation and IOLs Subcommittee. Microincisions in cataract surgery. *J Cataract Refract Surg.* 2014;40(9):1549–1557.

Alternative Technologies for Cataract Extraction

Laser Photolysis

Since the advent of phacoemulsification, alternative technologies have been developed to facilitate cataract extraction. The first laser system, the Dodick Photolysis system, a Q-switched Nd:YAG laser system (A.R.C. Laser Corp), was approved by the US Food and

Drug Administration (FDA) in 2000. This system generates laser shock waves at 200–400 ns that strike a titanium target at the end of the aspirating handpiece, thereby breaking up the lens nucleus.

Femtosecond Laser–Assisted Cataract Surgery

In 2010, the US FDA approved femtosecond lasers for cataract extraction. Well known to refractive surgeons, these Nd:glass lasers generate focused, ultrashort pulses (10^{-15} s) at a wavelength of 1053 nm (in the near-infrared region), creating cavitation bubbles within the tissues by photodisruption. Because femtosecond laser technology virtually eliminates collateral damage, it can be used to dissect tissue on a microscopic scale, enabling creation of a capsulotomy, lens fragmentation patterns, corneal relaxing incisions, and clear corneal incisions, if desired (Video 8-9).

VIDEO 8-9 Femtosecond laser treatment before cataract extraction.
Courtesy of Eric D. Snyder, MD.

Before femtosecond laser–assisted surgery, the treatment plan is entered into the system's computer. For a capsulotomy, the intended size and centration method are selected. For lens fragmentation, the pattern used to segment and soften the lens is chosen (ie, available patterns vary by machine). For corneal relaxing incisions, the optical zone, arc length, axis, and depth are selected. The laser can create either anteriorly penetrating corneal relaxing incisions or intrastromal (nonpenetrating) corneal relaxing incisions (see Chapter 9). For clear corneal incisions, the location, size, and wound architecture are selected.

After the eye has been dilated, the patient assumes a supine position. A patient interface docks the patient's eye to the laser unit. The system measures and maps the dimensions of the anterior segment with 3-dimensional spectral-domain optical coherence tomography (SD-OCT) or Scheimpflug imaging. The surgeon confirms the intended treatment protocol and ocular landmarks, including the proper axis orientation of any intended astigmatic treatment, and then activates the femtosecond laser by depressing the foot pedal. During lens fragmentation, gas released from the cavitation bubbles can accumulate between the nucleus and the capsule, creating a pneumodissection effect, which may reduce the need for subsequent hydrodissection. When the laser portion of the procedure is finished, the patient is undocked; some surgeons instill additional eyedrops at this point to address possible laser-induced miosis.

In the operating room, the patient is then prepped and draped for cataract surgery in the typical fashion and positioned beneath the operating microscope for cataract extraction using phacoemulsification (Video 8-10). If clear corneal incisions were created as part of the laser treatment, the surgeon dissects them open. The surgeon verifies that the capsulotomy is complete, carefully removes the anterior capsule with forceps, and may perform gentle hydrodissection and nucleus rotation before proceeding with nucleus removal. To titrate any anteriorly penetrating corneal relaxing incisions and increase their astigmatic effect, the surgeon may gently open them, either during surgery or in the postoperative period at the slit lamp. Methods of marking the intended axis of toric IOL alignment, including small astigmatically neutral corneal incisions or small tabs on the capsulotomy pattern, vary by laser platform.

VIDEO 8-10 Cataract extraction after femtosecond laser treatment.
Courtesy of Charles Cole, MD.

Potential complications related to femtosecond laser–assisted cataract surgery include subconjunctival hemorrhage from the patient interface; incomplete capsulotomy, which may lead to a radial capsular tear; and buildup of gas bubbles within the capsular bag, which can lead to posterior capsule rupture with aggressive hydrodissection.

Since the femtosecond laser was introduced into cataract surgery, its utility has been intensely debated within the ophthalmological community. Proponents of this approach extol its precision, reproducibility, and safety. Others have raised concerns about the higher costs involved and point out that similar results can be achieved by small-incision phacoemulsification as it is currently practiced.

Currently, 5 femtosecond laser technology platforms for cataract surgery are commercially available in the United States: Catalys (Johnson & Johnson Vision), LenSx (Alcon Laboratories), Lensar (LENSAR), Victus (Bausch + Lomb), and Femto LDV Z8 (Ziemer USA).

Outcomes of Cataract Surgery

Modern cataract surgery usually improves visual acuity and enhances subjective visual function. More than 90% of otherwise healthy eyes achieve a best-corrected visual acuity of 20/40 or better after surgery. When eyes with comorbid conditions such as diabetic retinopathy, glaucoma, and age-related macular degeneration are included, these rates are reported to be 85%–89%. A study of a large multicenter European database reported that approximately 93% of eyes achieved a postoperative spherical equivalent within 1.00 D of that predicted by preoperative biometry.

However, visual acuity is only 1 measure of the functional success of cataract surgery. Research tools have also been developed to assess how cataract progression and cataract surgery affect visual function (see Chapter 6). Prospective studies using these tools have shown that patients who undergo cataract surgery have substantial improvement in many quality-of-life parameters, including performance of activities in the community and the home, number of falls, mental health, driving ability, and life satisfaction.

Jaycock P, Johnston RL, Taylor H, et al. The Cataract National Dataset electronic multi-centre audit of 55,567 operations: updating benchmark standards of care in the United Kingdom and internationally. *Eye (Lond).* 2009;23(1):38–49.

Lundström M, Dickman M, Henry Y, et al. Risk factors for refractive error after cataract surgery: analysis of 282,811 cataract extractions reported to the European Registry of Quality Outcomes for cataract and refractive surgery. *J Cataract Refract Surg.* 2018;44(4):447–452.

Melles RB, Holladay JT, Chang WJ. Accuracy of intraocular lens calculation formulas. *Ophthalmology.* 2018;125(2):169–178.

Glossary of Fluidics and Phacodynamics Terminology

The following terms are commonly used in the discussion of fluidics and phacodynamics in phacoemulsification.

Aspiration flow rate (or flow rate) The rate of removal of fluid and lens material from the eye through the tubing, measured in milliliters per minute (mL/min); produced by depressing the foot pedal to position 2 and continuing in position 3. Flow occurs when the aspiration port is not completely occluded, and the rate of flow helps determine how quickly fragments approach the aspiration port.

Aspiration port The opening at the end of an instrument (eg, phaco tip or irrigation/aspiration handpiece) through which fluid and lens material are removed from the eye.

Compliance A measure of how easily aspiration tubing is deformed by vacuum forces. Compared with low-compliance tubing, high-compliance tubing collapses more easily as vacuum builds, leading to a greater surge once occlusion has been broken and the tubing rebounds to an uncollapsed state.

Followability A qualitative descriptor for how quickly and easily fragments are attracted to and held at the aspiration port. Distal followability (how quickly fragments are attracted to the aspiration port) is improved by increasing the aspiration flow rate. Proximal followability (how easily fragments are held at the aspiration port) is improved by increasing both aspiration flow rate (in the case of partial occlusion) and vacuum (in cases of partial and complete occlusion).

Infusion pressure The pressure of the fluid coming through the irrigation tubing. It is controlled either by the irrigation bottle height (on a gravity-based machine) or by the intraocular pressure (IOP) setting (on a saline bag compression-based machine).

Irrigation The influx of fluid into the eye, which is related to the infusion pressure.

Occlusion An obstruction of the aspiration port or aspiration tubing that causes vacuum to build until it reaches the machine's preset value or until the material is evacuated.

Rise time The time it takes for vacuum to build to a given level once the aspiration port has been occluded.

Surge (or postocclusion surge) An undesirable phenomenon that occurs when vacuum has built up because of an occlusion and the occlusion is suddenly broken, causing the fluid in the higher-pressure (positive) anterior chamber to rush into the lower-pressure (negative) aspiration tubing. When the sudden egress of fluid exceeds the influx capability of the irrigation line, sudden shallowing of the anterior chamber may occur, and the iris or posterior capsule may be drawn into the aspiration port. Surge can be minimized by increased infusion pressure (ie, increased irrigation), lower vacuum, low-compliance tubing of smaller diameter, a smaller aspiration port, coiled aspiration tubing, and occlusion-mode software (including automatic modification of irrigation and aspiration flow rate).

Vacuum The magnitude of negative pressure created in the aspiration tubing, measured in millimeters of mercury (mm Hg). Vacuum builds when the aspiration port is occluded, providing a gripping force; its strength determines how strongly particulate material will be held.

Vacuum limit The maximum level of vacuum that a pump can produce upon complete occlusion of the aspiration port.

Glossary of Ultrasonic Technology Terminology

The following terms are commonly used in reference to the ultrasonic technology of phacoemulsification.

Cavitation The formation of gas bubbles arising from the aqueous in response to pressure changes at the phaco tip. The bubbles expand and contract; implosion of the bubbles causes localized intense heat and pressure liberation at the tip, resulting in emulsification of lens material. Continuous cavitation, produced by continuous ultrasound delivery, is less efficient than transient cavitation, produced by intermittent ultrasound delivery.

Chatter This undesirable phenomenon occurs when the repulsive force of the ultrasonic stroke overcomes the vacuum, or "holding power." This process causes the nuclear fragments to be repelled by the ultrasonic tip until the vacuum reaches a level sufficient to neutralize this repulsive energy and once again hold the material. This back-and-forth movement of lens material from the tip impairs followability (see the Glossary of Fluidics and Phacodynamics Terminology). Chatter can be diminished by reducing the phaco power (ie, by decreasing the stroke length of the tip), thereby reducing the forces that push a fragment away from the tip.

Duty Cycle The ratio of power-on time to total power-on plus power-off time. For example, a 10 millisecond pulse of phaco power followed by a 30 millisecond rest interval would have a duty cycle of 25%.

Energy Power multiplied by time. Surgeons can reduce the amount of energy released inside the eye by decreasing either the phaco power or the length of time that the phaco power is on. Thus, energy and power are not the same.

Frequency The speed at which the phaco needle moves back and forth. The term *ultrasonic* is used for frequencies above the range of human audibility, or greater than 20,000 Hz. The frequency of phaco handpieces is between 27,000 and 60,000 Hz.

Piezoelectric crystal A type of transducer used in ultrasonic handpieces that transforms electrical energy into mechanical energy. Linear motion is generated when a tuned, highly refined crystal is deformed by the electrical energy supplied by the console.

Power The ability of the phaco needle to vibrate and cavitate the adjacent lens material. Power is noted as a linear percentage of the maximum stroke length of the phaco needle. Phaco power is produced when the foot pedal is in position 3.

Stroke length The linear distance that the tip traverses to impact the lens material. Among phaco devices, the stroke length varies from 0.05 to 0.10 mm (or 0.002 to 0.004 inch).

CHAPTER 9

Optimizing Refractive Outcomes of Cataract Surgery

This chapter includes a related video. Go to www.aao.org/bcscvideo_section11 or scan the QR code in the text to access this content.

Highlights

- Modern intraocular lenses (IOLs) are typically made of either acrylic (hydrophobic or hydrophilic) or silicone, are foldable and injectable, and have a biconvex aspheric optic with a square posterior edge.
- IOL-based strategies for correcting presbyopia include pseudophakic monovision, accommodating IOLs, multifocal IOLs, and extended depth of focus IOLs. Toric platforms of presbyopic IOLs are available.
- Approximately 40% of cataract surgery patients have 1.00 diopter (D) or more of preoperative keratometric astigmatism. Over 85% of adults have posterior corneal astigmatism that contributes against-the-rule corneal astigmatism.
- Each degree of toric IOL rotation away from the optimal axis reduces effective astigmatic correction by 3.3%. Toric IOL misalignments greater than 30° will increase the astigmatic refractive error of the eye.

Intraocular Lenses

Refractive correction has increasingly become a part of modern cataract surgery. Improvements in preoperative biometry, surgical techniques and instrumentation, intraocular lens (IOL) technology and calculations, and postoperative enhancement options have all yielded more accurate refractive outcomes following cataract surgery (see Chapter 7). IOLs have undergone remarkable development in the decades since their initial introduction. For discussion of the history of IOL design and development, see the Appendix in this volume. For additional detailed clinical discussion of IOLs and surgical presbyopia correction, see BCSC Section 3, *Clinical Optics and Vision Rehabilitation*, and Section 13, *Refractive Surgery*. For a discussion of cataract surgery and IOL selection in pediatric cases, see BCSC Section 6, *Pediatric Ophthalmology and Strabismus*.

Intraocular Lens Characteristics

Modern posterior chamber IOLs typically have the following characteristics (Table 9-1):

- are foldable and injectable
- are made from either silicone or acrylic materials
- have a biconvex aspheric optic with a square posterior edge
- are either single-piece or 3-piece

Foldable IOLs allow for a smaller incision size, which minimizes surgically induced corneal astigmatism and decreases postoperative wound complications. Injectable IOLs (either manually loaded into the injector cartridge or preloaded by the manufacturer) reduce exposure of the IOL to possible ocular surface contamination. Both silicone (which is hydrophobic) and acrylic (which can be either hydrophobic or hydrophilic) IOLs are suitable for the majority of patients.

Adherence of silicone oil to the surface of a silicone IOL can occur (Fig 9-1). Use of an IOL material other than silicone may be preferable in patients who will likely later require vitrectomy with silicone oil injection (eg, presence of proliferative diabetic retinopathy, retinal detachment in the fellow eye). Additionally, postoperative optic calcification of hydrophilic acrylic IOLs has been associated with exposure to air or gas. In patients who will be undergoing future intraocular surgeries that require the intraoperative use of gas (eg, endothelial or lamellar keratoplasty, vitrectomy), it may be advisable to consider a different material. Nd:YAG laser capsulotomy is not effective in treating this opacification, which may require IOL explantation.

Table 9-1 Modern IOL Characteristics

Characteristic	Benefit
Foldable	Allows for a smaller incision
Injectable	Minimizes exposure of IOL to ocular surface contamination
Aspheric optic	Improves contrast sensitivity by minimizing spherical aberration
Square posterior optic edge	Minimizes PCO
Biconvex optic	Allows for a thinner optic (and a smaller incision)

IOL = intraocular lens; PCO = posterior capsular opacification.

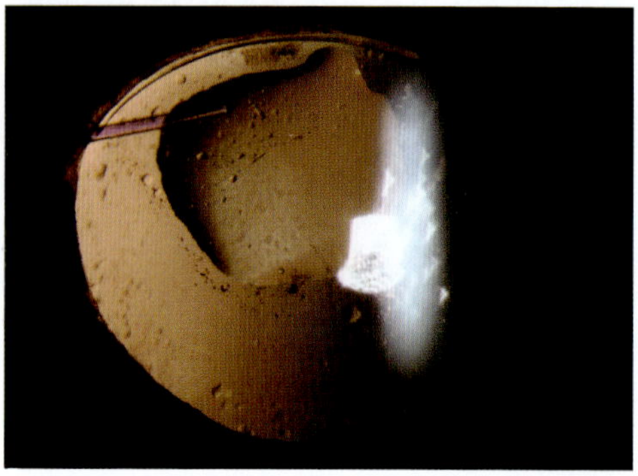

Figure 9-1 A large silicone oil droplet is adherent to the posterior surface of this 3-piece silicone intraocular lens (IOL). *(Courtesy of Christopher Kirkpatrick, MD and Anna Kitzmann, MD, Photographer: Toni Venckus, CRA. Available from https://webeye.ophth.uiowa.edu/eyeforum/atlas/pages/silicone-oil-drop-IOL.htm)*

IOL optic geometry has evolved from earlier plano-convex models to the newer biconvex design (see BCSC Section 3, *Clinical Optics and Vision Rehabilitation*). The addition of a square posterior optic edge design has reduced posterior capsular opacification (PCO) by blocking cell migration behind the optic (Fig 9-2). For more discussion of IOL design and PCO, including photos and illustrations, see Chapter 7 in BCSC Section 3, *Clinical Optics and Vision Rehabilitation.*

Most corneas have some degree of positive spherical aberration. The designs of older types of IOLs were spherical, adding positive spherical aberration to the optical system of the eye, thereby decreasing contrast sensitivity. Newer IOLs are aspheric, with varying degrees of zero or negative spherical aberration (ranging from 0 to –0.27 μm) to offset any positive spherical aberration of the cornea and thus improve contrast sensitivity. It should be noted that corneas with prior *hyperopic* laser in situ keratomileusis (LASIK) or photorefractive keratectomy (PRK) treatments often have *negative* spherical aberration, which can affect IOL selection. A decentered IOL that has any amount of positive or negative spherical aberration will induce coma.

Almost all modern IOLs also incorporate ultraviolet (UV)-absorbing chromophores into the material of the IOL that protects the retina from UV radiation. Some IOLs also incorporate blue-light filtering to attenuate blue-wavelength light (the optic of these IOLs therefore appears yellow to the surgeon). Proponents of these "blue-blocking" IOLs contend that they protect the macula from blue-light exposure; however, opponents claim that there is no evidence of benefit from blue-blocking IOLs, and they are concerned that these lenses might create problems with circadian rhythms or with mesopic or scotopic vision.

IOL technology has advanced, enabling it to address presbyopia and astigmatism, thereby reducing dependence on spectacles. The specialized IOL designs include accommodating, multifocal, extended depth of focus (EDOF), toric, and phakic IOLs. Toric IOLs are discussed later in this chapter in the section Modification of Preexisting Astigmatism. Phakic IOLs are discussed in BCSC Section 13, *Refractive Surgery.*

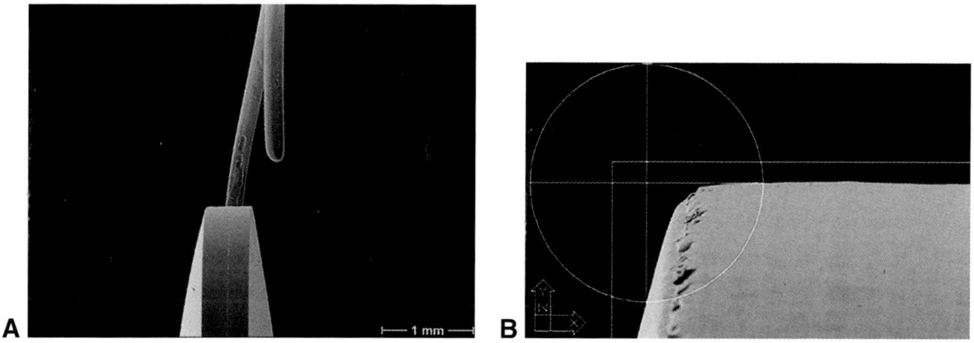

Figure 9-2 The actual geometry of the "square" posterior optic edge depends on the configuration of the optic and the IOL power. **A,** Scanning electron micrograph (SEM) shows the IOL at 25× magnification, with the posterior edge on the left. **B,** SEM shows the junction of the posterior surface with the lateral edge of the optic at 1000× magnification. Increasing the power of the IOL on the posterior surface increases the curvature of that surface and increases the obtuse angle of the intersecting surfaces. *(Courtesy of Werner L, Müller M, Tetz M. Evaluating and defining the sharpness of intraocular lenses: microedge structure of commercially available square-edged hydrophobic lenses.* J Cataract Refract Surg. *2008;34(2):310–317.)*

Mainster MA, Turner PL. Blue-blocking IOLs vs. short-wavelength visible light: hypothesis-based vs. evidence-based medical practice. *Ophthalmology.* 2011;118(1):1–2.
Srinivasan S. Intraocular lens opacification: What have we learned so far. *J Cataract Refract Surg.* 2018;44(11):1301–1302.

Presbyopia Correction

Many patients who undergo cataract surgery have both eyes corrected for emmetropia with monofocal IOLs and rely on spectacles for their intermediate- and near-vision tasks. However, there are also several surgical strategies for correcting presbyopia at the time of cataract surgery currently available in the United States. These strategies include pseudophakic monovision, accommodating IOLs, multifocal IOLs, and EDOF IOLs. Table 9-2 lists several examples of presbyopia-correcting IOLs currently available in the United States.

Pseudophakic Monovision

Pseudophakic monovision is a surgical technique in which different refractive targets are set for each eye. Typically, the dominant eye is targeted for emmetropia. The fellow eye is targeted for some degree of myopia. The term *modified monovision* (or *mini-monovision*) refers to a milder myopic target (eg, –0.50 to –1.50 diopters [D]), compared with “traditional” monovision (–1.50 to –2.50 D).

Hayashi K, Ogawa S, Manabe S, Yoshimura K. Binocular visual function of modified pseudophakic monovision. *Am J Ophthalmol.* 2015;159(2):232–240.

Accommodating IOLs

The accommodating lens was designed to improve distance, intermediate, and near acuity via the movement of its hinged haptics during the accommodative process. Currently, 1 accommodating IOL design (and a similar toric accommodating IOL) has been approved for use by the US Food and Drug Administration (FDA). The accommodating IOL provides some degree of improved intermediate vision (Fig 9-3). A possible mechanism of

Table 9-2 Examples of Presbyopia-Correcting Intraocular Lenses Available in the United States

Accommodating	Multifocal (Bifocal or Trifocal)	Extended Depth of Focus
Crystalens AO (Bausch + Lomb)	AcrySof IQ PanoptixTrifocal (Alcon Laboratories) AcrySof IQ ReSTOR (Alcon Laboratories) TECNIS Multifocal (Johnson & Johnson Vision) TECNIS Synergy (Johnson & Johnson Vision)	AcrySof IQ Vivity (Alcon Laboratories) TECNIS Symfony (Johnson & Johnson Vision)

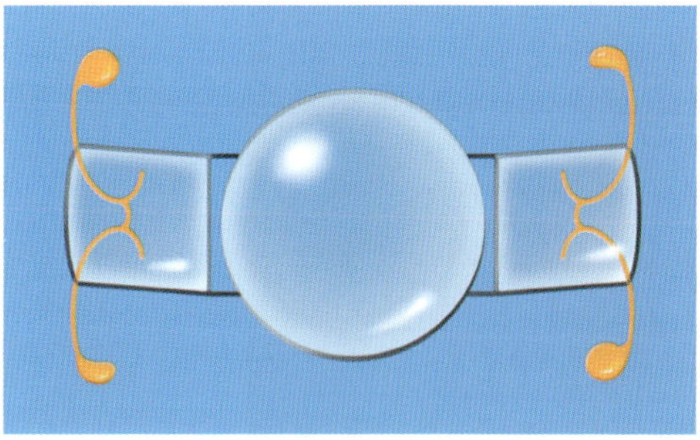

Figure 9-3 Accommodating IOL. *(Illustration courtesy of Mark Miller.)*

action that would explain this improvement is that this IOL provides some pseudoaccommodative depth of focus, because there is no clear clinical evidence that these "accommodating" IOLs change axial position in the eye during near-vision tasks.

Dhital A, Spalton DJ, Gala KB. Comparison of near vision, intraocular lens movement, and depth of focus with accommodating and monofocal intraocular lenses. *J Cataract Refract Surg.* 2013;39(12):1872–1878.

Multifocal IOLs

Multifocal IOLs (MFIOLs) achieve both distance and intermediate/near vision by dividing light into 2 or more focal points (Fig 9-4). This is achieved by either refractive or diffractive optics, or a combination of the 2. Several multifocal lenses (including toric MFIOLs) have been FDA-approved for use in the United States (Fig 9-5). Models are available in various power adds.

The advantage of MFIOLs is reduced dependence on spectacles. Disadvantages include reduction in contrast sensitivity (which patients may perceive as dimmer vision), the presence of glare and halos (particularly in mesopic or scotopic conditions), and the presence of multiple images. Lower-add MFIOLs (ie, with their "near" focal point farther from the eye) may reduce some of these symptoms compared to higher-add MFIOLs. Patients with preoperative hyperopia may be less bothered by some of the visual aberrations associated with these lenses than patients with preoperative myopia. It is important for the cataract surgeon to counsel patients receiving MFIOLs about the intended postoperative visual outcome and limitations; a specialized consent process can be used.

MFIOLs are most suitable for use in patients with excellent ocular health; they can cause reduced quality of vision and unsatisfactory outcomes in patients with ocular pathology, such as amblyopia or diseases of the cornea, optic nerve (eg, glaucoma), or macula. MFIOLs work best when implanted bilaterally and when minimal postoperative astigmatism can be achieved. Options for patients unhappy with their uncorrected visual outcome due to residual postoperative refractive error include spectacle or contact lens correction, keratorefractive surgery, or IOL exchange, preferably performed before capsular fibrosis increases the difficulty of explantation.

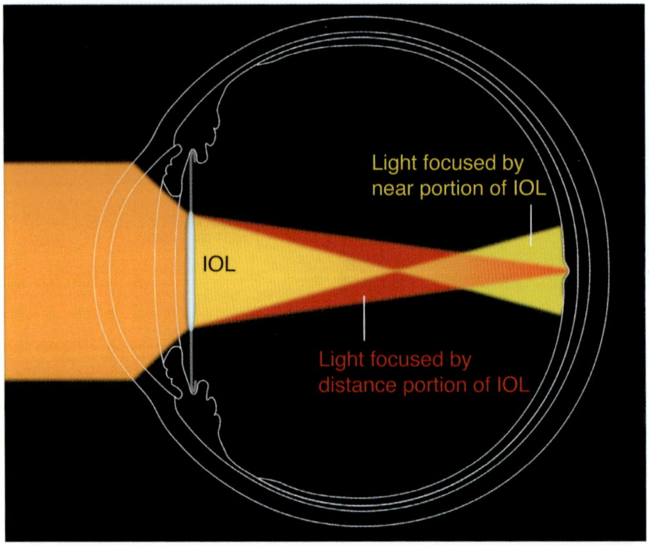

Figure 9-4 Diffractive optics of a multifocal (bifocal) IOL. Note the unfocused light rays hitting the retina, which can contribute to dysphotopsias. *(Illustration courtesy of Mark Miller.)*

Figure 9-5 Multifocal IOL. *(Illustration courtesy of Mark Miller.)*

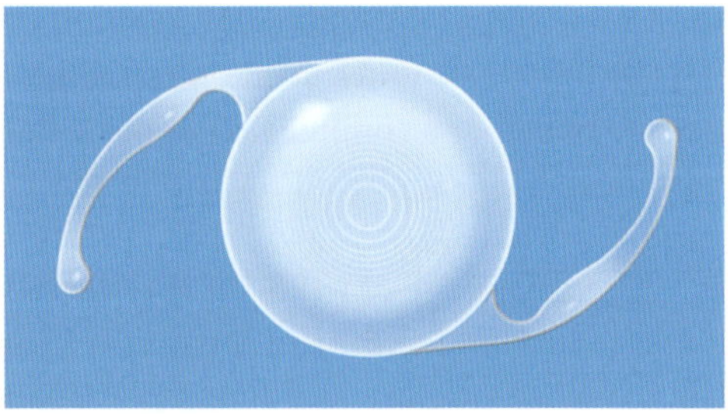

Braga-Mele R, Chang D, Dewey S, et al; ASCRS Cataract Clinical Committee. Multifocal intraocular lenses: relative indications and contraindications for implantation. *J Cataract Refract Surg.* 2014;40(2):313–322.

Extended Depth of Focus IOLs

Extended depth of focus (EDOF) IOLs are a class of presbyopia-correcting IOLs that can have various potential mechanisms of action. The FDA has approved 2 EDOF IOLs for use in the United States; these IOLs are also available in toric models.

Instead of 2 distinct focal points, EDOF IOLs create an elongated focal range (Figs 9-6, 9-7). They provide a range of vision from distance through intermediate, with a low level of dysphotopsias such as glare and halos. Some surgeons employ mini-monovision with EDOF IOLs, setting the nondominant eye for mild residual myopia (eg, –0.50 D) and the dominant

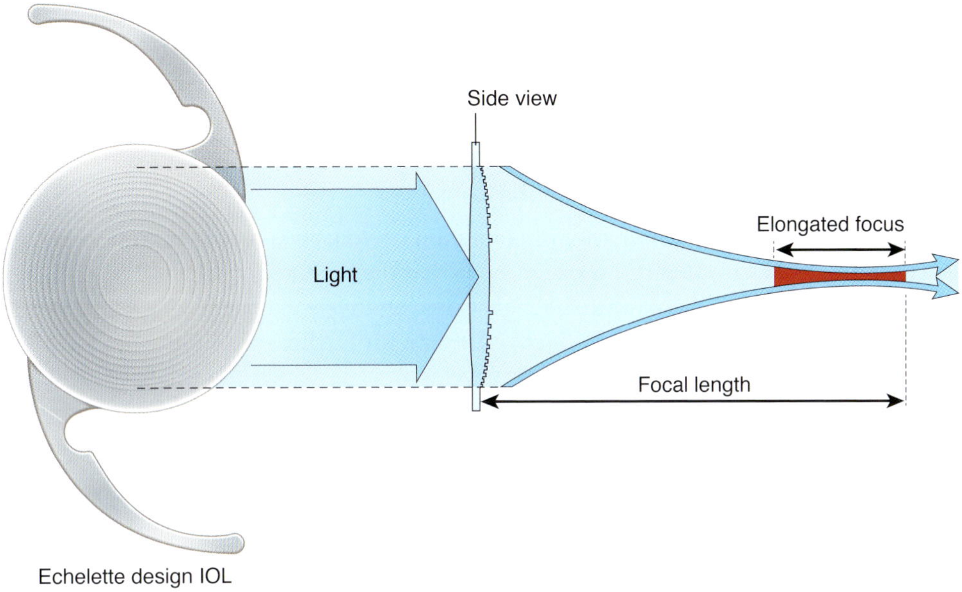

Figure 9-6 Extended depth of focus (EDOF) IOL. *(Illustration courtesy of Mark Miller.)*

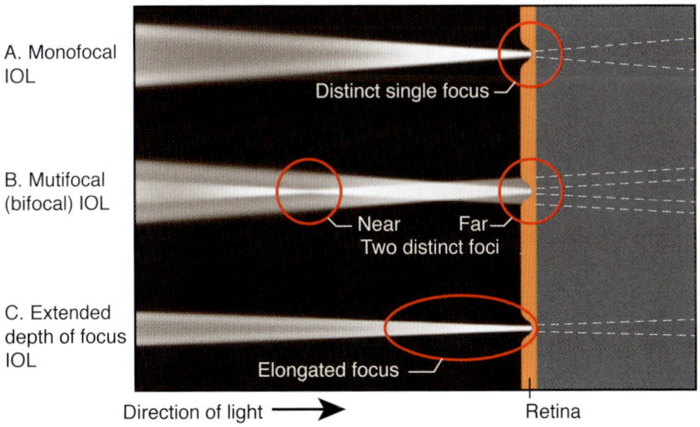

Figure 9-7 Comparison of focal points. **A,** Monofocal IOL. **B,** Multifocal (bifocal) IOL. **C,** EDOF IOL. *(Illustration courtesy of Mark Miller.)*

eye for emmetropia. These adjustments can enable the EDOF IOL to provide better near vision in the nondominant eye.

The advantages and disadvantages of EDOF IOLs are similar to those of MFIOLs (discussed in the previous section), including some loss of contrast sensitivity. As with MFIOLs, patient selection and counseling are critically important.

Cochener B; Concerto Study Group. Clinical outcomes of a new extended range of vision intraocular lens: International Multicenter Concerto Study. *J Cataract Refract Surg.* 2016;42(9):1268–1275.

Other Presbyopia-Correcting IOLs

There are other presbyopia-correcting IOLs available outside the United States or in development. These include other trifocal IOLs, rotationally asymmetric MFIOLs, and EDOF IOLs with different mechanisms of action (eg, the pinhole effect).

Postoperative Adjustment of Intraocular Lenses

The ability to adjust IOL power after implantation could help surgeons minimize postoperative refractive error. In 2017, the FDA approved the light-adjustable IOL. This 3-piece silicone IOL can be irradiated with UV light postoperatively to change its spherocylindrical power. See BCSC Section 13, *Refractive Surgery,* for further discussion.

Refractive indexing is a technique in development in which a specialized femtosecond laser system is used to change the refractive index of a material (eg, an acrylic IOL), thereby changing its optical power. This technique would enable the surgeon to adjust the IOL's spherocylindrical power postoperatively.

Sahler R, Bille JF, Enright S, Chhoeung S, Chan K. Creation of a refractive lens within an existing intraocular lens using a femtosecond laser. *J Cataract Refract Surg.* 2016;42(8):1207–1215.

Modification of Preexisting Astigmatism

Residual astigmatism after cataract surgery can impact visual function and patient satisfaction. Approximately 40% of cataract patients have 1.00 D or more of preoperative keratometric astigmatism. Therefore, correction of regular astigmatism during cataract surgery has increasingly become a priority for both patients and surgeons. For additional detailed discussions of astigmatism management, see BCSC Section 3, *Clinical Optics and Vision Rehabilitation*, and Section 13, *Refractive Surgery*.

Refractive astigmatism (eg, as found by manifest refraction) is a combination of total corneal astigmatism and lenticular astigmatism. Lenticular astigmatism, which is contributed by the cataract, is eliminated during cataract surgery. Thus, to manage astigmatism with cataract surgery, the surgeon addresses the total corneal astigmatism.

Total corneal astigmatism comprises both anterior and posterior corneal astigmatism. Anterior corneal astigmatism tends to drift from with-the-rule (steeper vertical meridian) toward against-the-rule (steeper horizontal median) with increasing age. In contrast, posterior corneal astigmatism does not tend to change with age. In over 85% of adults, the posterior cornea is steeper in the vertical meridian. Because the posterior cornea is a minus lens, this creates net plus refractive power horizontally, adding against-the-rule astigmatism to the total corneal astigmatism. The average magnitude of posterior corneal astigmatism is approximately 0.30–0.50 D, but there is considerable variation in the general population. Therefore, anterior corneal measurements alone will often overestimate with-the-rule astigmatism, and underestimate against-the-rule astigmatism, due to the unmeasured against-the-rule effect of the posterior cornea.

Anterior corneal astigmatism can be accurately measured by a variety of methods, including keratometry (manual or automated), topography, Scheimpflug imaging, or optical coherence tomography (OCT). It is best to combine keratometry with other imaging methods, because irregular corneal astigmatism or ectatic disease may not be apparent without the use of topography or tomography. Although accurately measuring *posterior corneal astigmatism* is difficult, Scheimpflug imaging, OCT, and light-emitting diode (LED)-based devices can be used. (See BCSC Section 3, *Clinical Optics and Vision Rehabilitation,* for further discussion of optical instruments.) Many surgeons employ regression formulas, such as the Abulafia-Koch formula, or theoretical formulas, such as the Barrett toric calculator, to account for the unmeasured effect of the posterior cornea.

Although the preoperative refractive cylinder is not a reliable indicator of total corneal astigmatism (due to the potential lenticular astigmatism), the manifest refraction can still provide suggestive information about the magnitude and axis of total corneal astigmatism because it necessarily incorporates the effect of the patient's posterior cornea.

Another key component to account for in preoperative planning to correct astigmatism is the surgically induced astigmatism (SIA) of the corneal incision(s) used during cataract surgery. A centroid value (ie, vectorial average) for SIA can be input into any of the available online toric calculators. A 2.4-millimeter (mm) temporal clear corneal incision has been shown to have a centroid value of approximately 0.10 D of flattening in the meridian of the incision, though the actual magnitude and meridian of SIA in any individual case can vary dramatically. Alternatively, surgeons may choose to use their personally calculated centroid SIA value, which has been based on a series of cases. If a larger incision is required, placing it across the steeper meridian may reduce preoperative astigmatism.

Abulafia A, Koch DD, Holladay JT, Wang L, Hill W. Pursuing perfection in intraocular lens calculations: IV. Rethinking astigmatism analysis for intraocular lens-based surgery: suggested terminology, analysis, and standards for outcome reports. *J Cataract Refract Surg.* 2018;44(10):1169–1174.

Abulafia A, Koch DD, Wang L, et al. New regression formula for toric intraocular lens calculations. *J Cataract Refract Surg.* 2016;42(5):663–671.

Hayashi K, Manabe S, Hirata A, Yoshimura K. Changes in corneal astigmatism during 20 years after cataract surgery. *J Cataract Refract Surg.* 2017;43(5):615-621.

Koch DD, Ali SF, Weikert MP, Shirayama M, Jenkins R, Wang L. Contribution of posterior corneal astigmatism to total corneal astigmatism. *J Cataract Refract Surg.* 2012;38(12):2080–2087.

Corneal Relaxing Incisions

Modern corneal relaxing incisions include the use of both astigmatic (or arcuate) keratotomies and limbal relaxing incisions (Fig 9-8). Both of these techniques employ partial-thickness arcuate incisions to reduce regular corneal astigmatism without altering the spherical equivalent power of the cornea. These incisions decrease the curvature of the incised steep meridian and increase the curvature of the meridian 90° away (a phenomenon known as *coupling*).

Although they were previously studied as a technique for correcting several diopters of astigmatism, corneal relaxing incisions are now most commonly used for treating lower amounts of astigmatism, and toric IOLs are used instead for treating higher amounts of astigmatism.

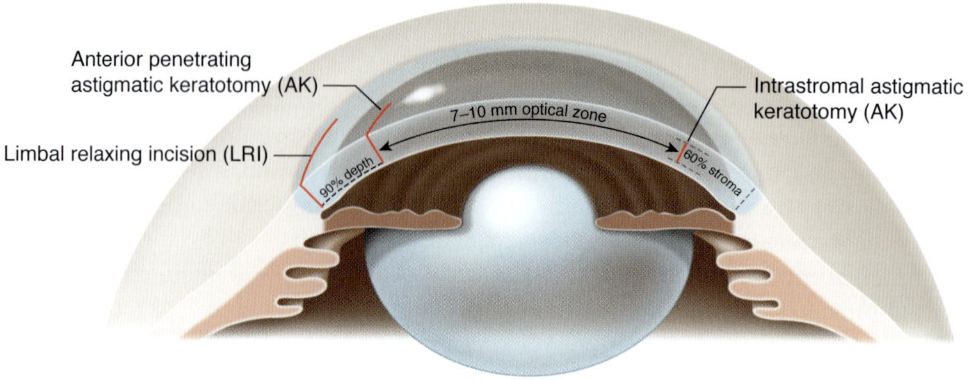

Figure 9-8 Corneal relaxing incisions. **A,** Limbal relaxing incision. **B,** Anterior penetrating astigmatic keratotomy. **C,** Intrastromal astigmatic keratotomy. *(Illustration courtesy of Mark Miller.)*

Astigmatic (arcuate) keratotomy

Astigmatic (or arcuate) keratotomies (AKs) can be single or paired. They are placed centered on the steep meridian of the cornea, typically in the 7–10 mm optical zone. If they are placed too close to the visual axis, glare and irregular astigmatism can be problematic.

AKs can be performed with a diamond blade or with a femtosecond laser platform. Femtosecond lasers can create AKs of a specified arc length, optical zone, and depth. Laser-created AKs that are placed to penetrate anteriorly can be manually opened later, if necessary, to "titrate" the astigmatic effect. Alternatively, the laser can also create intrastromal AKs (ie, AKs that do not penetrate the epithelial surface). Nomograms for both intrastromal and anterior-penetrating AKs have been created; existing nomograms have also been modified for use with the femtosecond laser.

Day AC, Lau NM, Stevens JD. Nonpenetrating femtosecond laser intrastromal astigmatic keratotomy in eyes having cataract surgery. *J Cataract Refract Surg.* 2016;42(1):102–109.

Roberts HW, Wagh VK, Sullivan DL, Archer TJ, O'Brart DPS. Refractive outcomes after limbal relaxing incisions or femtosecond laser arcuate keratotomy to manage corneal astigmatism at the time of cataract surgery. *J Cataract Refract Surg.* 2018;44(8):955–963.

Limbal relaxing incisions

Limbal relaxing incisions (LRIs) can be single or paired and are placed in the peripheral cornea near the limbus. LRIs are more peripheral than AKs, reducing the risk of glare or irregular astigmatism. However, their peripheral location also means that LRIs need to be longer than AKs for the same astigmatic effect.

These incisions are often performed with a diamond blade. Some surgeons place the cataract incision within 1 of the paired LRIs; others prefer to use a separate location. LRIs may also be done postoperatively in an office setting. Various LRI nomograms have been published (Tables 9-3 and 9-4 offer 2 examples), and some are available online (eg, www.lricalculator.com/).

Table 9-3 Donnenfeld LRI Nomogram

Astigmatism (Diopters)	LRI and Arc Length[a]
0.50	1 incision, 45°
0.75	2 incisions, 30° each
1.50	2 incisions, 60° each
3.00	2 incisions, 90° each

LRI = limbal relaxing incision.

[a] For against-the-rule astigmatism, increase arc length by 5°. For younger patients, increase arc length by 5°. For older patients, decrease arc length by 5°.

Data from LRI Calculator website; www.lricalculator.com. Accessed October 1, 2019.

Table 9-4 Nichamin Age- and Pachymetry-Adjusted LRI Nomogram

With-the-Rule[a]						
Preoperative Cylinder (Diopters)	20–30 yrs old	31–40 yrs old	41–50 yrs old	51–60 yrs old	61–70 yrs old	71–80 yrs old
0.75	40°	35°	35°	30°	30°	25°
1.00	45°	40°	40°	35°	35°	30°
1.25	55°	50°	45°	40°	35°	35°
1.50	60°	55°	50°	45°	40°	40°
1.75	65°	60°	55°	50°	45°	45°
2.00	70°	65°	60°	55°	50°	45°
2.25	75°	70°	65°	60°	55°	50°
2.50	80°	75°	70°	65°	60°	55°
2.75	85°	80°	75°	70°	65°	60°
3.00	90°	90°	85°	80°	70°	65°
Against-the-Rule[b]						
Preoperative Cylinder (Diopters)	20–30 yrs old	31–40 yrs old	41–50 yrs old	51–60 yrs old	61–70 yrs old	71–80 yrs old
0.75	45°	40°	40°	35°	35°	30°
1.00	50°	45°	45°	40°	40°	35°
1.25	55°	55°	50°	45°	40°	35°
1.50	60°	60°	55°	50°	45°	40°
1.75	65°	65°	60°	55°	50°	45°
2.00	70°	70°	65°	60°	55°	50°
2.25	75°	75°	70°	65°	60°	55°
2.50	80°	80°	75°	70°	65°	60°
2.75	85°	85°	80°	75°	70°	65°
3.00	90°	90°	85°	80°	75°	70°

Blade depth is set to 90% of the thinnest pachymetry.

[a] Steep corneal meridian at 45°–135°.

[b] Steep corneal meridian at 0°–44° or 136°–180°.

Data from LRI Calculator website; www.lricalculator.com. Accessed October 1, 2019.

Toric IOLs

Toric IOLs are designed to correct regular corneal astigmatism. In the United States, toric IOLs are available in optical powers that can correct from approximately 1.00 D to 4.00 D of corneal astigmatism. Accommodative IOLs, MFIOLs, and EDOF IOLs all also have toric platforms.

As discussed in the previous sections, careful preoperative measurements and calculation of total corneal astigmatism using a modern toric calculator are essential in order to account for the effect of the posterior cornea. Topography or tomography can help to rule out patients who may not be good candidates for corneal relaxing incisions or toric IOLs (eg, irregular astigmatism, corneal ectatic disease).

Preoperatively, the surgeon makes horizontal and/or vertical reference marks on the cornea while the patient is in the upright position. This positioning avoids misalignment errors from potential cyclotorsion of the eye when the patient is supine. The surgeon uses these reference marks to mark the cornea at the calculated axis for toric IOL alignment. Various marking devices, smartphone apps, and intraoperative alignment systems (which use preoperative reference images) are available to assist in proper alignment of the IOL. The toric IOL is then inserted into the capsular bag and rotated so that the IOL axis markings align with the calculated steep corneal meridian (Video 9-1; Fig 9-9).

VIDEO 9-1 Toric IOL implantation and positioning.
Courtesy of Cynthia S. Chiu, MD.
Go to www.aao.org/bcscvideo_section11 to access all videos in Section 11.

Unintentional postoperative rotation of the toric IOL can lead to suboptimal correction or even worsening of astigmatism. Each degree of toric IOL rotation away from the optimal meridian reduces the effect of astigmatism correction by 3.3%. Misalignments greater than 30° will therefore increase the astigmatic refractive error. If necessary,

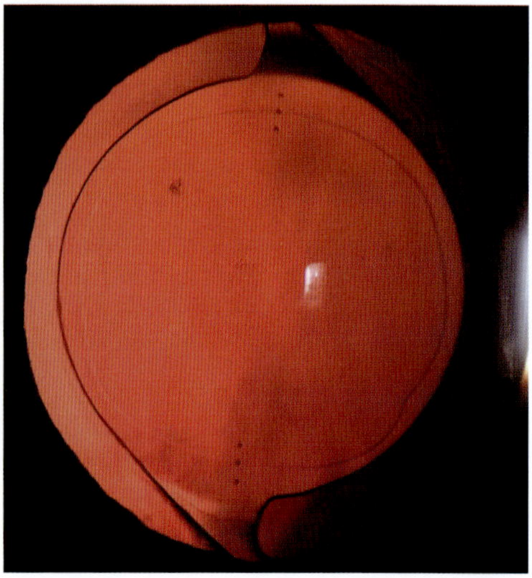

Figure 9-9 A toric IOL in vivo. The axis markings on the IOL are aligned with the calculated steep corneal meridian. *(Reprinted from* Journal of Cataract & Refractive Surgery, *Volume 40, Issue 12, Joshua C. Teichman, et al. Simple technique to measure toric intraocular lens alignment and stability using a smartphone, pp 1949–1952, Copyright 2014, with permission from Elsevier.)*

Table 9-5 Possible Risk Factors for Postoperative Toric IOL Rotation

Anatomic	Intraoperative	Postoperative
Long axial length	OVD retained behind the IOL	Incision leakage
High myopia	Incomplete overlap of anterior capsular rim and IOL optic	Ocular trauma
Large capsular bag	Polishing the anterior capsule	Vigorous physical activity
With-the-rule corneal astigmatism	Low spherical IOL power (ie, thin IOL optic)	

IOL = intraocular lens; OVD = ophthalmic viscosurgical device.

a second procedure to rotate the toric IOL to the correct meridian can be considered relatively early in the postoperative period, before capsular fibrosis and tenacious capsular adherence to the IOL occur.

Several factors have been implicated in case reports of postoperative toric IOL rotation (Table 9-5). Anatomically, longer axial length and larger capsular bag size likely increase the risk of postoperative rotation. Additionally, the lower spherical power IOLs needed for these myopic patients have thinner optics, which may take up less space in the capsular bag. Alignment of the toric IOL to correct with-the-rule corneal astigmatism may also increase the risk of postoperative rotation.

Intraoperatively, complete overlap of the anterior capsular rim with the toric IOL optic is desirable; some surgeons avoid polishing the anterior capsule in toric IOL cases to promote adherence between the anterior capsule and the IOL. Complete removal of the ophthalmic viscosurgical device (OVD), including from behind the IOL, may also help minimize the risk of postoperative toric IOL rotation.

Postoperative incision leakage, trauma, or vigorous physical activity may also contribute to IOL rotation. Insertion of a capsular tension ring (CTR) into the capsular bag may decrease the risk of postoperative IOL rotation, especially in high-risk cases. Despite any of these anecdotal prophylactic measures, postoperative toric IOL rotation may still occur.

Tilting of both toric and nontoric IOLs can contribute to postoperative astigmatic error. For example, horizontal tilting of an IOL around the vertical meridian (with the nasal IOL border tilted anteriorly, and the temporal IOL border tilted posteriorly) will induce against-the-rule astigmatism. Larger amounts of tilt and higher IOL powers will lead to greater induced astigmatism.

Intraoperative wavefront aberrometry may assist in more accurate IOL selection and placement, particularly in eyes that have undergone prior keratorefractive surgery. This technology uses infrared (IR) light and interferometry, both to obtain an aphakic refraction as soon as the cataract has been removed (while the patient is on the operating table) and to confirm proper alignment of the toric IOL. This process allows the surgeon either to rotate the lens to minimize astigmatism or to exchange it immediately if the power is not accurate.

Fram NR, Masket S, Wang L. Comparison of intraoperative aberrometry, OCT-based IOL formula, Haigis-L, and Masket formulae for IOL power calculation after laser vision correction. *Ophthalmology*. 2015;122(6):1096–1101.

Miyake T, Kamiya K, Amano R, Iida Y, Tsunehiro S, Shimizu K. Long-term clinical outcomes of toric intraocular lens implantation in cataract cases with preexisting astigmatism. *J Cataract Refract Surg*. 2014;40(10):1654–1660.

Wang L, Guimaraes de Souza R, Weikert MP, Koch DD. Evaluation of crystalline lens and intraocular lens tilt using a swept-source optical coherence tomography biometer. *J Cataract Refract Surg*. 2019;45(1):35–40.

CHAPTER 10

Intraoperative Challenges in Cataract Surgery

This chapter includes related videos. Go to www.aao.org/bcscvideo_section11 or scan the QR codes in the text to access this content.

Highlights

- Posterior capsule rupture is the most common serious intraoperative complication of phacoemulsification.
- Patients with intraoperative floppy iris syndrome have an increased risk of surgical complications.
- Because a continuous curvilinear capsulorrhexis (CCC) resists radial anterior capsule tears and helps stabilize the nucleus and the intraocular lens (IOL), any discontinuity of the CCC can complicate the remainder of the cataract extraction and IOL placement.
- In cases of posterior capsule rupture, vitreous loss can be reduced by reducing fluid inflow and stabilizing the anterior chamber with an ophthalmic viscosurgical device (OVD) prior to removing instruments from the main incision.
- Vitreous loss should be managed preferably with bimanual vitrectomy, not with pulling and external cutting.
- Expulsive suprachoroidal hemorrhage is one of the most devastating intraoperative complications and can result in vision loss.

Introduction

Complications of cataract surgery that result in permanent loss of vision are rare, thanks to the advent of modern surgical techniques and technology, in the hands of experienced cataract surgeons. Posterior capsule rupture is the most common serious *intraoperative* complication of phacoemulsification (reported in 0.3%–3.5% of cases). The incidence of severe adverse events after cataract surgery, including endophthalmitis, suprachoroidal hemorrhage, and retinal detachment, has declined over the past several decades. *Postoperative* complications are discussed in Chapter 11.

Minimizing intraoperative complications begins with surgical planning and preparation. As discussed in Chapters 7 and 12, it is critical to make sure that the patient is comfortable in order to avoid complications due to excessive or inadvertent patient motion. The function of instruments and devices to be used in the eye should always be checked prior to surgery. A loose cannula can become a projectile in the anterior chamber (Video 10-1); a retracted irrigation sleeve can slip external to the incision; or a detached irrigation tube from the phacoemulsification handpiece can cause a sudden collapse of the anterior chamber. Some complications are mild and self-limited; others are severe and vision-threatening (Table 10-1).

VIDEO 10-1 Projectile in anterior chamber.
Courtesy of Charles Cole, MD.
Go to www.aao.org/bcscvideo_section11 to access all videos in Section 11.

American Academy of Ophthalmology Cataract/Anterior Segment Panel, Hoskins Center for Quality Eye Care. Preferred Practice Pattern® Guidelines. *Cataract in the Adult Eye—2016.* American Academy of Ophthalmology; 2016. www.aao.org/ppp

Stein JD. Serious adverse events after cataract surgery. *Curr Opin Ophthalmol.* 2012;23(3): 219–225.

Corneal and Conjunctival Complications

Self-Limited Intraoperative Complications

Subconjunctival hemorrhages may occur due to conjunctival contact with stabilization instruments used while making clear corneal incisions, or from incidental conjunctival contact during other maneuvers. Conjunctival chemosis can result from balanced salt solution exiting the wounds underneath the conjunctiva, especially when a limbal or near-clear corneal incision has been made. Excessive subconjunctival fluid may cause liquid to pool over the cornea, inhibiting visualization. A small conjunctival peritomy can be created so that the fluid does not continue to accumulate. Intraoperative corneal abrasions can result from contact during draping, with an instrument during surgery or sloughing of epithelium in eyes with conditions such as epithelial basement membrane dystrophy.

Incision and Wound Complications

Proper incision construction and closure are critical in reducing surgical complications. An incision that is too large may result in fluid efflux and intraoperative shallowing of the anterior chamber. An incision that is too tight may restrict fluid influx, increasing the risk of corneal burn. Scleral, limbal, or corneal wound strength is only 10% of normal tissue strength at 1 week, increasing to just 40% by 8 weeks and 75%–80% of its original strength by 2 years. Some studies have suggested that sutureless clear corneal incisions may be responsible for an increased incidence of postoperative wound leakage and subsequent greater risk of endophthalmitis. More studies are needed to determine whether incision location or other confounding factors lead to an observed increased incidence of endophthalmitis.

Table 10-1 High-Risk Characteristics for Intraoperative Challenges and Complications

Preoperative Condition	Surgical Challenge	Complication
Dense brunescent nuclear cataract	Minimal cortex and epinucleus protecting capsule	PCR, VL
	Poor visualization due to intraoperative miosis	RLF
	Zonular laxity	Zonular dehiscence, IOL dislocation
	Increased ultrasound time	Corneal edema
	Increased risk of thermal and mechanical injury to cornea and iris	Incision/wound complications
High hyperopia (short axial length)	Shallow anterior chamber and higher risk of endothelial trauma	Corneal edema
	Iris trauma and prolapse	Iris defects
	Intraoperative suprachoroidal effusion (nanophthalmic eyes)	PCR, VL, RLF
High myopia	Deep anterior chamber	Lens–iris diaphragm retropulsion syndrome
Miotic pupil	Poor visualization	Iris damage, PCR, VL, RLF
Posterior polar cataract	Defective posterior capsule	PCR, VL, RLF
Posterior synechiae	Intraoperative miosis and decreased visualization	PCR, VL, RLF
	Iris bleeding	Hyphema
Prior intravitreal injections	Weakened or open posterior capsule	PCR, VL, RLF
Prior glaucoma surgery	Increased filtration through bleb during surgery with shallow anterior chamber	PCR, VL, RLF, corneal edema
	Zonular laxity	Zonular dehiscence, IOL dislocation
Prior keratorefractive surgery	Dehiscence of RK incision	Wound leakage, irregular astigmatism
Prior pars plana vitrectomy	Intraoperative anterior chamber depth fluctuations	PCR, VL, RLF
	Miosis	Iris damage
	Weakened lens capsule and zonules	IOL dislocation
Prior keratoplasty	Poor visualization	RLF
	Prior full-thickness corneal incisions	Wound leak, graft failure/rejection
Pseudoexfoliation	Zonular laxity	Zonular dehiscence, IOL dislocation
	Miosis	PCR, VL, RLF
	Decreased trabecular outflow	Elevated IOP
Use of tamsulosin and other α_{1a}-adrenergic antagonists	IFIS	PCR, VL, RLF
	Iris prolapse	Iris trauma/defects
White cataract	Difficulty visualizing and performing CCC	IOL dislocation
	Lens intumescence	Radial anterior capsule tear with extension to posterior capsule, VL, RLF

(Continued)

Table 10-1 *(continued)*

Preoperative Condition	Surgical Challenge	Complication
Zonular laxity or dehiscence	Phacodonesis	Vitreous prolapse around equator of lens, dropped nucleus
	Difficulty performing capsulorrhexis	IOL dislocation or decentration, capsule contraction/phimosis

CCC = continuous curvilinear capsulorrhexis; IFIS = intraoperative floppy iris syndrome; IOL = intraocular lens; IOP = intraocular pressure; PCR = posterior capsule rupture; RK = radial keratotomy; RLF = retained lens fragments; VL = vitreous loss.

Data from American Academy of Ophthalmology Cataract/Anterior Segment Panel, Hoskins Center for Quality Eye Care. Preferred Practice Pattern® Guidelines. *Cataract in the Adult Eye—2016.* American Academy of Ophthalmology; 2016. www.aao.org/ppp

All incisions should be checked to ensure closure at the end of the surgery. When gentle pressure is applied to the eye and to the edge of the incision with cellulose sponges, the incision should maintain integrity without leakage, and the eye should maintain a physiologic pressure. If the incision leaks, additional stromal hydration can be performed, or the incision can be closed with suture or tissue adhesive.

Prior corneal trauma or existing corneal incisions from laser in situ keratomileusis (LASIK), radial keratotomy (RK), or keratoplasty may become unstable during cataract surgery. It is important to avoid making incisions that interfere with or cross any existing incisions. Any wound dehiscence can be secured with sutures.

Endophthalmitis Study Group, European Society of Cataract & Refractive Surgeons. Prophylaxis of postoperative endophthalmitis following cataract surgery: results of the ESCRS multicenter study and identification of risk factors. *J Cataract Refract Surg.* 2007;33(6):978–988.

Thermal wound burn

Thermal injury to the incision may result in whitening of the corneal tissue, contraction, and wound gape (Fig 10-1). During phacoemulsification, heat may be transferred from the needle to the cornea because of inadequate cooling of the phaco tip. This can result from an insufficient inflow of coaxial irrigation fluid or from occlusion of outflow at the phaco tip or aspiration line by an ophthalmic viscosurgical device (OVD) or lens material. This complication is more common with a dispersive OVD, increased lens density, and use of continuous, rather than intermittent, ultrasound energy. Bimanual small-incision surgery raises the risk, because the phaco needle is in direct contact with the cornea without an irrigating jacket.

Friction produces heat, thereby causing the corneal collagen to contract at a temperature of 60°C or higher, which subsequently distorts the incision. If the distortion is significant, wound gape may occur with associated leakage. Although the overall incidence is low (0.037%–0.10%), the result of a wound burn is significant: these incisions are not usually self-sealing and thus require suturing, a sliding scleral flap, tissue adhesive, or

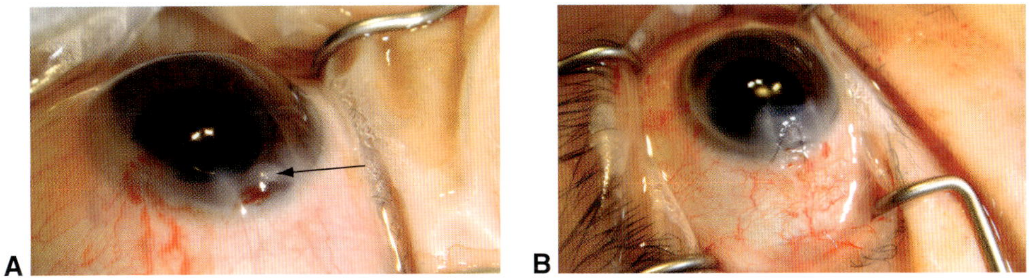

Figure 10-1 Thermal wound burn. **A,** Contraction and whitening of anterior corneal tissue *(arrow)* cause wound gape. **B,** Multiple sutures are required for closure. *(Courtesy of Uday Devgan, MD.)*

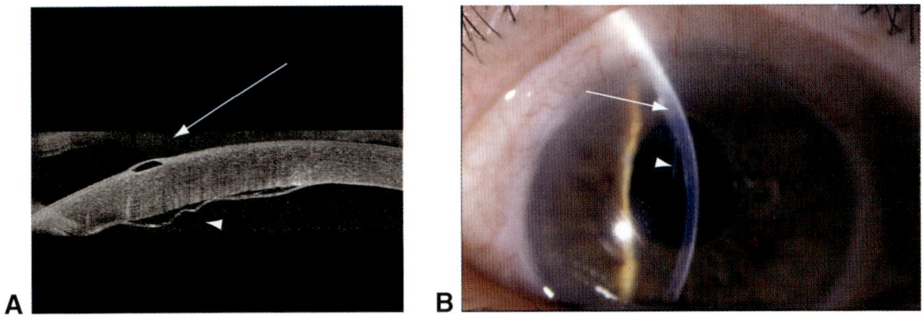

Figure 10-2 Descemet membrane detachment. **A,** Optical coherence tomography (OCT) of the anterior segment. Note the epithelial bullae *(arrow)* anterior to detachment *(arrowhead)*. **B,** Slit-lamp photograph of corneal edema superiorly *(arrow)*. The detached membrane is reflected inferiorly *(arrowhead)*. *(Part A courtesy of Benjamin Currie, MD; part B courtesy of Thomas L. Steinemann, MD.)*

patch grafts for adequate closure. Postoperatively, induced astigmatism is a significant concern.

Descemet Membrane Detachment

Descemet membrane detachment can occur when an instrument or IOL is introduced through the incision or when fluid or an OVD is inadvertently injected between the Descemet membrane and the corneal stroma. This complication results in stromal swelling and localized epithelial bullae (Fig 10-2). Small detachments may resolve spontaneously; otherwise, the membrane may be reattached with air or an expansile gas (eg, sulfur hexafluoride [SF_6] or perfluoropropane [C_3F_8]) tamponade in the anterior chamber. Larger detachments can be sutured back into place under gas or an OVD.

Anterior Segment Complications

Intraoperative Floppy Iris Syndrome

Intraoperative floppy iris syndrome (IFIS) refers to the intraoperative triad of iris billowing and floppiness, iris prolapse into the incisions, and progressive pupillary miosis. Especially when unexpected, IFIS results in a higher rate of surgical complications, including iris trauma, posterior capsule rupture, and vitreous loss. IFIS was originally associated solely with the use of tamsulosin, a selective α_{1a}-adrenergic antagonist, but now has also been reported with the use of other selective and nonselective α-adrenergic antagonists, such as doxazosin, terazosin, alfuzosin, and silodosin. IFIS may also occur following the use of some antipsychotic agents, such as chlorpromazine, or other drugs and supplements with α-adrenergic antagonist activity (Table 10-2). Drugs that are selective α_{1a}-adrenergic antagonists seem to have a greater effect on the iris dilator muscle than do nonselective drugs.

Tamsulosin is most commonly used to treat lower urinary tract symptoms associated with benign prostatic hypertrophy but is also used to treat patients with renal stones and women with urinary retention. Doxazosin, terazosin, prazosin, and labetalol (which is both an α-adrenergic antagonist and a β-adrenergic antagonist) are used to treat hypertension. IFIS may occur in patients who have had no apparent exposure to α-adrenergic antagonists, and it has been reported more commonly in patients with hypertension but not diabetes mellitus. There is no correlation with adrenergic antagonist dosage or duration of therapy, and discontinuing the medication preoperatively seems to have no effect on the degree of IFIS.

It is important to question all preoperative patients about their use of α-adrenergic antagonists. Since 2005, the US Food and Drug Administration (FDA) has required that these medications be labeled with a precautionary statement about IFIS and cataract surgery.

Many surgeons employ intracameral irrigation with 0.5–1.0 mL of buffered, preservative-free lidocaine 0.75% solution mixed with preservative-free epinephrine 1:4000 or phenylephrine 1.5%. Because these solutions must be compounded, mixing errors and subsequent toxic anterior segment syndrome (TASS) may occur. Preservative-free and bisulfite-free epinephrine is available in the United States (through 503B compounding pharmacies);

Table 10-2 Medications Associated With Intraoperative Floppy Iris Syndrome

Selective α_{1a}-adrenergic antagonists
Tamsulosin (Flomax)
Silodosin (Rapaflo)
Tamsulosin and dutasteride (Jalyn)
Nonselective α_1-adrenergic antagonists
Alfuzosin (Uroxatral)
Doxazosin (Cardura)
Prazosin (Minipress)
Terazosin (Hytrin)
Other drugs with α-adrenergic antagonist activity
Chlorpromazine (Thorazine)
Donepezil (Aricept)
Labetalol (Normodyne, Trandate)
Mianserin
Naftopidil
Rispiridone (Risperdal)
Zuclopenthixol

in addition, epinephrine stabilized with bisulfite has been used successfully when diluted in a ratio of at least 1:4 with balanced salt solution. Also available in the United States is a commercial solution of unpreserved ketorolac and phenylephrine used as an additive to the irrigation solution. Despite these interventions, significant miosis and/or iris prolapse still occurs intraoperatively in some patients (Video 10-2). See the section Small Pupil in Chapter 12 for further discussion and management options.

VIDEO 10-2 Intraoperative floppy iris syndrome.
Courtesy of Tom Oetting, MD; The University of Iowa.

PROPOSED INTERVENTIONS TO REDUCE THE INTRAOPERATIVE EFFECTS OF IFIS

- use of preoperative atropine
- intracameral injection of α-adrenergic agonists, such as phenylephrine or epinephrine
- addition of phenylephrine and ketorolac to the balanced salt infusion bottle
- avoidance of incisions that are too short, too posterior, or too wide
- use of iris hooks or pupil expansion rings for stabilization
- use of bimanual microincision surgical techniques
- employment of highly retentive OVDs to "viscodilate" the pupil and maintain a concave iris near the incisions
- discontinuation of fluid inflow prior to withdrawal of instruments to prevent fluid and iris egress
- use of low-flow settings to minimize anterior chamber turbulence and eliminate a higher pressure gradient posterior to the iris

Femtosecond Laser–Associated Miosis

The use of a femtosecond laser for lens fragmentation and creation of incisions prior to phacoemulsification can result in pupillary miosis by a different mechanism than IFIS. Compared to control cataract surgery patients, aqueous humor concentrations of cytokines and prostaglandin E_2 (PGE_2) are elevated following femtosecond laser treatment.

Preoperative use of topical nonsteroidal anti-inflammatory drugs (NSAIDs) mitigates the rise in PGE_2 levels after femtosecond laser treatment, and reduces, but does not eliminate, the associated miosis. Femtosecond laser–induced pupillary miosis may be managed by the same strategies listed for IFIS (see sidebar above).

Chang DF. Intraoperative floppy iris syndrome. *Focal Points: Clinical Modules for Ophthalmologists.* American Academy of Ophthalmology; 2010, module 11.

Jun JH, Hwang KY, Chang SD, Joo CK. Pupil-size alterations induced by photodisruption during femtosecond laser-assisted cataract surgery. *J Cataract Refract Surg.* 2015;41(2):278–285.

Jun JH, Yoo YS, Lim SA, Joo CK. Effects of topical ketorolac tromethamine 0.45% on intraoperative miosis and prostaglandin E_2 release during femtosecond laser-assisted cataract surgery. *J Cataract Refract Surg.* 2017;43(4):492–497.

Lens–Iris Diaphragm Retropulsion Syndrome

Lens–iris diaphragm retropulsion syndrome (LIDRS) is characterized by posterior displacement of the lens–iris diaphragm with a marked deepening of the anterior chamber, posterior iris bowing, and pupil dilation. It occurs more commonly in highly myopic eyes and in eyes that have undergone previous vitrectomy. LIDRS results from a high level of infusion pressure in the anterior chamber with a reverse pupillary block; it may cause stress on the zonular apparatus and considerable discomfort for patients under topical anesthesia. Surgery may be more difficult in eyes with LIDRS due to the excessively deep anterior chamber. Lifting the iris off the anterior capsule is usually sufficient to break the pupillary block and restore normal anterior chamber depth. LIDRS is also discussed in Chapter 12 in the section Conditions Associated With Extremes in Axial Length.

Iridodialysis and Iris Trauma

Iridodialysis, the tearing of the iris at its root or insertion, may occur at the time of insertion of the phaco tip or IOL. Traction on the iris root during phacoemulsification or irrigation/aspiration (I/A) can cause a tear and subsequent hyphema. If the iridodialysis is small or insignificant, it can be left alone. More extensive iridodialysis that could cause optical problems or be cosmetically significant may require surgical reattachment by suturing the iris to the sclera (Fig 10-3).

Chronic mydriasis or iris damage from surgery or trauma may cause the patient to experience excessive glare, particularly if the pupillary light response is inadequate or if the edge of the IOL is not covered. An iris defect may be repaired by a variety of techniques, including:

- a McCannel suture technique with a Siepser sliding knot (see Chapter 11 for a discussion of dislocated IOLs)
- a single-pass 4-throw pupilloplasty (Video 10-3)
- pupillary cerclage (Video 10-4) or the implantation of artificial iris devices to alleviate symptoms or address a patient's cosmetic concerns
- postoperative use of an iris-colored contact lens as a nonsurgical alternative

VIDEO 10-3 Iris repair with single-pass 4-throw pupilloplasty.
Courtesy of Jason Leng, MD.

VIDEO 10-4 Iris repair with pupillary cerclage.
Courtesy of Jason Leng, MD.

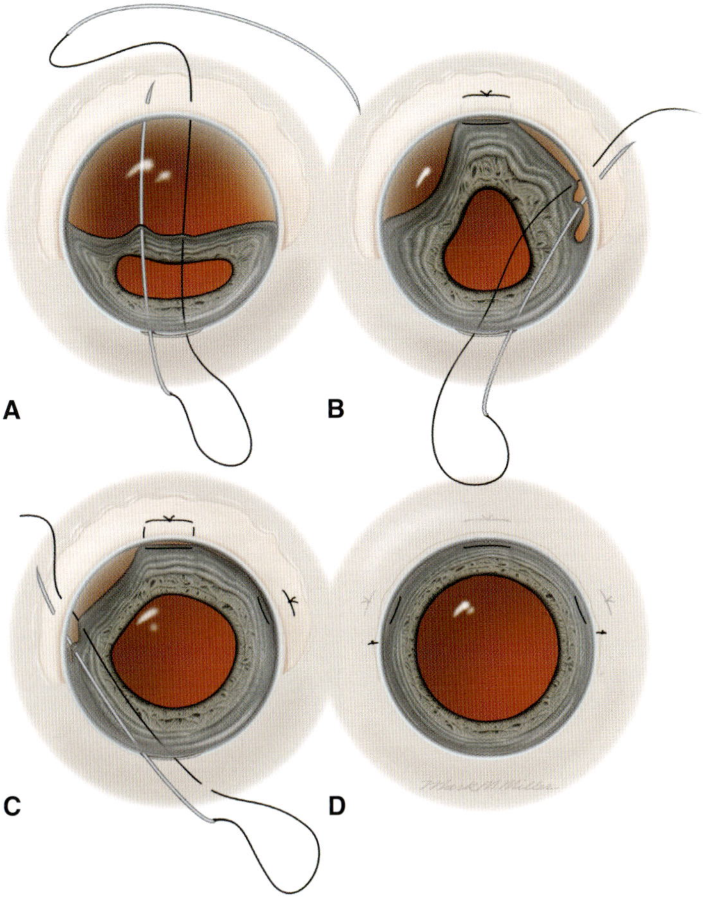

Figure 10-3 Iridodialysis repair. *(Figure developed by Natalie Afshari, MD, and illustrated by Mark Miller.)*

Cyclodialysis

Cyclodialysis, the separation of the ciliary body from its insertion at the scleral spur, may occur as a result of trauma or surgical manipulation of intraocular tissue (Fig 10-4). Gonioscopic examination shows a deep-angle recess with a gap between the sclera and the ciliary body (Fig 10-5). Repair of a cyclodialysis cleft is often indicated if hypotony results. Closure may be achieved with laser photocoagulation at the site of cyclodialysis; if this is ineffective, it may be necessary to reattach the ciliary body with sutures (Video 10-5). A significant and sudden elevation in IOP may occur as a result of cyclodialysis closure. For further discussion of cyclodialysis, see BCSC Section 10, *Glaucoma.*

VIDEO 10-5 Closure of a cyclodialysis cleft.
Courtesy of Arsham Sheybani, MD.

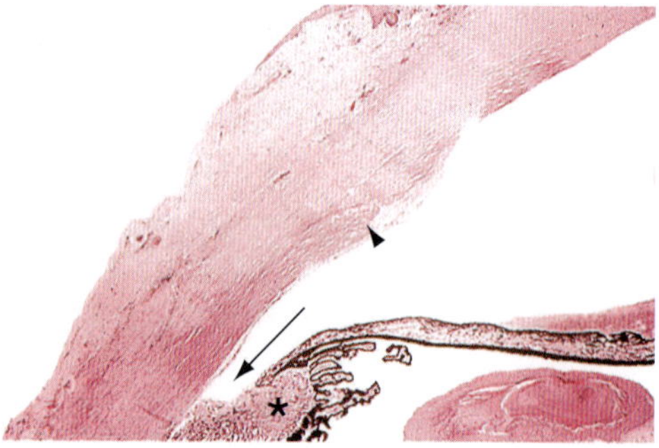

Figure 10-4 Pathology of cyclodialysis. Detachment of ciliary body muscle *(asterisk)* from the scleral spur *(arrowhead)* resulting in a cyclodialysis cleft *(arrow)*. *(© 2019 American Academy of Ophthalmology.)*

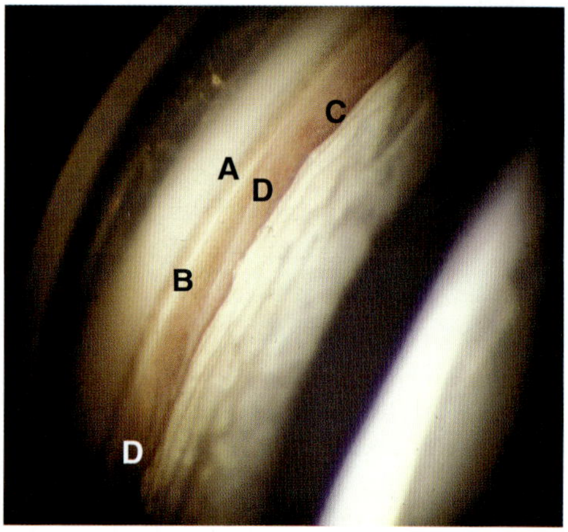

Figure 10-5 Goniophotograph of cyclodialysis. **A,** Trabecular meshwork. **B,** Scleral spur. **C,** Ciliary body band. **D,** Area of separation of ciliary band from sclera. *(Courtesy of Hans E. Grossniklaus, MD. © 2019 American Academy of Ophthalmology.)*

Intraoperative Shallow or Flat Anterior Chamber

During extracapsular cataract extraction (ECCE) or phacoemulsification, the anterior chamber may become shallow because of inadequate infusion, leakage through an oversized incision, external pressure on the globe, "positive vitreous pressure," fluid misdirection syndrome, suprachoroidal effusion, or suprachoroidal hemorrhage. If the reason for loss of normal chamber depth is not apparent, the surgeon first reduces aspiration, then raises the infusion bottle height, and checks the incision. If the incision is too large, the surgeon may partially suture it in order to keep the chamber formed. External pressure on the globe can be relieved by readjusting the surgical drapes or the eyelid speculum. "Positive vitreous pressure," or forward displacement of the lens–iris diaphragm, occurs more commonly in patients who are obese or who have thick necks, in patients with pulmonary disease such as chronic obstructive pulmonary disease (COPD), and in patients experiencing a level of anxiety or discomfort that may lead them to squeeze their eyelids or perform a Valsalva maneuver. Placing obese patients in a reverse Trendelenburg position may alleviate the pressure. Intravenous mannitol can be used to reduce the vitreous volume and deepen the anterior chamber in selected cases.

If the reason for the loss of anterior chamber depth or the elevated IOP is unknown, it is important to check the red reflex to evaluate for the possibility of a suprachoroidal hemorrhage or effusion. In these situations, the eye typically becomes very firm, and the patient becomes agitated and reports experiencing pain. The surgeon should immediately close the incisions and confirm the diagnosis by examining the fundus with an indirect ophthalmoscope or fundus lens. If the hemorrhage or effusion is significant, the operation should be postponed until the pressure has decreased. (See the section Suprachoroidal Effusion or Hemorrhage, later in this chapter, and BCSC Section 12, *Retina and Vitreous.*)

In *posterior fluid misdirection syndrome,* irrigation fluid infused into the anterior chamber may be misdirected into the vitreous cavity through intact zonular fibers or through a zonular or capsular tear, causing an increase in the vitreous volume with subsequent forward displacement of the lens and shallowing of the anterior chamber. The fluid may accumulate in the retrolental space or dissect posteriorly along the vitreoretinal interface. If gentle posterior pressure on the lens or reinflation of the capsular bag with OVD does not alleviate the fluid accumulation, an intravenous infusion of mannitol and waiting at least 20 minutes may allow the anterior chamber to deepen. If suprachoroidal effusion or hemorrhage has been ruled out, the surgeon can insert a 20- to 23-gauge needle through the pars plana into the vitreous by direct visualization, gently aspirate fluid vitreous, and deepen the anterior chamber with irrigation fluid or OVD. Alternatively, vitreous aspiration may be performed with a cutting/aspirating pars plana vitrectomy tip inserted through a sclerotomy 3.5 mm behind the limbus, combined with infusion of balanced salt solution or injection of additional OVD into the anterior chamber.

A shallow or flat anterior chamber can also occur postoperatively; see Chapter 11 for further discussion.

Anterior Capsule Tears

A continuous curvilinear capsulorrhexis (CCC) is an integral step in phacoemulsification surgery (see Chapter 8). Any discontinuity in the CCC can complicate the remainder of the phacoemulsification procedure. Occasionally during a CCC, the capsulorrhexis (also spelled capsulorhexis) may extend toward the periphery (ie, larger than the intended diameter). A "Little maneuver" can be used to rescue an errant anterior capsulorrhexis in such cases (see Video 10-6 and sidebar).

VIDEO 10-6 Little capsulorrhexis rescue maneuver.
Courtesy of Tom Oetting, MD; The University of Iowa.

If it is not possible to complete the CCC, several options are available; these maneuvers can be facilitated with intraocular scissors, microforceps, and the generous use of OVDs to maintain a fully deep anterior chamber. One option would be to create a second tear with a cystotome near the origin of the first tear and extend it in the opposite

HOW TO PERFORM A LITTLE CAPSULORREXIS RESCUE MANEUVER

1. Completely fill the anterior chamber with OVD.
2. Using an instrument or OVD, unfold the anterior capsule flap and lay it flat against the lens cortex.
3. Using capsulorrhexis forceps, grasp the edge of the flap as close to the root of the tear as possible.
4. Pull the flap back circumferentially in the direction from which it came while applying traction in the horizontal plane of the capsule to maintain tension.
5. Apply inward traction to pull the flap centrally.
6. Refold the flap forward and safely complete the capsulorrhexis.

Little BC, Smith JH, Packer M. Little capsulorhexis tear-out rescue. *J Cataract Refract Surg.* 2006;32(9):1420–1422.

direction until it "meets up" with the original tear. Another option would be to convert to a *"can-opener" capsulotomy* (see the Appendix).

Other causes of anterior capsule tears may occur during surgery. In eyes with white intumescent cataracts, the anterior capsule may suddenly split, creating an "Argentinian flag sign" in capsules that have been stained with trypan blue (see Chapter 12). During a femtosecond laser capsulotomy, a radial tear may occur if a complete capsulotomy is not created before removing the capsule remnant. During phacoemulsification, contact of the phaco tip with the capsule may result in a tear in the capsule. In eyes with a discontinuous capsulorrhexis, care must be taken during each subsequent step of the surgery to make sure that the anterior capsule tear is not extended to the posterior capsule, because of the higher risk of vitreous loss and retained lens fragments (see the sidebar Interventions for a Discontinuous Capsulorrhexis). If extension past the equator to the posterior capsule does occur, it should be managed as a capsule rupture (see the sidebar Management of Posterior Capsule Rupture later in this chapter).

INTERVENTIONS FOR A DISCONTINUOUS CAPSULORRHEXIS

- use of a push-pull instrument (eg, a Kuglen hook) to retract the iris and check the extent of a radial tear
- hydrodissection and hydrodelineation, performed gently and without excessive pressure
- use of "low-flow" phacoemulsification settings (ie, lower infusion pressure, vacuum, and aspiration flow rate) to minimize fluctuations of anterior chamber depth
- liberal use of OVD to prevent anterior chamber collapse

- avoidance of aspirating "tags" of anterior capsule, which can cause extension of the tear, during aspiration of the cortex. Prior to IOL insertion, the extent of the anterior capsule tear can be checked with a push-pull instrument after an OVD is placed.
- if a 1-piece acrylic IOL is used, placement of the haptics so that they are not located in the area of the anterior capsule tear, to avoid uveitis-glaucoma-hyphema (UGH) syndrome (see Chapter 11)
- placement of a monofocal IOL to avoid potential postoperative complications. A toric or presbyopia-correcting IOL may be able to be placed within the capsule if the haptics will not be in the position of the tear, but rotation and centration, and intended visual correction, may be affected.
- placement of a 3-piece IOL into the ciliary sulcus, unless there is concomitant zonular compromise

Posterior Capsular Rupture

If posterior capsule rupture occurs during surgery, it is important to reduce fluid inflow and stabilize the anterior segment with an OVD prior to withdrawing any instrument from the main incision in order to minimize the risk of vitreous prolapse.

Causes of posterior capsule rupture include

- *extension of an anterior capsular radial tear* (see discussion in previous section)
- *intraoperative capsular block syndrome,* in which excessive pressure within the capsule causes blowout of the posterior capsule. This occurs during hydrodissection and may be more likely with
  - posterior polar cataract
  - preexisting capsule defects, such as those resulting from intravitreal injections or trauma
  - dense cataracts with a small capsulorrhexis
  - femtosecond laser treatment in which gas bubbles build up behind the nucleus
- *contact with the phacoemulsification or I/A tip.* Risk of this increases with
  - higher flow settings
  - poor visualization, for example in eyes with IFIS or miotic pupil
  - dense nucleus with minimal epinuclear shell
  - anterior chamber fluctuations and postocclusion surge (see Chapter 8)
  - "posterior pressure," for example with choroidal effusion or Valsalva maneuver
- *contact with an intraocular instrument,* such as a cannula, chopper, or manipulator
- *rapid insertion and unfolding of an IOL*

After a posterior capsule rupture, lens material may enter the posterior segment, and vitreous may prolapse into the anterior segment. The location and size of the tear determine the appropriate response. A small rupture in the posterior capsule during emulsification of the nucleus can be managed by alteration of the surgical technique. The surgeon can compartmentalize the vitreous with a dispersive OVD and use low-flow, low-vacuum settings to remove the remaining nuclear and cortical material. Full occlusion of the aspiration port and use of minimal phaco power reduce the risk of aspiration of vitreous or further damage to the capsule.

If a small tear appears in the posterior capsule during aspiration of the cortex and the vitreous face remains intact, the surgeon can attempt to remove the residual cortex without expanding the tear. Using low-flow I/A and compartmentalizing the vitreous with an OVD help avoid disruption of the vitreous face. Some surgeons prefer a manual dry-aspiration technique, which involves using a cannula attached to a handheld syringe to remove the residual cortex after a capsular rupture, thereby avoiding any pressure from irrigation. After the anterior chamber is stabilized with the use of an OVD, capsulorrhexis forceps may be employed to convert the posterior capsule tear into a round posterior capsulorrhexis that will resist extending equatorially.

If most of the nucleus remains and the capsular tear is large, further attempts at phacoemulsification should be abandoned. To extract the remaining nuclear fragments mechanically, the surgeon can enlarge the incision and remove the nucleus with a lens loop or spoon in a manner that minimizes vitreous traction and further damage to the capsule. Insertion of a second instrument or lens glide behind the nuclear remnant may help prevent the remnant from being dislocated into the vitreous. Alternatively, an OVD can be introduced posterior to the fragment in an effort to float it anteriorly, or the nucleus can be elevated into the anterior chamber with an instrument or nuclear spear. Retrieval of nuclear fragments from the deep vitreous is not recommended.

If vitreous prolapse occurs, it is best to remove all vitreous from the anterior chamber during the initial surgery. Doing so will facilitate the removal of residual cortex and the subsequent placement of an IOL. In addition, a vitrectomy can reduce the chance of vitreoretinal traction or vitreous adherence to the IOL, the iris, or the incision. Vitreous loss during cataract surgery is associated with an increased risk of retinal detachment, cystoid macular edema, and endophthalmitis.

The vitreous may be stained with unpreserved or washed triamcinolone for better visualization. It is important to avoid manually externalizing and cutting vitreous through the incision, because this causes excessive vitreoretinal traction, which increases the risk of retinal tears and retinal detachment. A 2-port bimanual anterior vitrectomy can be performed with separate infusion and aspirating/cutting instruments inserted through new, properly sized limbal incisions (Fig 10-6A; Video 10-7). Alternatively, the aspiration/cutting instrument may be placed through a pars plana incision while irrigation is continued through the limbus (Fig 10-6B; Video 10-8), directing flow posteriorly and reducing the amount of vitreous that migrates into the anterior segment, thereby decreasing vitreoretinal traction.

VIDEO 10-7 Bimanual anterior vitrectomy.
Courtesy of Arsham Sheybani, MD.

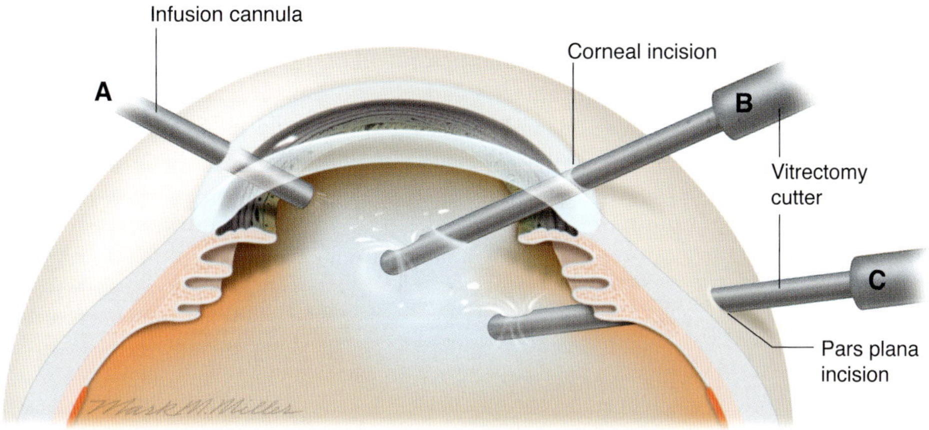

Figure 10-6 Bimanual anterior vitrectomy. Infusion cannula **(A)** through corneal incision. A corneal incision may be used for a vitrectomy cutter **(B).** Alternatively, a pars plana incision may be used for the vitrectomy cutter **(C).** *(Figure developed by Natalie Afshari, MD, and illustrated by Mark Miller.)*

VIDEO 10-8 Bimanual anterior vitrectomy with pars plana incision.
Courtesy of Charles Cole, MD.

MANAGEMENT OF POSTERIOR CAPSULE RUPTURE

- Maintain a normotensive globe and prevent anterior chamber collapse.
- Avoid intraoperative vitreous traction.
- Compartmentalize the lens and vitreous with an OVD.
- Attempt removal of lens fragments only if they are visible and easily accessible.
- Using either a bimanual limbal or pars plana approach, perform an anterior vitrectomy until no vitreous is seen anterior to the capsule.
- Insert an IOL only when safe and indicated—preferably a posterior chamber lens placed in the ciliary sulcus or fixated to iris or sclera, or an anterior chamber lens with prophylactic peripheral iridectomy.
- Adjust the lens power appropriately for the position and type of IOL used.
- Perform a watertight incision closure and remove the OVD.
- If posteriorly dislocated lens fragments are present, arrange a prompt referral to a vitreoretinal surgeon for removal.
- Disclose and discuss all surgical complications with the patient.

IOL Placement with Posterior Capsule Rupture

If posterior capsule support for intracapsular placement of the IOL is inadequate, the surgeon should attempt to preserve the anterior capsule and capsulorrhexis to enable placement of the IOL optic in the capsular bag with the haptics placed in the ciliary sulcus ("optic capture"; Fig 10-7A). Generally, a 3-piece IOL with a total diameter greater than 12.5 mm may be inserted into the ciliary sulcus with or without optic capture. In certain

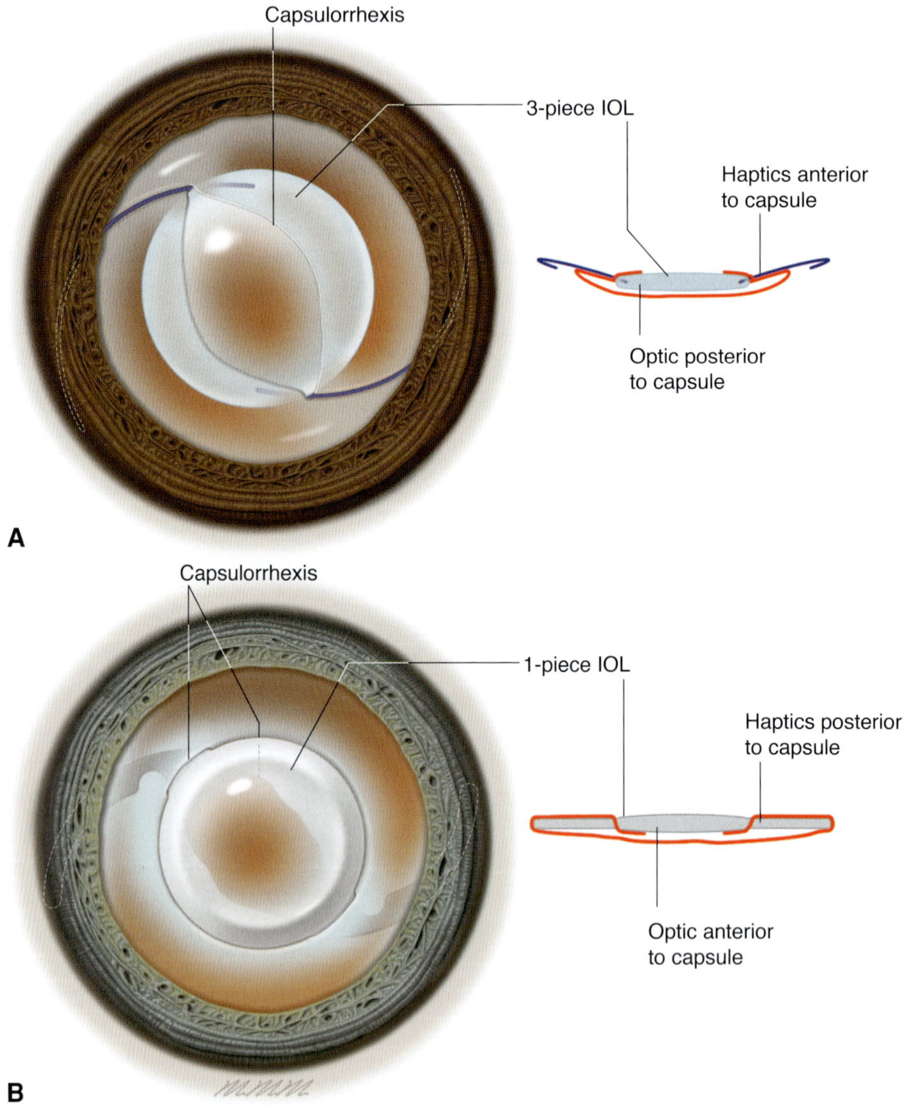

Figure 10-7 Intraocular lens (IOL) capture. **A,** IOL optic capture. A 3-piece IOL with haptics in the sulcus. The optic is "captured" within the capsule so that the anterior capsule edge is anterior to the optic. **B,** IOL reverse optic capture. A 1-piece IOL with the optic in the sulcus. The optic is "captured" by capsulorrhexis so that the anterior capsule edge is anterior to the haptics. *(Figure developed by Natalie Afshari, MD, and illustrated by Mark Miller.)*

situations, a single-piece acrylic IOL may be safely placed in the ciliary sulcus by *reverse optic capture* (Fig 10-7B). In reverse optic capture, the haptics of the IOL are placed within the capsule, while the optic is captured through the anterior capsule into the sulcus. To avoid possible UGH syndrome, the haptics of the single-piece acrylic IOL must be fully contained within the capsule; otherwise, a 3-piece lens is recommended.

If capsular integrity is insufficient, the surgeon may substitute an anterior chamber lens. A posterior chamber IOL (PCIOL) may also be used in the absence of capsular support by suturing the haptics to the iris or by fixing the haptics to the sclera through the ciliary sulcus. Several techniques for IOL fixation are discussed in detail in Chapter 11. If significant lens material remains in the posterior chamber, it can be approached via a pars plana vitrectomy performed by a vitreoretinal surgeon.

Hemorrhage

Retrobulbar Hemorrhage

Retrobulbar hemorrhages vary in intensity and are more common with retrobulbar anesthetic injections than with peribulbar injections, with an incidence of 0.44%–0.74% following retrobulbar injection.

Venous retrobulbar hemorrhages are usually self-limited and tend to spread slowly. *Arterial retrobulbar hemorrhages* occur more rapidly and are associated with taut orbital swelling, marked proptosis, elevated IOP, reduced mobility of the globe, inability to separate the eyelids, and massive ecchymosis of the eyelids and conjunctiva. This type of retrobulbar hemorrhage causes an increase in orbital volume and associated orbital pressure, which can restrict the vascular supply to the globe. Large orbital vessels may be occluded. Tamponade of the smaller vessels in the optic nerve may occur, resulting in severe vision loss from anterior ischemic optic neuropathy and subsequent optic atrophy, despite the absence of obvious retinal vascular occlusion.

Ophthalmologists can often make the diagnosis of retrobulbar hemorrhage by observing the rapid onset of eyelid and conjunctival ecchymosis and tightening of the orbit. The diagnosis can be confirmed by tonometry revealing elevated IOP. Ophthalmoscopy may reveal pulsation or occlusion of the central retinal artery in severe cases.

Treatment of acute retrobulbar hemorrhage consists of maneuvers to lower the intraocular and orbital pressure as quickly as possible, such as the following:

- digital massage
- intravenous osmotic agents
- aqueous suppressants
- lateral canthotomy and cantholysis
- localized conjunctival peritomy (to allow egress of blood)

The planned surgery should be postponed until the IOP and mobility of the globe and eyelids are normal. To reduce the risk of a recurrent retrobulbar hemorrhage, it may be advisable to use another form of anesthesia for the second attempt at surgery.

In addition to retrobulbar hemorrhage, potential complications of retrobulbar injections include central retinal artery occlusion, ischemic optic neuropathy, toxic neuropathy or myopathy, diplopia, ptosis, and inadvertent subdural injections with possible central nervous system depression and apnea. Ischemic complications are more common if epinephrine is used in the anesthetic. (See BCSC Section 1, *Update on General Medicine,* and Section 6, *Pediatric Ophthalmology and Strabismus.*)

Intraoperative Hemorrhage

Iris manipulation, such as lysis of posterior synechiae, sphincterotomies, or pupil expansion or stretching may result in intraoperative hemorrhage and early postoperative hyphema. Surgical trauma to the iris, iris root, and ciliary body can cause significant bleeding. Hemorrhage may also originate from the angle structures when cataract surgery is combined with minimally invasive glaucoma surgery (MIGS; see also BCSC Section 10, *Glaucoma*). Resolution of hemorrhage may take longer if vitreous is mixed with the blood. (See the section Hyphema in Chapter 11.)

Suprachoroidal Effusion or Hemorrhage

Suprachoroidal effusion with or without suprachoroidal hemorrhage usually occurs intraoperatively but may also occur later in cases with prolonged postoperative hypotony. Suprachoroidal effusion typically presents as a forward prolapse of ocular structures, including iris, lens diaphragm, and vitreous, generally accompanied by a change in the red reflex. Clinically, suprachoroidal effusion may be difficult to differentiate from suprachoroidal hemorrhage. Patient agitation and pain followed by an extremely firm globe suggest suprachoroidal hemorrhage. Suprachoroidal effusion and suprachoroidal hemorrhage have been associated with

- hypertension
- arteriosclerotic cardiovascular disease
- tachycardia
- obesity
- high myopia
- glaucoma
- advanced age
- nanophthalmos
- choroidal hemangioma associated with Sturge-Weber syndrome
- chronic ocular inflammation

Fortunately, both suprachoroidal effusion and suprachoroidal hemorrhage are much less likely with small-incision phacoemulsification than with larger-incision surgery because of the relatively closed system formed by the small, self-sealing incisions. The relatively tight fit of the phaco tip in the incision prevents prolonged hypotony and reduces intraoperative fluctuations in IOP.

Suprachoroidal effusion may be a precursor to suprachoroidal hemorrhage. Exudation of fluid from choroidal vasculature ultimately stretches veins or arteries that supply the choroid after coursing through the sclera. If suprachoroidal hemorrhage occurs in this situation, it is presumably a result of disruption of 1 or more of these taut blood vessels (see also BCSC Section 12, *Retina and Vitreous*).

Expulsive Suprachoroidal Hemorrhage

Expulsive suprachoroidal hemorrhage, a rare but serious condition, generally occurs intraoperatively in eyes with hypotony. The hemorrhage usually presents as a sudden increase in IOP accompanied by acute onset of pain and the following:

- darkening of the red reflex
- incision gape
- iris prolapse
- expulsion of the lens, vitreous, and bright red blood

The instant any suprachoroidal effusion or hemorrhage is recognized, the surgeon must close the incision with sutures or digital pressure. Prolapsed vitreous is excised and uveal tissue reposited, if possible. After the wound is securely closed, the surgeon may consider posterior sclerotomies to allow the escape of suprachoroidal blood to decompress the globe, enable repositioning of prolapsed intraocular tissue, and facilitate permanent closure of the cataract incision. Drainage of suprachoroidal blood may be achieved by performing sclerotomies in 1 or more quadrants, 5–7 mm posterior to the limbus (Video 10-9). Sclerotomies for choroidal hemorrhage are also discussed in BCSC Section 12, *Retina and Vitreous*. Elevated IOP serves both to stop bleeding and to expel suprachoroidal blood. Once there is optimal clearance of blood from the suprachoroidal space, the sclerotomies may be left open to allow further drainage postoperatively. It may be necessary to repeat the drainage procedure 7 days or more after an expulsive hemorrhage in cases of residual suprachoroidal blood that threatens ocular integrity or vision. These procedures may lower dangerously elevated IOPs and restore appropriate anatomical relationships within the eye, but they carry some risk that bleeding will recur.

VIDEO 10-9 Drainage of suprachoroidal hemorrhage.
Courtesy of Christina Weng, MD.

If the incision can be closed without posterior sclerotomies, more rapid tamponade of the bleeding vessel can be achieved. Most surgeons would then terminate the operation and observe the patient for 7–14 days to allow clotting and liquefaction of the hemorrhage, while managing elevated IOP medically. Referral to a vitreoretinal surgeon for management and subsequent drainage of choroidal hemorrhage may be considered. It is important to inform the patient of the guarded prognosis for restoration of vision.

CHAPTER 11

Postoperative Surgical Course and Complications

This chapter includes related videos. Go to www.aao.org/bcscvideo_section11 or scan the QR codes in the text to access this content.

Highlights

- Treatment of a retained lens fragment depends on the location of the fragment, the presence of corneal edema, the degree of inflammation, and the effect on intraocular pressure (IOP).
- Dislocated or decentered intraocular lenses (IOLs) have various surgical options for correction.
- Opacification of the posterior capsule occurs frequently after cataract surgery; it can appear months to years after cataract surgery and is commonly treated with Nd:YAG capsulotomy.
- Toxic anterior segment syndrome is a sterile inflammation that is caused by toxic substances such as residue on instruments and may mimic endophthalmitis.
- Despite numerous studies showing a reduced incidence of endophthalmitis with the use of intracameral antibiotics at the completion of cataract surgery, no antibiotics are currently approved by the US Food and Drug Administration for this indication.
- Cystoid macular edema (CME) is a common cause of decreased vision that occurs weeks to months following cataract extraction. It is associated with increased perifoveal capillary permeability and accumulation of fluid in the inner nuclear and outer plexiform layers of the retina.

Introduction

In uncomplicated phacoemulsification, the postoperative course generally allows for rapid vision rehabilitation over several weeks:

- *Symptoms:* Foreign-body sensation and photosensitivity are common immediately after surgery. Fluctuations in vision may occur. Topical lubrication may alleviate these symptoms.

- *Signs:* The corneal incisions are typically Seidel-negative. There may be irregular epithelium or small epithelial defects at the incisions. Corneal edema is variable and may have a marked effect on visual acuity. Ideally, the anterior chamber is deep, with mild to moderate cellular reaction. Make sure the intraocular lens (IOL) is well positioned and stable. If present, ptosis is generally minimal (particularly if a block was used).
- *Course:* Typically, the patient's vision stabilizes, and the pain and photosensitivity decrease over several days to weeks. Although further refractive changes may occur later, most patients are prescribed postoperative spectacles by 2–6 weeks after uncomplicated cataract surgery.

Although the ophthalmologist strives to attain excellent results during both cataract surgery and the postoperative course, complications do occur, even in the best of hands. Therefore, recognizing and appropriately treating any complications are critical to a successful outcome.

Postoperative occurrences and complications of cataract surgery include the following:

- corneal edema (0.03%–5.18% of cases)
- retained lens fragments (0.45%–1.70% of cases)
- IOL dislocation (0.19%–1.10% of cases)
- posterior capsule opacification (common; increases with time after surgery)
- endophthalmitis (0.04%–0.20% of cases)
- clinically apparent cystoid macular edema (1.2%–3.5% of cases)
- retinal detachment (approximately 0.7% of cases in first postoperative year)

Corneal Complications

Corneal Edema

Stromal and/or epithelial edema due to multiple etiologies may occur throughout the postoperative period (Table 11-1). Edema due to surgical trauma and acute endothelial decompensation from underlying dystrophy, as well as epithelial edema due to elevated intraocular pressure (IOP), may be seen early. Toxic substances inadvertently introduced into the anterior chamber can also cause acute endothelial dysfunction as well as early diffuse corneal edema, referred to as *toxic anterior segment syndrome* (*TASS;* discussed later in this chapter). Late postoperative inferior corneal edema may occur because of small nuclear fragments retained in the anterior chamber angle. These fragments may be noticed on initial postoperative examinations, or they may be identified up to years later if they migrate into the anterior chamber from a secluded location in the posterior chamber. Vitreocorneal touch or adherence may contribute to persistent corneal edema after cataract surgery complicated by vitreous prolapse. Significant chronic corneal edema from loss of endothelial cells results in bullous keratopathy (discussed later in this chapter), which is associated with reduced vision, ocular irritation, foreign-body sensation, epiphora, and occasionally infectious keratitis.

In its early stages, corneal edema after cataract surgery can be managed with topical hypertonic drops, corticosteroids, and/or aqueous suppressants. A bandage (therapeutic)

Table 11-1 Principal Causes of Corneal Edema After Cataract Surgery

Causes of Early Postoperative Corneal Edema
Surgical effects
Mechanical energy from phacoemulsification
Instruments
Intraocular lens (IOL)
Irrigating solutions
Lens fragments
Prior or prolonged intraocular surgery
Corneal endothelial diseases
Fuchs dystrophy
Low endothelial cell density
Descemet membrane detachment
Chemical or toxic effects
Toxic anterior segment syndrome
Preservatives in intraocular solutions
Residual toxic chemicals on instruments (eg, detergents, dried solutions)
Improper concentrations of intraocular solutions (eg, antibiotics, anesthetics, irrigating solutions)
Osmotic damage
Direct toxicity
Elevated intraocular pressure
Inflammation
Causes of Early or Late Postoperative Corneal Edema
IOL-related factors
IOL–endothelial touch
Uveitis-glaucoma-hyphema syndrome
Rigid anterior chamber IOL
Endothelial contact
Flat chamber centrally
Wound leak
Ciliary block (aqueous misdirection)
Suprachoroidal effusion or hemorrhage
Flat chamber peripherally
Pupillary block
Iris bombé
Vitreous touch
Retained foreign material
Nuclear fragments
Particulate matter
Membranous ingrowth
Epithelial or fibrous ingrowth
Endothelial proliferation
Brown-McLean syndrome

Adapted with permission from Steinert RF. *Cataract Surgery.* 3rd ed. Saunders; 2010:596.

contact lens may be used if necessary. Edema from surgical trauma generally resolves completely within 4–6 weeks. When epithelial edema is due to elevated IOP, lowering the pressure medically or via aqueous release from the paracentesis site often results in rapid resolution.

Removing all vitreous from the anterior chamber during complicated cataract surgery decreases the risks of corneal edema as well as cystoid macular edema (CME) and retinal detachment. When vitreous prolapse with corneal touch or incarceration in the wound is recognized postoperatively and corneal edema or CME develops, an anterior vitrectomy or Nd:YAG laser vitreolysis may be indicated. In more advanced cases with prolonged corneal edema, keratoplasty combined with vitrectomy may be indicated.

Brown-McLean syndrome

Brown-McLean syndrome, a condition of unknown etiology after intracapsular cataract extraction (ICCE) (and, in rare instances, extracapsular cataract extraction [ECCE] or phacoemulsification), is characterized by peripheral corneal edema with a clear central cornea. The edema usually starts inferiorly and progresses circumferentially, sparing the central 5–7 mm. Central cornea guttae frequently appear, and punctate brown pigment on the endothelium often underlies the edematous areas. In rare cases, Brown-McLean syndrome progresses to clinically significant central corneal edema.

Incision and wound complications

Intraoperative incision complications are discussed in Chapter 10 in this volume.

Signs of *postoperative* wound leakage include decreased vision, hypotony, corneal striae, shallow anterior chamber, hyphema, choroidal folds, choroidal effusion, macular edema, and optic nerve edema. A Seidel test, ultrasound biomicroscopy, or anterior segment optical coherence tomography (OCT) may help diagnose or confirm subtle cases. Small leaks in the early postoperative period may be asymptomatic and self-limited.

Medical treatment may include prophylactic topical antibiotics, cycloplegia, aqueous inhibitors, patching, decreased or discontinued corticosteroid therapy, or a collagen shield or bandage contact lens. Surgical repair is indicated in more serious cases with persistent shallowing of the anterior chamber, iris prolapse, prolonged hypotony, choroidal effusion, or macular edema. Suturing of the wound is usually sufficient, but an amniotic membrane graft or tissue adhesives such as cyanoacrylate or hydrogel glue may be used.

A wound leak under a conjunctival flap may lead to an inadvertent filtering bleb, which may require surgical intervention. Efforts to promote wound healing and cicatrization of the bleb include cryotherapy, diathermy, chemical cauterization with trichloroacetic acid, or injection of an autologous blood patch. In chronic cases, it may be necessary to excise the bleb/conjunctiva and search for a fistula, which can be scraped free of invading epithelium or excised and covered with a scleral patch graft if necessary, followed by resuturing of the wound.

Late postoperative wound dehiscence may be spontaneous or secondary to trauma. Smaller incisions have decreased the occurrence of wound dehiscence. Traumatic wound rupture is often accompanied by extrusion of intraocular contents and almost always requires urgent surgical repair.

Corneal Melt

Keratolysis, or sterile melting of the cornea (Fig 11-1), may occur after cataract extraction. It is most frequently associated with preexisting tear film abnormalities resulting from

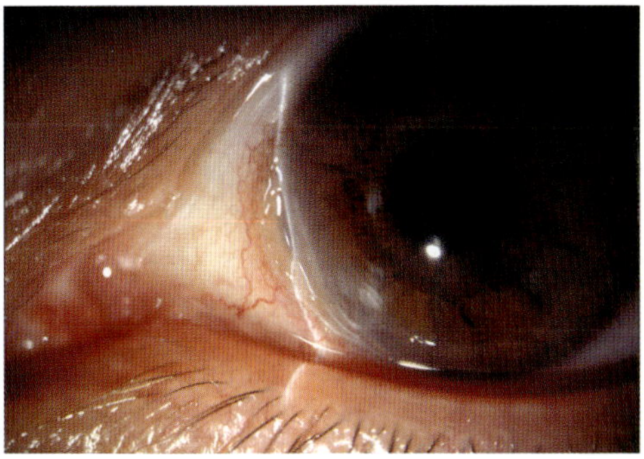

Figure 11-1 Corneal melt. *(Courtesy of Thomas L. Steinemann, MD.)*

keratoconjunctivitis sicca and autoimmune diseases such as Sjögren syndrome, rheumatoid arthritis, or graft-vs-host disease. Keratitis may be exacerbated by the chemical or mechanical stress of surgery or the topical medications used perioperatively.

Stromal melting has been reported with the postoperative use of topical nonsteroidal anti-inflammatory drugs (NSAIDs), due in part to the epithelial toxicity and hypoesthesia that these drugs can induce. NSAID-associated stromal melting is more likely to occur in patients with keratoconjunctivitis sicca, systemic autoimmune disease, or collagen vascular disease.

Frequent perioperative use of nonpreserved topical lubricants, punctal plug placement, or lateral tarsorrhaphy may lessen morbidity in eyes with preexisting tear film abnormalities. Persistent epithelial defects accompanied by stromal dissolution require intensive treatment with nonpreserved topical lubricants. It is important to minimize the use of preserved topical medications to reduce their toxic effect on the corneal epithelium. Additional treatments to encourage epithelialization and arrest stromal melting include punctal occlusion, bandage contact lenses, autologous serum eyedrops, collagenase inhibitors such as acetylcysteine 10% or hydroxyprogesterone 1%, and systemic matrix metalloproteinase inhibitors such as doxycycline.

If the disease continues to progress despite medical therapy, a commercially available temporary amniotic membrane graft may be considered. In advanced recalcitrant cases, lamellar or penetrating keratoplasty may be necessary. Corneal melting may recur even with grafted tissue. For the treatment of any underlying autoimmune disease, systemic immunosuppressive therapy may be necessary.

Induced Astigmatism

Localized change in corneal curvature may result from corneal burns produced by the phaco tip or, more commonly, from surgical incisions. Most well-constructed peripheral corneal, limbal, or scleral incisions that are less than 3 mm wide will induce less than 1.00 diopter (D) of astigmatism, usually flattening in the meridian of the incision. Larger incisions closer to the corneal apex or those that require suture closure are more likely to induce astigmatism. Tight radial sutures may steepen corneal curvature in the meridian of the suture.

The astigmatism induced by larger sutured incisions, such as those used in ICCE, ECCE, and secondary IOL implantation, may decrease by several diopters over time as the sutures dissolve or relax. When suture removal is needed to modulate astigmatism, waiting 6–8 weeks postoperatively is preferred. When more than 1 suture must be removed, it is preferable to cut adjacent sutures in a series of visits rather than all at once. Removal of too many sutures too early in the postoperative period may result in either significant corneal flattening in the meridian of the incision or wound dehiscence.

Other Anterior Segment Complications

Epithelial or Fibrous Ingrowth

Epithelial ingrowth (or *downgrowth*) is a rare complication of intraocular surgery (Fig 11-2) or trauma. It is characterized by the growth of epithelium intraocularly with proliferation over the corneal endothelium, trabecular meshwork, and/or iris surfaces. Epithelial cells introduced into the anterior chamber during surgery may adhere to intraocular structures and proliferate as a cellular mass or membrane. Alternatively, a sheet of epithelium from the ocular surface may grow through a wound or incision. Signs of epithelial ingrowth include elevated IOP, clumps of cells floating in the anterior chamber, a grayish retrocorneal membrane (usually with overlying corneal edema), an abnormal iris surface, and pupillary distortion. Green laser burns applied to the membrane on the iris surface will appear white if epithelial cells are present, which helps confirm the diagnosis.

Fibrous ingrowth (Fig 11-3) is more prevalent than epithelial ingrowth. Fibrovascular tissue, rather than epithelial cells alone, proliferates from a penetrating wound. Fibrous ingrowth progresses more slowly than epithelial ingrowth and may be self-limited. It is a common cause of corneal graft failure and may result in the formation of peripheral anterior synechiae (PAS) and secondary angle-closure glaucoma.

Risk factors for both epithelial and fibrous ingrowth include trauma, prolonged inflammation, wound dehiscence, delayed wound closure, vitreous incarceration, and Descemet

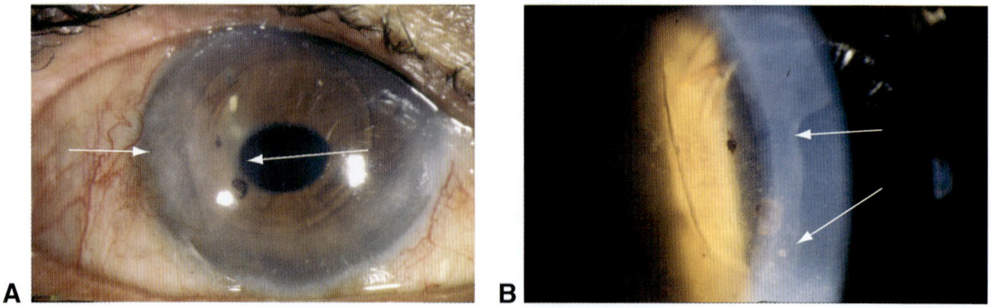

Figure 11-2 Epithelial ingrowth. **A,** Clinical photograph shows extent of epithelial ingrowth *(arrows)*. **B,** Slit-lamp photograph shows anterior extent of epithelial ingrowth *(arrows)*. *(Courtesy of Thomas L. Steinemann, MD.)*

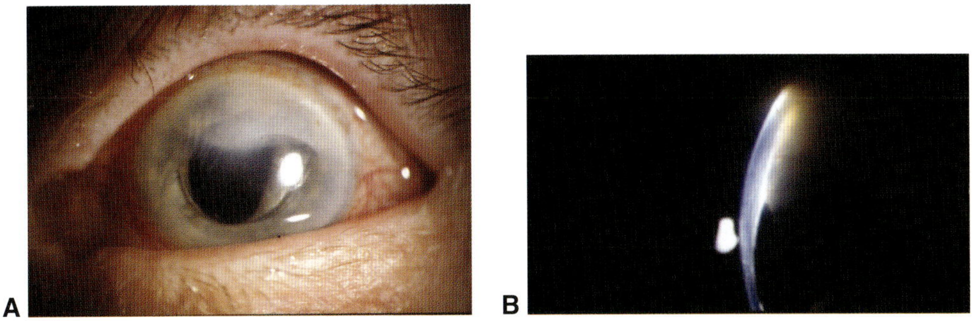

Figure 11-3 Fibrous ingrowth. **A,** Clinical photograph. **B,** Slit-lamp photograph. *(Courtesy of Thomas L. Steinemann, MD.)*

membrane tears. Many surgical treatments, including membrane excision and fistula repair, have been suggested, but none has been uniformly successful. Local application of cryotherapy or 5-fluorouracil has been effective. Elevated IOP is often difficult to control with medical therapy, and filtering procedures or tube shunt surgery may be necessary, as discussed in BCSC Section 10, *Glaucoma.*

Shallow or Flat Anterior Chamber

Intraoperative shallowing of the anterior chamber is discussed in Chapter 10.

During the postoperative period, a flat anterior chamber may permanently damage ocular structures. Prolonged apposition of the iris to angle structures can result in PAS formation and chronic angle-closure glaucoma. Corneal contact with the vitreous or an IOL can result in endothelial cell loss and chronic corneal edema. Postoperative shallow or flat anterior chambers can be classified according to their etiology and level of IOP (Table 11-2).

Patients with ocular hypotension (IOP below 10 mm Hg) and a shallow chamber may be asymptomatic, especially when a leaking incision is plugged by iris incarceration, allowing re-formation of the anterior chamber. Slow or intermittent leaks may still allow a formed anterior chamber. Performing a Seidel test and carefully comparing the chamber depth in the surgical eye with that of the fellow eye may help the surgeon identify subtle cases of incisional leaks. (For a discussion of the evaluation and management of an incisional leak, see the section "Incision and wound complications" earlier in this chapter.)

Surgical exploration with re-formation of the anterior chamber and repair of the incision is indicated if no improvement occurs within 24–48 hours, if an obvious wound gape is present, if the iris is prolapsed out of the incision, or if intraocular structures such as the IOL are in contact with the corneal endothelium.

Pupillary block with a shallow anterior chamber may occur from various causes. Early, it may follow a resolved incision leak. Later, postoperative uveitis with iridovitreal or iridocapsular synechiae may be the cause. Failure to perform a peripheral iridectomy

Table 11-2 Causes of Postoperative Flat or Shallow Anterior Chamber According to IOP Level

Associated With Low IOP in the Early Postoperative Period
Incision leak
Choroidal detachment
Ciliary body detachment
Associated With Low IOP in the Late Postoperative Period
Cyclodialysis
Retinal detachment
Filtering bleb formation
Uveitis
Associated With Normal or Elevated IOP
Anterior chamber IOL without patent PI
Pupillary block
Malignant glaucoma
Capsular block syndrome
Suprachoroidal hemorrhage

IOL = intraocular lens; IOP = intraocular pressure; PI = peripheral iridectomy.

after placement of an anterior chamber IOL (ACIOL) may also be associated with early or late postoperative pupillary block. When initial attempts at pupillary dilation fail to deepen the anterior chamber and lower the pressure, a laser peripheral iridotomy is usually effective.

Elevated IOP

A mild, self-limited rise in IOP is common after cataract surgery. However, a significant and sustained elevation may require timely management.

Ophthalmic viscosurgical devices (OVDs) retained in the eye after cataract surgery are frequently responsible for early postoperative IOP elevation, which peaks 4–6 hours after surgery. The large molecules of the viscoelastic material can impair aqueous outflow through the trabecular meshwork. Even when all apparent OVDs have been removed from the anterior chamber, residual OVDs can lodge in the posterior chamber or behind the lens implant. In general, IOP elevation usually does not last more than a few days and is amenable to medical treatment.

Marked IOP elevation in the early postoperative period may be temporarily managed by applying gentle pressure on the posterior lip of a preexisting paracentesis incision to release a small amount of aqueous humor. Caution is advised when performing this procedure in the setting of capsule rupture or zonular dialysis because vitreous strands may become incarcerated in the paracentesis. In addition, the surgeon may consider instilling povidone-iodine 5% solution or a topical antibiotic. Topical and/or systemic pressure-lowering agents should also be administered, as IOP reduction after aqueous release is short-lived, with the IOP likely to rise again within 1–2 hours of decompression.

After cataract surgery, elevated IOP without angle closure may also be caused by hyphema, TASS, endophthalmitis, retained lens material (phacolytic or phacoanaphylactic reactions), uveitis, iris pigment release, preexisting glaucoma, corticosteroid use, vitreous in the anterior chamber, or ghost cell glaucoma. Angle-closure glaucoma may be due to pupillary block, malignant glaucoma, epithelial ingrowth, neovascular glaucoma, or PAS. Treatment of the underlying cause of IOP elevation is indicated.

Malignant glaucoma

Malignant glaucoma (also known as *ciliary block glaucoma, aqueous misdirection,* or *vitreous block*) has been described as a ciliolenticular block induced by anterior movement of the lens–iris interface, poor vitreous fluid conductivity (increased resistance to fluid movement through the vitreous), and choroidal expansion. These factors cause the central and peripheral portions of the anterior chamber to become very shallow and lead to a secondary elevation of IOP due to angle obstruction. Malignant glaucoma occurs most commonly after intraocular surgery in eyes with prior angle-closure glaucoma, but it can also occur in small eyes with open angles.

Malignant glaucoma must be differentiated from pupillary block glaucoma, capsular block, suprachoroidal hemorrhage, and choroidal detachment. Unlike pupillary block, malignant glaucoma is not relieved by iridectomy but requires either intense medical therapy or more aggressive surgical therapy.

Medical treatment consists of cycloplegia and aqueous suppression, as well as hyperosmotic agents (eg, oral glycerin or intravenous mannitol). Use of miotics is not recommended because they can worsen malignant glaucoma by exacerbating anterior displacement of the lens–iris interface.

Surgical intervention consists of Nd:YAG laser irido-zonulo-hyaloidotomy and occasionally vitrectomy to disrupt the anterior vitreous face and vitreous–ciliary body interface, in effect establishing a unicameral eye with an open channel for aqueous to circulate into the anterior chamber. (See also BCSC Section 10, *Glaucoma.*)

Kaplowitz K, Yung E, Flynn R, Tsai JC. Current concepts in the treatment of vitreous block, also known as aqueous misdirection. *Surv Ophthalmol.* 2015;60(3):229–241.

Varma DK, Belovay GW, Tam DY, Ahmed II. Malignant glaucoma after cataract surgery. *J Cataract Refract Surg.* 2014;40(11):1843–1849.

Hyphema

Hyphema in the immediate postoperative period usually originates from the incision or the iris. The risk of hyphema is greater in patients with pseudoexfoliation syndrome, anterior segment neovascularization, Fuchs heterochromic uveitis, or vascular tufts at the pupillary margin. Combined minimally invasive glaucoma surgeries may cause hyphema postoperatively.

Hyphema is commonly mild and resolves spontaneously. When it is prolonged, the major complications are elevated IOP and corneal blood staining. IOP should be monitored closely and initially treated medically, although it may be difficult to control if the blood is mixed with the OVD used during the procedure. Resolution may take longer if the blood has mixed with vitreous. Surgical evacuation is occasionally necessary.

Hyphema occurring months to years after surgery is usually the result of incision vascularization or erosion of vascular tissue in the iris or ciliary body by an IOL haptic or optic edge. Laser photocoagulation of the bleeding vessel, often performed through a goniolens, may stop the bleeding or prevent rebleeding. To reduce the risk of continued or recurrent bleeding, antiplatelet or anticoagulation therapy may be withheld, if medically possible, until the hyphema resolves. Occasionally, an IOL that comes in contact with the iris or angle structures and causes recurrent intraocular hemorrhage (uveitis-glaucoma-hyphema syndrome, discussed later in this chapter) must be repositioned or exchanged.

Retained Lens Fragments

During cataract extraction, lens fragments may remain in the anterior chamber angle or in the posterior chamber behind the iris, or they may migrate into the vitreous cavity when zonular dehiscence or posterior capsule rupture occurs. Retained lens fragments are thought to occur more frequently in the anterior segment with phacoemulsification than with ECCE; the reported postoperative prevalence is 0.45%–1.70%, but the actual rates may be higher because of unrecognized cases. During phacoemulsification, intraocular turbulence may force small lens fragments to lodge in the angle or behind the iris, out of the surgeon's view. Femtosecond laser–assisted cataract surgery can also create many small nuclear fragments, some of which may be retained behind the iris. Dispersive OVDs may trap and retain more lens fragments than cohesive OVDs.

Patients with retained lens fragments present with varying degrees of inflammation, depending on the size of the lens fragment, the type of lens material, the time elapsed since surgery, and the patient's individual response. Clinical signs of retained lens material include uveitis, elevated IOP, corneal edema, and vitreous opacities. With persistent postoperative inflammation but no lens fragment seen on slit-lamp examination, gonioscopy is indicated to look for a retained lens particle.

Retained cortical lens material or nuclear fragments do not necessarily require surgical intervention. In general, cortical material is better tolerated and more likely to be reabsorbed over time than is nuclear material, which, even in small amounts, persists longer and is more likely to incite a significant inflammatory reaction, corneal edema, or elevated IOP.

Inflammation can be controlled with corticosteroid and nonsteroidal anti-inflammatory drops. Elevated IOP can be treated with aqueous suppressants. Surgical intervention may be necessary to remove residual lens fragments in the following situations:

- presence of a large or visually significant amount of lens material
- increased inflammation not readily controlled with topical medications
- medically unresponsive elevated IOP resulting from inflammation
- corneal edema
- associated retinal detachment or retinal tears

For retained lens fragments in the anterior chamber with an intact posterior capsule, simple irrigation/aspiration or viscoexpression of the residual material may be performed through the original phacoemulsification incision.

The reported incidence of intravitreal retained lens fragments is between 0.1% and 1.6%. When lens material has migrated into the vitreous cavity through a defect in the zonular fibers or posterior capsule, referral to a vitreoretinal surgeon for pars plana vitrectomy and removal of the lens material is indicated. If necessary, the vitreoretinal surgeon can delay intervention for more than a week after cataract surgery without jeopardizing a successful outcome.

Modi YS, Epstein A, Smiddy WE, Murray TG, Feuer W, Flynn HW Jr. Retained lens fragments after cataract surgery: outcomes of same-day versus later pars plana vitrectomy. *Am J Ophthalmol.* 2013;156(3):454-459.e1.

Vanner EA, Stewart MW. Vitrectomy timing for retained lens fragments after surgery for age-related cataracts: a systematic review and meta-analysis. *Am J Ophthalmol.* 2011;152(3): 345–357.e3.

Vitreous Prolapse in the Anterior Chamber

Vitreous in the anterior chamber may lead to chronic intraocular inflammation, corneal edema, glaucoma, and CME. The pupil may be distorted by vitreous adherent to the incision. Inflammation, symptoms of glare due to an exposed IOL edge, and patient dissatisfaction with the appearance of the iris may prompt intervention. In symptomatic patients, Nd:YAG laser vitreolysis or anterior vitrectomy may be considered when the response to topical anti-inflammatory therapy is inadequate. If the vitreous extends through the incision to the ocular surface, a vitrectomy is warranted. The exposed vitreous may act as a wick, enabling bacteria to enter the eye and increasing the risk of endophthalmitis. In cases of suspected corneal compromise, a posterior vitrectomy approach may be preferable to an anterior approach to reduce surgical trauma to the cornea.

Postoperative IOL Complications

Decentration and Dislocation

The reported incidence of symptomatic decentration or dislocation of an IOL after uncomplicated cataract surgery is 0.19%–3.00%. The decentered or dislocated IOL may be either inside the capsule (intracapsular) or outside it (extracapsular) (Fig 11-4). The most common cause of intracapsular IOL malposition is zonular degradation associated with pseudoexfoliation syndrome. Insufficient zonular support may also be associated with trauma, previous vitreoretinal surgery, capsular contraction, retinitis pigmentosa, high myopia, uveitis, or congenital conditions that affect zonular integrity. Asymmetric bag/sulcus haptic positions (ie, 1 haptic in the capsular bag and 1 in the sulcus) aggravated by capsular fibrosis and contraction may also tilt or decenter an IOL. The most common cause of extracapsular IOL malposition is sulcus placement of an inadequately sized IOL, such as a smaller 3-piece IOL designed for intracapsular placement. Additional causes include a decentered or oversized capsulorrhexis, localized zonular defects, capsular defects, and IOL haptic damage.

Decentration of an IOL can cause unwanted glare and reflections or multiple images if the edge of the lens is within the pupillary space. When an aspheric, multifocal, or accommodating lens is decentered, the effect of the lens is diminished. Decentration of an aspheric lens with negative spherical aberration (used to counteract the positive spherical aberration of the cornea) results in greater higher orders of aberration (eg, coma) than decentration of a spherical lens. However, a decentered aspheric lens with zero spherical aberration correction causes less coma than a decentered spherical lens. Therefore, when postoperative IOL decentration is a significant concern, the surgeon may consider implanting an aspheric IOL with zero spherical aberration correction. Decentration of any

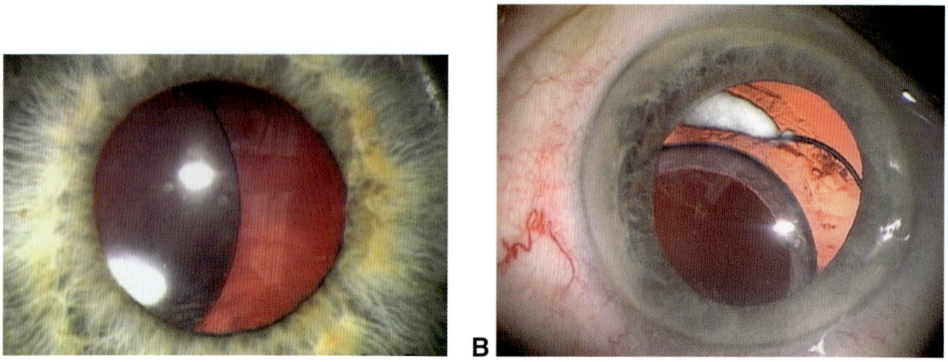

A B

Figure 11-4 Intraocular lens (IOL) dislocation. **A,** Extracapsular (out-of-the-bag) dislocation. **B,** Intracapsular (in-the-bag) dislocation. *(Part A reprinted from Dorey MW, Condon GP. Management of dislocated intraocular lenses.* Focal Points: Clinical Modules for Ophthalmologists. *American Academy of Ophthalmology; 2009, module 9:2. Part B reprinted with permission from Gimbel HV, Condon GP, Kohnen T, Olson RJ, Halkiadakis I. Late in-the-bag intraocular lens dislocation: incidence, prevention, and management.* J Cataract Refract Surg. *2005;31(11):2193–2204. © 2005, Elsevier.)*

posterior chamber intraocular lens (PCIOL) may lead to pupillary capture or uveitis-glaucoma-hyphema (UGH) syndrome owing to contact with uveal tissue.

Minor decentration may be treated with miotics to constrict the pupil over the IOL optic; in cases of pigment dispersion or recurrent hyphema, treatment with cycloplegic agents can reduce iris chafing by the IOL optic or haptics. Laser pupilloplasty may be used to realign the pupillary aperture with the IOL optical center. This procedure may be particularly useful with multifocal lenses. Severe cases of IOL decentration or dislocation are managed with IOL repositioning, stabilization with sutures, or exchange.

An extracapsular decentered IOL may be rotated and repositioned into a stable axis if there is sufficient support. Many extracapsular and selected intracapsular 3-piece IOL dislocations can be managed with peripheral iris suture fixation using a McCannel suture or Siepser sliding knot technique with a nonabsorbable monofilament suture, such as 9-0 or 10-0 polypropylene (Video 11-1; Fig 11-5). Iris fixation has some advantages over scleral fixation, including decreased risks of late suture erosion or breakage, IOL tilting, intraocular hemorrhage, and endophthalmitis. Disadvantages include possible posterior iris pigment chafing, pupil distortion, pseudophacodonesis, and hyphema. One-piece uniplanar acrylic IOLs are not suitable for secondary sulcus or iris fixation because of chafing of the iris pigment (Fig 11-6) and possible development of UGH syndrome.

VIDEO 11-1 Iris fixation of IOL.
Courtesy of Charles Cole, MD.
Go to www.aao.org/bcscvideo_section11 to access all videos in Section 11.

When irregular capsular fibrosis decenters an IOL placed in the capsular bag, deformation of the haptics may limit rotation for surgical recentering of the IOL. In such cases, the IOL haptics may need to be moved into the ciliary sulcus or the lens replaced. When the optic is removed before implantation of a new IOL, haptics fixated in the capsular bag or sulcus can be either amputated and left in place or slipped out of a fibrous cocoon.

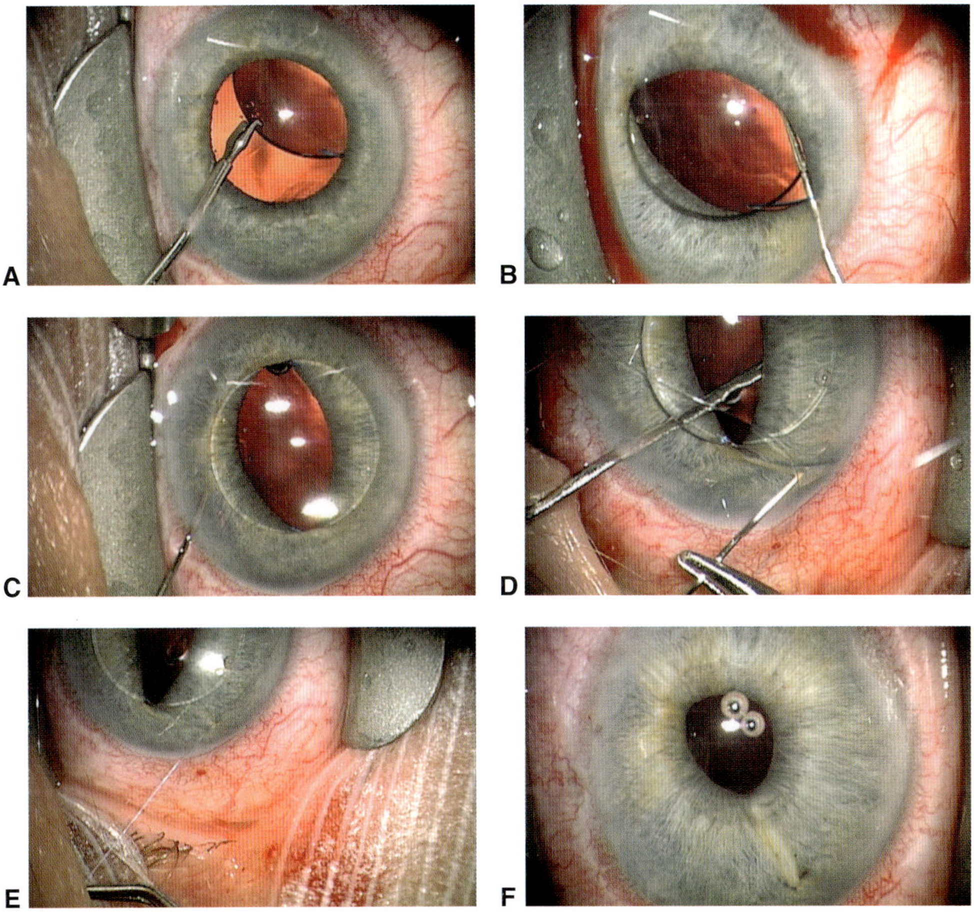

Figure 11-5 Peripheral iris suture fixation technique for IOL dislocation out of the capsular bag. **A,** The IOL is grasped and rotated with microsurgical forceps. **B,** Iris hooks are used to bring the optic above the iris plane. **C,** Optic capture by the pupil is completed through the addition of acetylcholine to induce miosis. **D,** The needle has been passed through a paracentesis incision, then through the iris and behind the haptic, and then back out through the iris and distal clear cornea. **E,** A Siepser sliding knot is used to secure the haptic to the peripheral iris. **F,** After both haptics are secured, the optic is prolapsed back into the posterior chamber. The sutures are minimally visible at the 5- and 10-o'clock positions. *(Parts A–C and F reprinted with permission from Condon GP. Following a posterior capsular rent, the sulcus-fixated intraocular lens has become decentered. How should I proceed? In: Chang DF, ed.* Curbside Consultation in Cataract Surgery: 49 Clinical Questions. *Slack; 2007:227–232. Part D courtesy of Garry P. Condon, MD.)*

Severe pseudophacodonesis or intracapsular (in-the-bag) dislocation of an IOL due to zonular loss may be managed with haptic fixation to the sclera. There are many ab externo (Fig 11-7) and ab interno (Fig 11-8) approaches and suture configurations, including scleral suture fixation (Video 11-2), intrascleral haptic fixation in Scharioth tunnels, also called "glued IOL" technique (Fig 11-9; Video 11-3), and intrascleral flanged haptic fixation, also referred to as Yamane technique (Fig 11-10; Videos 11-4, 11-5). For sutureless techniques, IOLs with haptics made of material such as polyvinylidene fluoride are preferable, as the polymethyl methacrylate (PMMA) haptics of a 3-piece

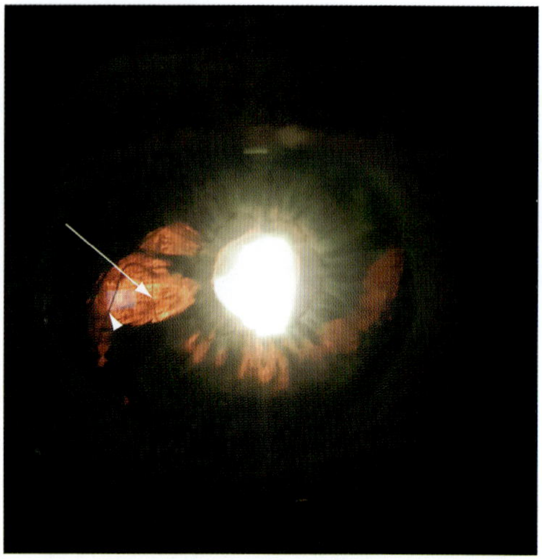

Figure 11-6 Transillumination defects of the iris from sulcus placement of a uniplanar 1-piece acrylic IOL. An *arrow* points out the optic edge; an *arrowhead* denotes the haptic edge. *(Courtesy of Charles Cole, MD.)*

foldable IOL can be brittle and prone to kinking or breaking with manipulation. A concurrent anterior vitrectomy is often necessary. Iris retractors may be used for better visualization or to stabilize the haptics during suturing. To prevent erosion through the conjunctiva, sutures through the scleral wall can be buried in a partial-thickness scleral groove or covered by a scleral flap. The scleral flap can be created through a conjunctival incision or a tunnel incision dissected posteriorly from the limbus (eg, Hoffman pockets; Video 11-6).

When dislocation of the IOL is complete, pars plana vitrectomy techniques are required to retrieve the lens or lens–capsule complex and elevate it safely into the anterior segment for fixation to the iris or sclera by a variety of techniques. In some cases, the implant may be removed altogether and replaced with either an ACIOL (see Chapter 8) or an iris- or scleral-fixated PCIOL.

Suture breakage and subluxation of scleral-fixated sutured IOLs occurring 3–9 years after implantation with 10-0 polypropylene fixation sutures have been reported. Double-fixation techniques and thicker 9-0 polypropylene or CV-8 Gore-Tex sutures (off-label use; W.L. Gore & Associates) are currently recommended for scleral fixation of IOLs. Other complications of sutured IOLs include vitreous or suprachoroidal hemorrhage, lens tilting, CME, retinal tears or detachment, suture erosion, and endophthalmitis. (See also BCSC Section 12, *Retina and Vitreous.*)

An ACIOL may be associated with decentration, iris tucking, UGH syndrome, corneal edema, or pseudophacodonesis, which will prompt repositioning of the lens or IOL exchange with either a differently sized flexible ACIOL or, preferably, a PCIOL. An ACIOL associated with pseudophakic bullous keratopathy is treated by endothelial keratoplasty, usually in combination with IOL exchange.

When an iris-supported lens becomes dislocated or associated with corneal edema or UGH syndrome, IOL exchange is warranted, if possible.

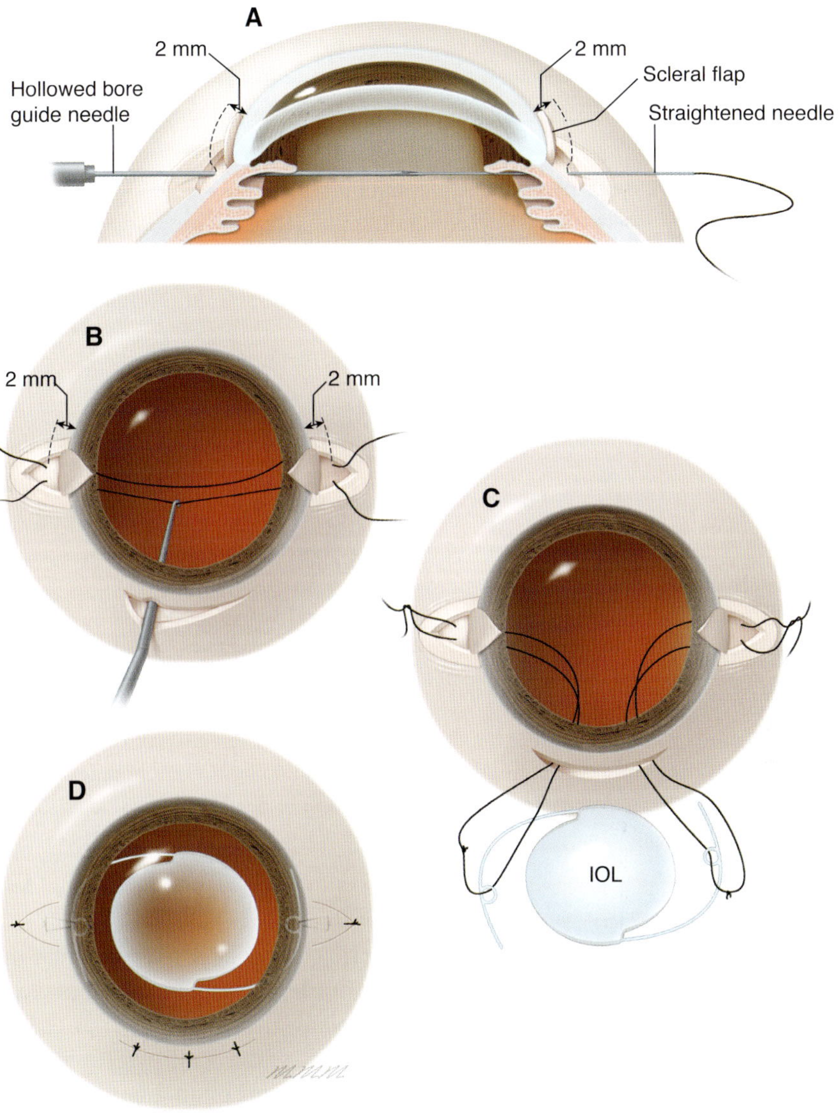

Figure 11-7 Illustration showing ab externo scleral fixation technique. **A,** Scleral flaps are created 180° apart. A single-armed suture on a straightened needle is passed under the scleral flap approximately 2 mm posterior to the limbus. The suture needle is retrieved by a hollow-bore guide needle under the opposite scleral flap. This process is repeated from the opposite direction. **B,** The 2 suture loops are externalized through the main limbal incision. **C,** The cut suture ends are tied to eyelets of the IOL haptic. The IOL is internalized through the limbal incision, and the sutures are tied under the scleral flaps. **D,** The limbal incision, scleral flaps, and conjunctiva are closed. *(Illustration courtesy of Mark Miller.)*

VIDEO 11-2 Ab externo IOL fixation (sutured).
Courtesy of The University of Iowa; Jesse Vislisel, MD; and Kenneth M. Goins, MD.

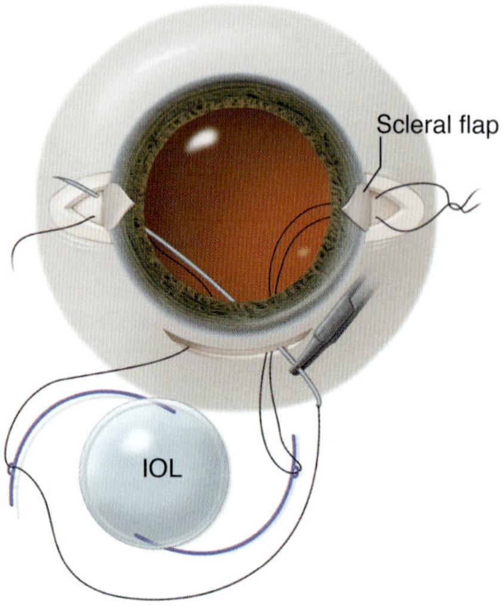

Figure 11-8 Illustration of ab interno IOL fixation. Double-armed sutures are secured to the eyelets of the IOL haptics. The needles are passed under the iris to exit the eye 1.5 mm posterior to the limbus under the scleral flaps. After the IOL is internalized, the sutures are tightened to center the IOL and tied under the scleral flaps. *(Illustration courtesy of Mark Miller.)*

Agarwal A, Jacob S, Kumar DA, Agarwal A, Narasimhan S, Agarwal A. Handshake technique for glued intrascleral haptic fixation of a posterior chamber intraocular lens. *J Cataract Refract Surg.* 2013;39(3):317–322.

Jacob S. Management of late lens implant and capsule dislocation. *Focal Points: Clinical Practice Perspectives.* American Academy of Ophthalmology; 2017, module 3.

Yamane S, Sato S, Maruyama-Inoue M, Kadonosono K. Flanged intrascleral intraocular lens fixation with double-needle technique. *Ophthalmology.* 2017;124(8):1136–1142.

Pupillary Capture

Postoperative pupillary capture of the IOL optic can occur for various reasons, such as formation of synechiae between the iris and underlying posterior capsule, improper placement of the IOL haptics, shallowing of the anterior chamber, or anterior displacement of the PCIOL optic. The last of these is associated with placement of nonangulated IOLs in the ciliary sulcus, upside-down placement of an angulated IOL so that it vaults anteriorly, excessive Soemmering ring formation, or asymmetric capsule contraction. Placement of a posteriorly angulated PCIOL in the capsular bag and creation of an anterior capsulorrhexis smaller than the lens optic decrease the likelihood of pupillary capture.

Pupillary capture may be simply a cosmetic concern. If the condition is chronic and the patient is asymptomatic, it can be left untreated. Surgical repositioning of an IOL may be indicated if pupillary capture causes glare, photophobia, chronic uveitis, unintended myopia, or monocular diplopia. In an acute pupillary capture, pharmacologic manipulation of the pupil with the patient in the supine position sometimes frees the optic. If conservative management fails, surgical intervention may be required to free the iris, lyse synechiae, manage capsule contraction or residual lens proliferation, and reposition the lens (Fig 11-11).

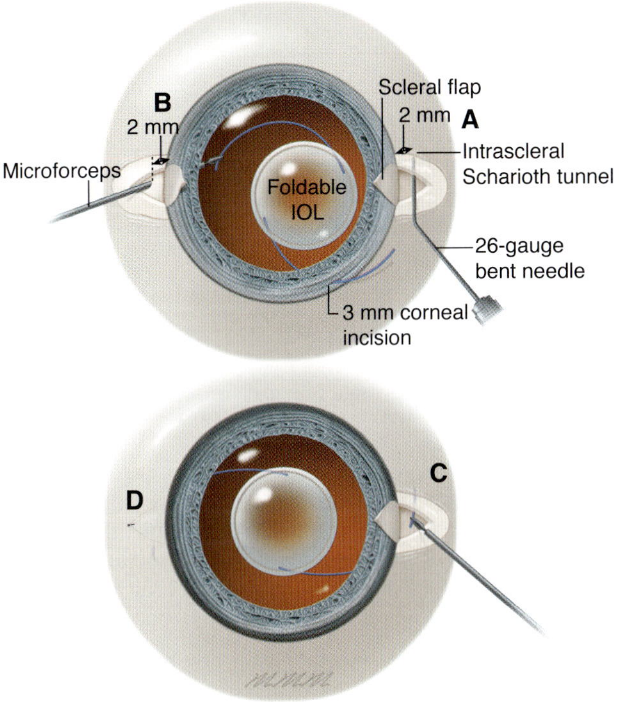

Figure 11-9 Illustration of intrascleral glued haptic IOL fixation. **A,** Scleral flaps are created 180° apart. Intrascleral Schariot tunnels are created parallel to the limbus with a bent 26-gauge needle. **B,** A 3-piece foldable IOL is injected into the eye while a microforceps is used to grasp the leading haptic and externalize it. Similarly, the trailing haptic is then externalized under the opposite scleral flap. **C,** The haptics are tucked into intrascleral tunnels. **D,** The flaps and conjunctiva are sealed with tissue glue. *(Illustration courtesy of Mark Miller.)*

VIDEO 11-3 Intrascleral haptic fixation with Scharioth tunnel (glued).
Courtesy of The University of Iowa; Jesse Vislisel, MD; and A. Tim Johnson, MD, PhD.

Capsular Block Syndrome

Postoperative capsular block syndrome (CBS) is caused by the intracapsular accumulation of liquefied material posterior to the nucleus or IOL and subsequent occlusion of the anterior capsulotomy. Early postoperative CBS may occur when residual OVD becomes trapped within the capsular bag, between the posterior capsule and the posterior surface of the IOL, causing a myopic shift in the refractive error from anterior displacement of the lens optic. Anterior displacement of the iris diaphragm with shallowing of the anterior chamber may also occur, which must be differentiated from a ciliary block mechanism. If left untreated, CBS may lead to posterior synechiae and secondary glaucoma. Nd:YAG laser anterior capsulotomy peripheral to the optic or posterior capsulotomy releases the trapped fluid, with resultant posterior movement of the IOL optic to its intended position, deepening of the anterior chamber, and resolution of the myopic shift.

Late postoperative CBS may occur years after surgery with the accumulation of a turbid or milky fluid between the posterior capsule and the IOL that is consistent with the

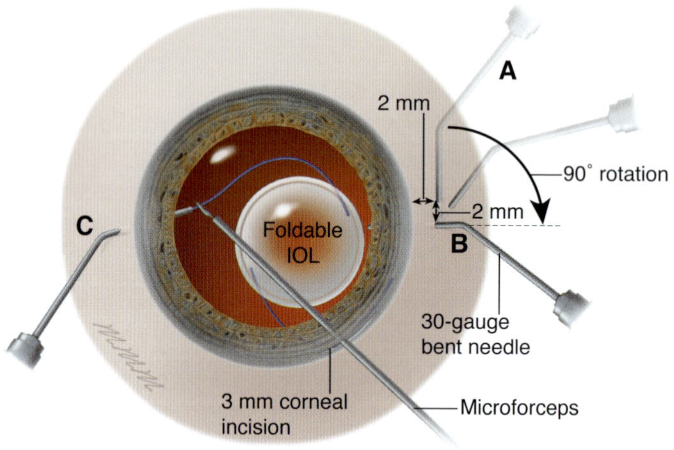

Figure 11-10 Illustration of intrascleral flanged haptic IOL fixation (Yamane technique). **A,** Transconjunctival scleral tunnels (180° apart) are made parallel to the limbus 2 mm posterior to the limbus with thin-walled (wide-bore) 30-gauge needles. Each tunnel is approximately 2 mm long. **B,** The needles are turned perpendicular *(arrow)* to the limbus to enter the eye. **C,** The leading haptic of a 3-piece foldable IOL is guided into the bore of the needle with microforceps under direct visualization. The same is done for the trailing haptic, and both are simultaneously externalized where noncontact thermal cautery is used to create a flange prior to replacement into the sclera (not shown; see Video 11-4). *(Illustration courtesy of Mark Miller.)*

VIDEO 11-4 Ab externo flanged-haptic IOL fixation, Yamane technique.
Courtesy of Charles Cole, MD.

VIDEO 11-5 Double-needle intrascleral flanged haptic IOL fixation, Yamane technique.
Courtesy of Wesley Green, MD, and Arsham Sheybani, MD.

VIDEO 11-6 Ab externo IOL reposition with Hoffman pockets.
Courtesy of Jason Leng, MD.

by-products of trapped, residual lens epithelial cells (Fig 11-12). Myopic shift is uncommon in these cases, and the patient may be asymptomatic. Nd:YAG laser posterior capsulotomy usually resolves this condition without complications.

Uveitis-Glaucoma-Hyphema Syndrome

UGH syndrome was first described in the context of rigid or closed-loop ACIOLs, as described in the Appendix. In modern surgery, it may also occur in patients with posterior chamber lenses owing to contact between lens haptics and uveal tissue in the posterior

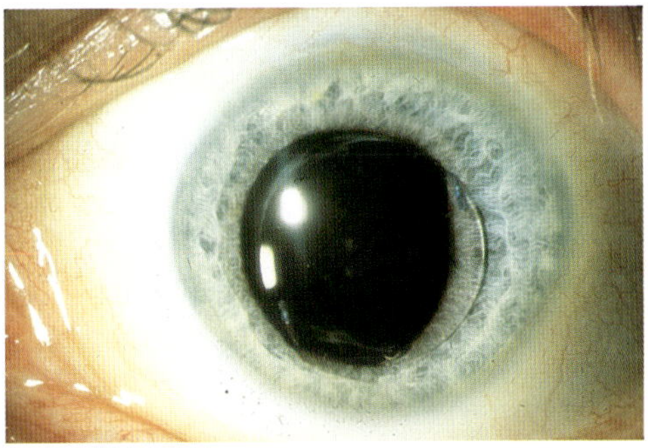

Figure 11-11 Pupillary capture by an angulated posterior chamber IOL in a patient who was assaulted 2 months after lens implantation surgery. *(Courtesy of Steven I. Rosenfeld, MD.)*

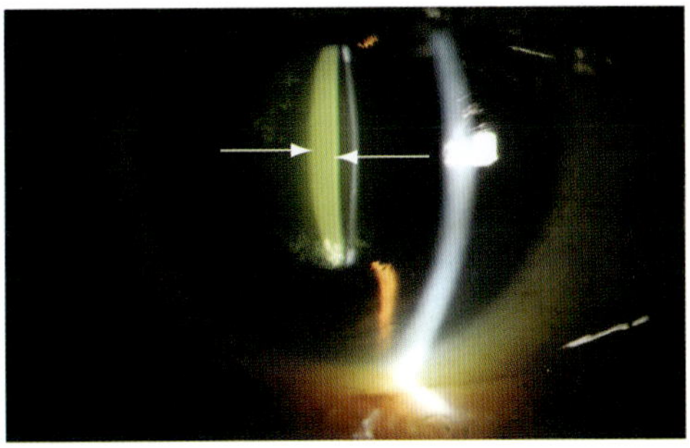

Figure 11-12 Late postoperative capsular block. *Arrows* show the posterior edge of the IOL and the posterior capsule containing turbid fluid. *(Courtesy of Chad Brasington, MD.)*

chamber. Single-piece acrylic IOL haptics should not be placed in the sulcus because of the high risk of UGH syndrome. The classic triad or individual components of the syndrome may also occur as a result of inappropriate IOL sizing, contact between the implant and vascular structures or the corneal endothelium, or defects in implant manufacturing.

Uveitis, glaucoma, and/or hyphema may respond to treatment with cycloplegics and topical anti-inflammatory or ocular hypotensive medications. If medical therapy does not sufficiently address the findings or if inflammation threatens either retinal or corneal function, IOL removal must be considered. This procedure may be complicated because of inflammatory scars, particularly in the anterior chamber angle or posterior to the iris. If such scarring is present, the surgeon may need to amputate the haptics from the optic and remove the lens piecemeal, rotating the haptic material out of the synechial tunnels to minimize trauma to the eye. In some cases, it is safer to leave portions of the haptics in place. Early lens explantation may reduce the risk of corneal decompensation and CME.

Pseudophakic Bullous Keratopathy

Certain IOL designs, particularly iris-clip lenses (iris-fixated lenses with the optic anterior to the iris) and closed-loop flexible anterior chamber lenses as described in the Appendix, have been associated with an increased risk of corneal decompensation. Iris-clip lenses have been shown to contact the corneal endothelium during eye movement, whereas closed-loop ACIOLs are associated with endothelial cell loss, thought to be due to chronic inflammation and contact between the lens and peripheral corneal endothelial cells. Thus, these 2 lens types are no longer in clinical use.

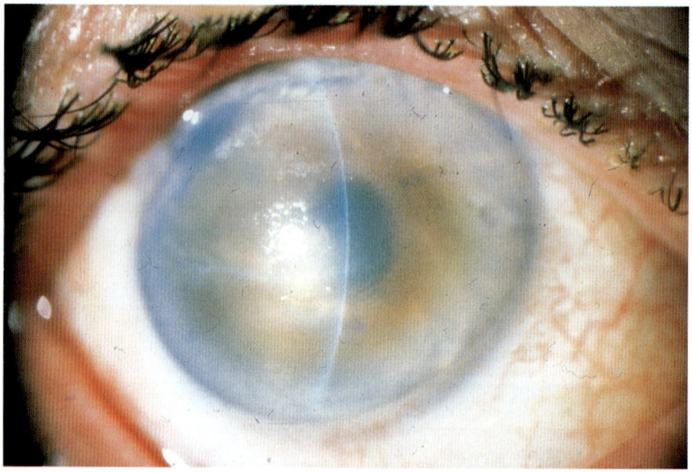

Figure 11-13 Pseudophakic bullous keratopathy. *(Courtesy of Karla J. Johns, MD.)*

With modern phacoemulsification and current IOLs, risk of corneal decompensation is increased with prolonged surgical time using high ultrasound energy, excessive use of ultrasound in the anterior chamber (as opposed to the iris plane or within the capsule), and inadequate protection of the corneal endothelium with OVDs (Fig 11-13). Underlying corneal endothelial dysfunction such as Fuchs corneal dystrophy also increases the risk of postoperative corneal edema. The surgeon can use OVDs to protect the corneal endothelium and avoid contacting the endothelium with instruments or lens particles.

Initial treatment of pseudophakic bullous keratopathy entails controlling postoperative inflammation while avoiding elevated IOP. As discussed earlier in this chapter (see the section Corneal Edema), topical hypertonic sodium chloride drops or ointment can be a conservative short-term treatment to decrease corneal edema. A bandage contact lens and topical antibiotics may be necessary for ruptured bullae.

Decreased vision, recurrent keratitis, and pain are possible indications for endothelial keratoplasty, which has been very successful in restoring clear corneas and improving vision. Bullae and associated pain may also be alleviated with phototherapeutic keratectomy, cautery of Bowman layer, anterior stromal micropuncture, or corneal crosslinking. When comfort is the primary goal in the eye with little or no vision potential, a Gundersen conjunctival flap or amniotic membrane graft is an option; neither of these carries the greater risks of keratoplasty. (See also BCSC Section 8, *External Disease and Cornea.*)

IOL Opacification

Several types of IOLs have developed opacities or discoloration, either immediately after implantation or progressively over the years. Five general processes of IOL opacification have been identified:

1. deposits or precipitates on the surface of or in the IOL
2. influx of water in hydrophobic optic material (glistenings)

3. staining of the IOL by capsular dyes or medications
4. IOL coating by substances such as ophthalmic ointment or silicone oil
5. progressive degradation of the IOL material (eg, snowflake degeneration in PMMA IOLs)

Calcium deposition within or on the surface of hydrophilic acrylic lenses can degrade quality of vision, and IOL explantation may be required. Calcium deposits on silicone lenses have been reported in eyes with asteroid hyalosis, usually after posterior capsulotomy.

Glistenings are fluid-filled microvacuoles that form within an IOL optic in an aqueous environment. They are observed within all IOL materials but are associated primarily with certain hydrophobic acrylic IOLs. Glistening formation and intensity increase with time. Although their appearance may be striking on slit-lamp examination, glistenings have not been shown to affect best-corrected visual acuity. Although studies have documented a negative effect on contrast sensitivity at high spatial frequency, IOL explantation for glistenings is rarely reported.

IOL explantation has been required when interlenticular opacification occurred between piggyback PCIOLs, especially when both lenses were made of hydrophobic acrylic material and were placed in the capsular bag. Using IOLs made of 2 different materials, enlarging the capsulorrhexis, and placing 1 lens in the capsular bag and 1 in the sulcus may reduce the incidence.

Colin J, Praud D, Touboul D, Schweitzer C. Incidence of glistenings with the latest generation of yellow-tinted hydrophobic acrylic intraocular lenses. *J Cataract Refract Surg.* 2012;38(7):1140–1146.

Espandar L, Mukherjee N, Werner L, Mamalis N, Kim T. Diagnosis and management of opacified silicone intraocular lenses in patients with asteroid hyalosis. *J Cataract Refract Surg.* 2015;41(1):222–225.

IOL Glare and Dysphotopsia

In addition to lens decentration and opacification of the IOL or capsule, glare can result when the diameter of the IOL optic is smaller than the diameter of the scotopic pupil. Optics with a square-edge design and multifocal IOLs are more likely to produce glare and halos, even when well centered. When the pupil is dilated, spherical aberration may cause some degree of distortion or glare under scotopic conditions even when the iris covers the edge of the lens optic. Aspheric IOLs may reduce some of these phenomena and improve contrast sensitivity. Although spherical aberration of the cornea varies in the population and changes with keratorefractive surgery, various aspheric and spherical IOLs can be matched to the degree of corneal asphericity (see Chapter 9).

Patients with diffractive or refractive multifocal IOLs are more likely to experience glare, decreased contrast sensitivity, or loss of desired multifocality with minor IOL decentration, altered pupil diameter or position, or posterior capsule opacity. An accommodating lens may vault anteriorly (a condition known as *Z syndrome*) because of misplaced haptics or asymmetric capsular contraction. This syndrome can often be managed by posterior capsulotomy, but the lens may need to be surgically repositioned or explanted. Toric IOLs must be located on a precise axis for maximal astigmatic correction. These lenses may need to be repositioned if they are placed improperly or rotate postoperatively. Refer to Chapter 9 for further discussion of toric IOLs, including risk factors for postoperative toric IOL rotation.

Dysphotopsias are abnormal visual symptoms related to light rays interacting with IOL optics (see BCSC Section 3, *Clinical Optics and Vision Rehabilitation*). Current research indicates that a central neuroadaptive component may also be involved in patient perceptions of dysphotopsia.

Positive dysphotopsia is

- described as glare, streaks, flashes, arcs, or halos of light in the midperiphery
- more common with truncated square-edge IOLs and those manufactured from higher-index materials, as well as with multifocal IOLs

Negative dysphotopsia is

- described as an arcuate dark or dim crescent-shaped region, usually in the temporal visual field
- likely to occur in the routine setting of a PCIOL centered in the capsular bag with the anterior capsule edge overlapping the lens optic
- possible with any type of IOL placed within the capsular bag
- more common with acrylic, square-edge optics with a higher index of refraction

In susceptible eyes, temporal light rays may interact with the nasal lens edge and overlying anterior capsule, causing a shadow (penumbra) on the nasal retina. This effect is more common with a miotic or nasally located pupil and may be relieved with dilation or by blocking light from the temporal side.

Although negative dysphotopsia symptoms are common in the early postoperative period (approximately 15% of all patients), they improve over time in most patients, presumably because of neuroadaptation or anterior capsule opacification. Only approximately 3% of patients report symptoms at 1 year postoperatively. Thus, initially, observation is advised. For patients with prolonged symptoms and compromised vision, surgery may be necessary. In most cases, repositioning of the optic anterior to the capsulorrhexis by reverse optic capture through the capsulorrhexis (with the haptics in the capsular bag) or sulcus fixation of an appropriate PCIOL is successful. However, when reverse optic capture is performed at the time of initial IOL implantation with cataract surgery, the reported rate of posterior capsule opacification requiring Nd:YAG laser posterior capsulotomy by 3 months postoperatively is 100%. Implantation of a piggyback IOL in the ciliary sulcus, partial nasal anterior capsulotomy, or truncation of the nasal optic within the capsular bag has also been successful in some cases.

Masket S, Fram NR, Cho A, Park I, Pham D. Surgical management of negative dysphotopsia. *J Cataract Refract Surg*. 2018;44(1):6–16.

Werner L. Glistenings and surface light scattering in intraocular lenses. *J Cataract Refract Surg*. 2010;36(8):1398–1420.

Unexpected Refractive Results

Cataract surgery and IOL implantation can provide patients with desirable refractive outcomes. See Chapter 9 and BCSC Section 13, *Refractive Surgery*, for a discussion of cataract surgery as a refractive procedure.

Unintended postoperative refractive errors may be the result of a preoperative error in the measurement of axial length or in the keratometry readings. Choosing the correct IOL power is difficult in patients with high hyperopia, high myopia, or prior vitrectomy; patients undergoing simultaneous penetrating keratoplasty; patients with silicone oil in the vitreous cavity; and patients who have had prior refractive surgery (see Chapter 6). The surgeon's failure to confirm the proper IOL at the time of surgery may result in implantation of an incorrect lens.

Unexpected postoperative refractive results may be due to inversion of an angulated IOL or placement of the lens in the sulcus when it was calculated for placement in the capsular bag, either of which results in anterior displacement and changes the effective power of the IOL. It is important to address other potential causes of an anterior or posterior shift in IOL position, such as posterior capsule rupture, capsular block, or malignant glaucoma. Mislabeling or manufacturing defects are the cause of these problems only in rare cases. If the visual acuity is less than expected early in the postoperative course and is confirmed by refraction, incorrect lens power may be suspected. Regardless of the source of the error, medical record documentation and full disclosure to the patient are necessary.

If the magnitude of the postoperative refractive error produces symptomatic ametropia, anisometropia, or patient dissatisfaction, there are several options that the surgeon can consider:

- refraction for glasses or contact lens wear
- IOL exchange
- insertion of a piggyback IOL
- secondary keratorefractive procedure

Capsular Opacification and Contraction

Posterior Capsule Opacification

The most common late occurrence after cataract surgery by means of ECCE or phacoemulsification is posterior capsule opacification (PCO). In addition, contracture of a continuous curvilinear capsulorrhexis may occlude the visual axis because of anterior capsule fibrosis and phimosis.

Capsular opacification stems from the continued viability of lens epithelial cells that remain after removal of the nucleus and cortex. Opaque secondary membranes are formed by proliferating lens epithelial cells, fibroblastic metaplasia, and collagen deposition. Lens epithelial cells proliferate in several patterns. Sequestration of nucleated bladder cells *(Wedl cells)* in a closed space between the adherent edges of the anterior and posterior capsule results in a doughnut-shaped configuration, referred to as a *Soemmering ring.* If the epithelial cells migrate out of the capsular bag, translucent globular masses resembling fish eggs *(Elschnig pearls)* form on the edge of the capsular opening. These pearls can fill the pupil or remain hidden behind the iris. Histologic examination shows that these "fish eggs" are nucleated bladder cells, identical to those proliferating within the capsule of a Soemmering ring but usually lacking a basement membrane. If the epithelial cells migrate across the anterior or posterior capsule, they may cause capsular wrinkling and opacification. These lens epithelial cells are capable of undergoing metaplasia with conversion to myofibroblasts. These cells can produce a matrix of fibrous and basement membrane collagen. Contraction of this collagen matrix causes wrinkles in the posterior capsule, with resultant distortion of vision and glare.

The reported incidence of PCO varies widely but has been diminishing as a result of modern IOL designs and placement. Older studies reported that the frequency of Nd:YAG laser capsulotomy varied between 3% and 53% within 3 years of cataract surgery. More recent clinical series with a 3- to 5-year follow-up of cases with either hydrophobic acrylic or silicone square-edge design show PCO rates up to 5%. IOL design is now considered the dominant factor both in inhibiting posterior migration of lens epithelial cells and in influencing the rate of PCO. The IOL material also has a modest effect on opacification rates. Hydrogel IOLs are associated with the highest rate, followed by PMMA, then silicone; IOLs made of hydrophobic acrylic material are associated with the lowest rate. Compared to round-edge optics, the truncated square-edge optic design is associated with lower rates of PCO in both silicone and acrylic IOLs, although these lenses may increase the incidence of undesirable optical reflections and positive dysphotopsias. See BCSC Section 3, *Clinical Optics and Vision Rehabilitation,* for further discussion of IOL design.

Other factors thought to increase PCO rate include:

- younger age of the patient
- history of intraocular inflammation
- pseudoexfoliation syndrome
- anterior capsulorrhexis that does not cover 360° of the IOL edge
- incomplete cortical cleanup
- round-edge design of the IOL optic
- time elapsed since surgery
- presence of silicone oil

There seems to be no difference in PCO rates with prolonged use of postoperative topical corticosteroids or NSAIDs.

Rönbeck M, Zetterström C, Wejde G, Kugelberg M. Comparison of posterior capsule opacification development with 3 intraocular lens types: five-year prospective study. *J Cataract Refract Surg.* 2009;35(11):1935–1940.

Anterior Capsule Fibrosis and Phimosis

Capsular fibrosis is associated with clouding of the anterior capsule. If a substantial portion of the IOL optic is covered by the opaque anterior capsule, including portions exposed through the undilated pupil, the patient may experience symptoms such as glare, especially at night because of physiologic mydriasis in darkness, or a perception that vision has become cloudy or hazy. The term *capsular phimosis* describes the postoperative contraction of the anterior capsule opening as a result of circumferential fibrosis. Phimosis produces symptoms similar to and often more pronounced than those of fibrosis alone.

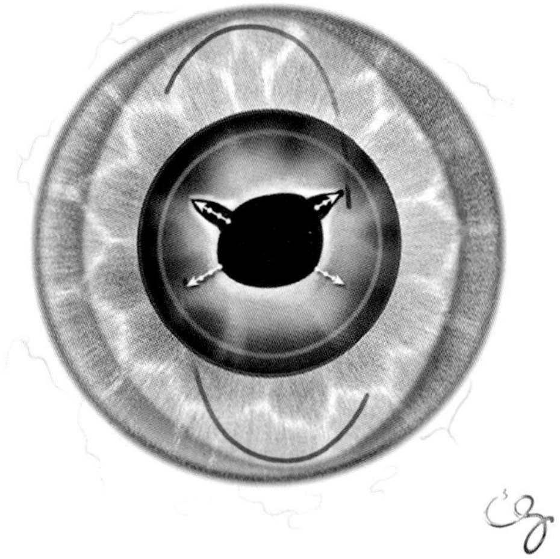

Figure 11-14 Illustration of Nd:YAG laser anterior capsulotomy. Multiple radial anterior capsulotomies *(arrows)* can relieve anterior capsule phimosis and traction on the zonular fibers. *(Illustration by Christine Gralapp.)*

Fibrosis and anterior capsule contraction occur more frequently with smaller capsulorrhexis openings, underlying pseudoexfoliation syndrome, and abnormal or asymmetric zonular support (eg, penetrating or blunt trauma, Marfan syndrome, or surgical trauma). Anterior capsule contraction may contribute to late pseudophacodonesis or in-the-bag IOL subluxation due to stress on the zonular apparatus.

Anterior capsule contraction, but not PCO, may be reduced with anterior capsule polishing to remove residual lens epithelial cells. Capsular phimosis can be treated with several radial Nd:YAG laser anterior capsulotomies to release the annular contraction, reduce the traction on the zonule, and enlarge the anterior capsule opening (Fig 11-14). This procedure is performed similar to Nd:YAG laser posterior capsulotomy, with care taken to not defocus too far posteriorly and damage the underlying IOL with laser pitting. In general, the anterior capsule tissue or a fibrotic ring is tougher and thus requires more laser power than does the posterior capsule.

Nd:YAG Laser Capsulotomy

The Nd:YAG laser is used to treat secondary opacification of the posterior capsule and/or contraction of the anterior capsule. Alternatively, intraocular surgical cleaning of the capsule may be performed during concurrent anterior segment surgery to maintain an intact posterior capsule if desired. To reduce the possibility of vitreous prolapse around the IOL and into the anterior chamber, posterior capsulotomy would ideally be delayed if possible until there is adequate apposition and fusion of the anterior and posterior capsules peripheral to the lens optic. Otherwise, the ideal time to treat symptomatic posterior capsule opacity with posterior capsulotomy has not been established.

In addition to capsulotomy, the Nd:YAG laser can be used for vitreolysis, synechiolysis, iris cystotomy, iridotomy, anterior hyaloidotomy for malignant glaucoma, removal of precipitates and membranes from an IOL surface, and fragmentation of retained cortical material.

Indications

The success rate of Nd:YAG laser posterior capsulotomy exceeds 95%. Indications for Nd:YAG capsulotomy include the following:

- visual acuity symptomatically decreased as a result of PCO
- a hazy posterior capsule preventing a clear view of the ocular fundus required for diagnostic and therapeutic purposes
- monocular diplopia, a Maddox rod–like effect, or glare caused by wrinkling of the posterior capsule or by encroachment of a partially opened posterior capsule into the visual axis
- contraction of anterior capsulotomy (capsular phimosis) causing encroachment on the visual axis, excessive traction on the zonular fibers, or alteration of the lens optic position
- capsular block syndrome

Contraindications

Contraindications for Nd:YAG laser capsulotomy include the following:

- inadequate visualization of the posterior capsule
- a patient who is unable to remain still or hold fixation during the procedure (use of a contact lens or retrobulbar anesthesia may enhance the feasibility of a capsulotomy in such patients)
- active intraocular inflammation, uncontrolled glaucoma, high risk of retinal detachment, and suspected CME (all relative contraindications)

Procedure

The center of the visual axis, usually 3–4 mm in diameter, is the desired site for posterior capsulotomy. Dilation is not always necessary for the procedure, but it may be helpful when a larger opening is desired.

A high plus-powered anterior segment laser lens may improve ocular stability and enlarge the cone angle of the beam, reducing the depth of focus. The smaller focus diameter facilitates the laser pulse puncture of the capsule, and structures in front of and behind the point of focus are less likely to be damaged.

Capsulotomy can be performed in a spiral (Fig 11-15A), cruciate (Fig 11-15B), or inverted D–shaped pattern, beginning in the periphery to reduce the likelihood of central optic pitting until ideal energy levels and focus have been established. Occasional IOL dislocation into the vitreous has been reported after capsulotomy, particularly with silicone plate–haptic lenses. Constructing the capsulotomy in a spiraling circular pattern, rather than in a cruciate pattern, creates an opening that is less likely to extend radially, reducing the risk of dislocation. Also, the diameter of the capsulotomy should not exceed that of the IOL optic.

When minimal laser energy is applied, the anterior vitreous face may remain intact. A ruptured anterior vitreous face will usually not result in anterior chamber prolapse by the barrier effect of a PCIOL, although in rare instances vitreous strands can migrate around the lens and through the pupil.

Any PCIOL can be damaged by laser energy, but the threshold for lens damage appears to be lower for silicone than for other materials. The surgeon focuses the laser just behind

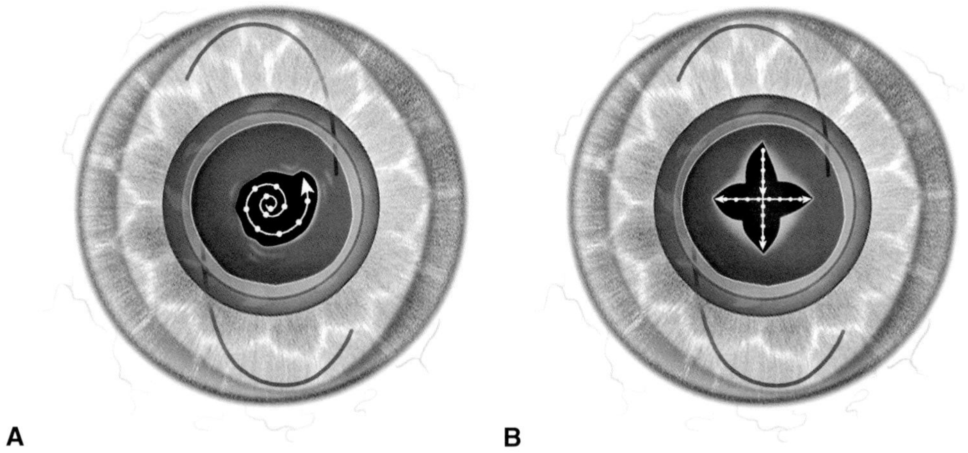

Figure 11-15 Illustrations of Nd:YAG laser posterior capsulotomy. **A,** A spiral pattern *(arrow)* may reduce the risk of radial tears. **B,** A cruciate pattern *(arrows)* or inverted D–shaped pattern (not shown) with an inferior flap hinge allows for initial punctures in the periphery and may help reduce the risk of central IOL laser damage. *(Illustration by Christine Gralapp.)*

the posterior capsule; pulses too far behind the IOL will be ineffective. The safest approach is to focus the laser beam slightly behind the posterior surface of the capsule for the initial application and then move anteriorly for subsequent applications until the desired puncture is achieved.

In cases of anterior capsule contraction, multiple relaxing incisions of the fibrotic ring relieve the contracting force and create a larger optical opening (see Fig 11-14).

Occasionally, the Nd:YAG laser is insufficient to address exceptionally dense fibrosis, which may require surgical manipulation with a discission knife, vitrectomy handpiece, or scissors.

Complications

Complications of Nd:YAG laser capsulotomy include:

- transient or long-term elevated IOP
- CME
- retinal detachment
- hyphema
- damage to or dislocation of the IOL
- corneal edema
- corneal abrasions (from the focusing contact lens for the laser surgery)

Transient elevation of IOP occurs in a substantial number of patients, with pressure levels peaking 2–3 hours after surgery. This elevation is likely due to obstruction of the outflow pathways by debris scattered by the laser treatment. It is more common in eyes with vitreous prolapse, those without in-the-bag fixation of the IOL, or those with preexisting glaucoma. Such elevation responds quickly to topical glaucoma medications, which can be continued for 3–5 days after the procedure.

To reduce the risks of postprocedure IOP spikes, inflammation, and CME following any type of laser capsular surgery, many surgeons prescribe prophylactic preoperative and postoperative ocular hypotensive medications (α-adrenergic agonist or β-blocker drops), as well as either topical corticosteroids or NSAIDs, although there is insufficient evidence to uniformly recommend these prophylactically in patients without additional risk factors. In patients with a history of CME or in high-risk patients such as those with diabetic retinopathy, the prophylactic use of topical corticosteroids or NSAIDs may be beneficial.

Nd:YAG laser capsulotomy may increase the risk of retinal detachment; the reported incidence is 0%–3.6%. Approximately 50%–75% of retinal detachments after cataract extraction occur within 1 year of surgery or within 6 months of capsulotomy, often in association with posterior vitreous detachment (PVD). In many cases, it is difficult to ascertain whether the retinal detachment is related to the capsulotomy or to the cataract surgery itself or whether it is simply a consequence of a naturally occurring PVD. Factors that increase the risk of retinal detachment after Nd:YAG capsulotomy include axial myopia, male sex, young age, trauma, vitreous prolapse, a family history of retinal detachment, and preexisting vitreoretinal pathology. It is important to instruct all patients to promptly report any new symptoms suggesting a PVD or retinal tear.

American Academy of Ophthalmology Cataract/Anterior Segment Panel. Preferred Practice Pattern® Guidelines. *Cataract in the Adult Eye.* American Academy of Ophthalmology; 2016. www.aao.org/ppp

Diplopia

A thorough discussion of diplopia is presented in BCSC Section 6, *Pediatric Ophthalmology and Strabismus,* and in Section 5, *Neuro-Ophthalmology.* There are 2 types of diplopia, monocular and binocular, which can be easily differentiated by covering the eyes. If the diplopia is present only with both eyes open, then it is binocular. If it is still present with only 1 eye open, then it is monocular. As it pertains to cataract surgery, monocular diplopia generally results from optical aberrations in the operative eye. Binocular diplopia results from ocular misalignment or anisometropia (Table 11-3). It is important to document preoperative ocular misalignment, which is present in 13%–16% of patients undergoing cataract surgery. Regarding intractable binocular diplopia, a 2008 study of patients found that the most common cause was extraocular muscle restriction or paresis in the anesthetic block group and decompensation of a preexisting phoria in the topical group.

Corneal topography may be useful in determining a corneal cause of diplopia. OCT may help exclude macular causes of monocular diplopia. Treatment of monocular diplopia is directed at the source, as is treatment of persistent binocular diplopia. Disruption of fusion and anisometropia may be managed by proper optical correction with a prism and slab-off bifocal if necessary. Cataract surgery on the contralateral eye or contact lens correction may be required. If a muscle paresis/restriction is present, prism correction often is adequate; however, referral to a specialist in strabismus may be necessary.

Table 11-3 Causes of Postoperative Diplopia

Monocular	Binocular
Keratitis (eg, keratitis sicca)	Extraocular muscle damage (eg, myotoxicity from local anesthetic or bridle suture placement)
Uncorrected refractive error (eg, astigmatism)	Nerve toxicity from local anesthetic
Corneal edema	Decompensated phoria
Irregular corneal epithelium (eg, corneal abrasion or epithelial basement membrane dystrophy)	Nerve palsy (may be unrelated to surgical procedure)
Keratoconus	Disruption of binocular fusion (eg, from anisometropia)
Posterior capsule wrinkle or opacification	
IOL decentration or opacification	
Macular pathology: ERM, macular edema, maculopathy	

ERM = epiretinal membrane; IOL = intraocular lens.

Inflammatory and Infectious Complications

Postoperative Uveitis

After cataract extraction, nearly all eyes exhibit some degree of intraocular inflammation. With uncomplicated cataract surgery and the use of postoperative topical corticosteroids and/or NSAIDs, most eyes are typically free of inflammation by 3–4 weeks postoperatively. Complicated cases requiring manipulation of intraocular tissues (eg, iris stretching, sphincterotomy, iridectomy, or repair), involving vitreous loss or prolapse, or requiring sulcus fixation of an IOL may have a more prolonged recovery. Increased inflammation may also be seen in children; in patients with diabetes mellitus; in patients who have had previous surgery, pseudoexfoliation syndrome, or pigment dispersion syndrome; and with long-term miotic use.

Low-grade inflammation lasting more than 4 weeks raises the possibility of chronic infection, retained lens fragments, or other causes of chronic inflammation such as IOL malposition. The presence of vitritis or a hypopyon warrants investigation to determine the source of inflammation and to rule out an infectious cause. In patients who have persistent uveitis without a history of inflammation, investigation for a possible microbial endophthalmitis is also indicated. Chronic uveitis after cataract surgery has been associated with low-grade infections with bacterial pathogens, including *Propionibacterium acnes* and *Staphylococcus epidermidis.* Such patients may have an unremarkable early postoperative course and lack the classic findings of acute endophthalmitis. Weeks or months after surgery, however, they develop chronic uveitis that is variably responsive to topical corticosteroids. This condition is usually associated with granulomatous keratic precipitates and, less commonly, with hypopyon. A localized focus of infection sequestered within the capsular bag may occasionally be observed (Fig 11-16).

Diagnosis of endophthalmitis requires a high level of clinical suspicion, coupled with examination and cultures of appropriate specimens of aqueous, vitreous, and (where

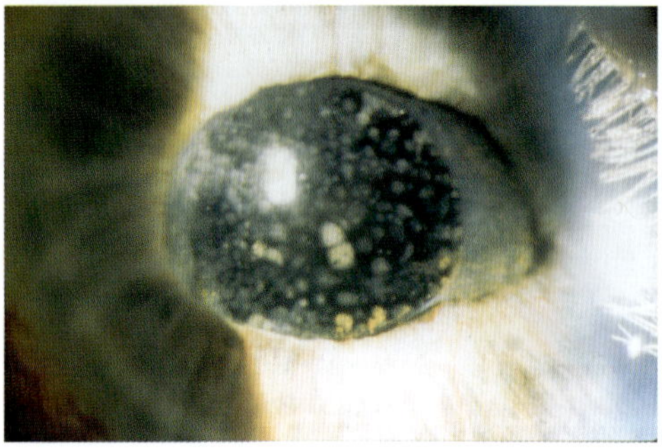

Figure 11-16 *Propionibacterium acnes* on a lens capsule. *(Courtesy of Thomas L. Steinemann, MD.)*

applicable) retained lens material that may harbor a nidus of infection. Appropriate intravitreal antibiotic therapy is indicated. If this treatment fails, the clinician may need to search for and remove any visible focus of infection in order to sterilize the eye. In some cases, total removal of the residual capsule and IOL is necessary.

Patients with preexisting uveitis may have excessive postoperative inflammation but generally do well with small-incision cataract surgery with IOL implantation in the capsular bag. Some surgeons prefer acrylic IOL material over silicone in patients with preexisting uveitis or a risk of chronic inflammation.

Management of chronic uveitis focuses on the cause. Surgery is used for correction of mechanical issues with IOL malposition, vitreous incarceration, or retained lens fragments. If no obvious etiology can be found, prolonged use of topical or subconjunctival corticosteroids is indicated, with continued efforts to identify a cause.

Toxic Anterior Segment Syndrome

Toxic anterior segment syndrome (TASS) is an acute sterile postoperative inflammation. The symptoms and signs of TASS may mimic those of infectious endophthalmitis and include photophobia, severe reduction in visual acuity, corneal edema, and marked anterior chamber reaction, occasionally with hypopyon (Fig 11-17). However, TASS presents within 12 to 48 hours of surgery, whereas acute infectious endophthalmitis typically develops 3–10 days postoperatively. Other potentially distinguishing features of TASS include diffuse, limbus-to-limbus corneal edema; anterior chamber fibrinous exudate;

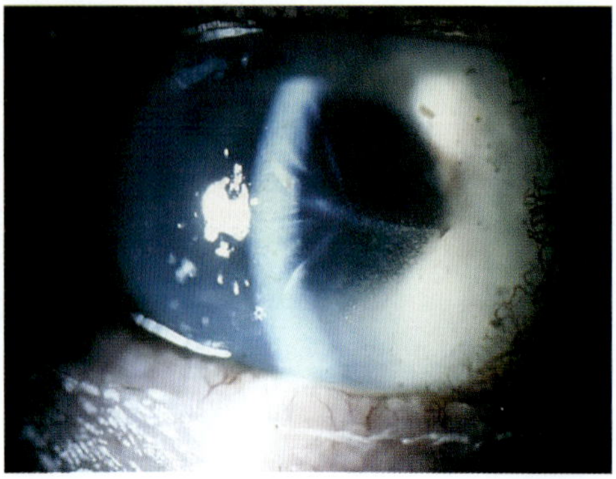

Figure 11-17 Toxic anterior segment syndrome. *(© 2019, American Academy of Ophthalmology.)*

a dilated, irregular, or nonreactive pupil; and elevated IOP. The pathologic changes are limited to the anterior chamber. Pain is typically much milder than that experienced with an infection. When endophthalmitis is suspected, diagnostic and therapeutic interventions (described later in this chapter) are indicated.

TASS is thought to be caused by the inadvertent introduction of a substance toxic to the corneal endothelium or uvea. A 2018 report by a TASS task force showed the risk factors to be inadequate flushing and rinsing of handpieces, use of enzymatic detergents, and use of ultrasonic baths. Ultrasonic baths are susceptible to contamination with gram-negative bacteria and may result in residue on instruments of heat-stable bacterial endotoxin. It is necessary to properly clean and maintain ultrasound baths, if they are used.

RECOMMENDATIONS FOR AVOIDING TASS

- Use preservative-free and bisulfite-free medications.
- Properly mix and dose any intracameral antibiotics, anesthetics, or other medications.
- Thoroughly flush ophthalmic viscosurgical devices (OVDs) from ophthalmic instruments.
- Thoroughly flush all handpieces and reusable cannulas to remove debris.
- Avoid the use of enzymes and detergents in the cleaning of ophthalmic instruments.
- Avoid the use of ultrasound water baths for cleaning ophthalmic instruments.
- Properly clean and maintain autoclave steam sterilizer systems.
- Follow strict protocol for general cleaning and sterilization of ophthalmic instruments.
- Separate ophthalmic instruments from other surgical instruments for cleaning and sterilization.

Other causes of TASS include surgical glove residue or talc on instruments or IOLs; use of a denatured OVD; substitution of sterile water for balanced salt solution; intraocular use of inappropriate irrigating solutions, antibiotics, or anesthetics; and inadvertent introduction of substances into the anterior chamber. Subconjunctival antibiotic injections and topical ophthalmic ointments applied with patching have been reported to enter the anterior chamber through corneoscleral incisions. Skin cleansers containing chlorhexidine gluconate have caused irreversible corneal edema and opacification when they come into contact with the endothelium. Clusters of TASS due to irrigation fluids tainted with bacterial endotoxin have also been reported. Ideally, all solutions used intracamerally are free of stabilizers and preservatives and buffered to physiologic osmolarity and pH.

Treatment of TASS consists of intensive topical corticosteroids until the inflammation subsides. A brief course of systemic corticosteroids may be beneficial. Frequent follow-up is necessary to monitor IOP and to reassess for signs of bacterial infection.

Bodnar Z, Clouser S, Mamalis N. Toxic anterior segment syndrome: update on the most common causes. *J Cataract Refract Surg.* 2012;38(11):1902–1910.

Chang DF, Mamalis N; Ophthalmic Instrument Cleaning and Sterilization Task Force. Guidelines for the cleaning and sterilization of intraocular surgical instruments. *J Cataract Refract Surg.* 2018;44(6):765–773.

Mamalis N. Toxic anterior segment syndrome (TASS). *Focal Points: Clinical Modules for Ophthalmologists.* American Academy of Ophthalmology; 2009, module 10.

Endophthalmitis

Endophthalmitis is a rare but dreaded complication of cataract surgery that may lead to severe loss of vision or loss of the eye. The symptoms of endophthalmitis include mild to severe ocular pain, vision loss, floaters, and photophobia. Early diagnosis and prompt treatment are essential, because delayed treatment can substantially alter the visual prognosis. Recent large retrospective studies of the incidence of endophthalmitis after cataract surgery reveal rates between 0.04% and 0.20%. Factors that increase the risk of infection include diabetes mellitus, older age, male sex, complicated or prolonged surgery, vitreous loss, posterior capsule rupture, wound leaks, and possibly the use of clear corneal incisions.

Prevention

To reduce the incidence of postoperative endophthalmitis, it is important to use preoperative povidone-iodine skin prep, povidone-iodine 5% drops, careful eyelid and eyelash draping, and sterile technique. Meticulous attention to watertight incision closure is also important in preventing endophthalmitis, particularly when clear corneal incisions are used. Prophylactic preoperative and postoperative topical antibiotics are often prescribed for cataract surgery, although no randomized clinical studies support this practice.

In 2006, the Endophthalmitis Study Group of the European Society of Cataract and Refractive Surgeons (ESCRS) conducted a prospective, randomized, partially masked cataract surgery study and reported that the endophthalmitis rate was 0.07% in patients given intracameral cefuroxime 1 mg at the conclusion of surgery compared with a rate of 0.34% in patients given topical levofloxacin drops alone. The ESCRS also reported a 5.88-fold increase in risk with the use of clear corneal incisions instead of scleral tunnels.

A report based on outcomes of more than 600,000 consecutive cataract surgeries performed between 2014 and 2016 at Aravind Hospitals in India showed a decrease in endophthalmitis rates from 0.07% without intracameral antibiotics to 0.02% with intracameral moxifloxacin. In the phacoemulsification group, the incidence decreased from 0.07% to 0.01% with intracameral moxifloxacin.

Although the practice is not universally accepted, many surgeons use an intraocular antibiotic such as preservative-free moxifloxacin, cefuroxime, or vancomycin at the conclusion of cataract surgery. Although no commercially available preservative-free antibiotics are currently marketed for intracameral use in the United States, multiple 503B compounding pharmacies provide medications for intraoperative use. Surgeons must consider the reduction in endophthalmitis rates against the risk of TASS from dilutional errors for intraocular medications. The use of intraocular vancomycin for prophylaxis has decreased since reports of vancomycin-associated hemorrhagic occlusive retinal vasculitis (HORV; see the discussion of HORV later in this chapter).

See BCSC Section 12, *Retina and Vitreous,* for additional discussion of endophthalmitis.

Endophthalmitis Study Group, European Society of Cataract & Refractive Surgeons. Prophylaxis of postoperative endophthalmitis following cataract surgery: results of the ESCRS multicenter study and identification of risk factors. *J Cataract Refract Surg.* 2007;33(6):978–988.

Haripriya A, Chang DF, Ravindran RD. Endophthalmitis reduction with intracameral moxifloxacin prophylaxis: analysis of 600 000 surgeries. *Ophthalmology.* 2017;124(6):768–775.

Shorstein NH, Winthrop KL, Herrinton LJ. Decreased postoperative endophthalmitis rate after institution of intracameral antibiotics in a Northern California eye department. *J Cataract Refract Surg.* 2013;39(1):8–14.

Diagnosis

Infectious endophthalmitis may present in an acute form or a more indolent or chronic form. *Acute* endophthalmitis, defined as inflammation occurring within 6 weeks of surgery, typically develops 3–10 days postoperatively and runs a fulminant course. The hallmark of acute endophthalmitis is vitreous inflammation, but other signs include eyelid or periorbital edema, ciliary injection, chemosis, anterior chamber inflammation, hypopyon, decreased visual acuity, corneal edema, and retinal hemorrhages (Fig 11-18).

Acute infectious endophthalmitis must be differentiated from TASS (discussed earlier in this chapter). The clinical presentation is often diagnostic, but occasionally the clinician may be able to diagnose sterile endophthalmitis only by excluding possible infectious causes with appropriate aqueous and vitreous cultures.

In contrast, *chronic* endophthalmitis may develop weeks or months after surgery. It may be characterized by chronic iridocyclitis or granulomatous uveitis and is often

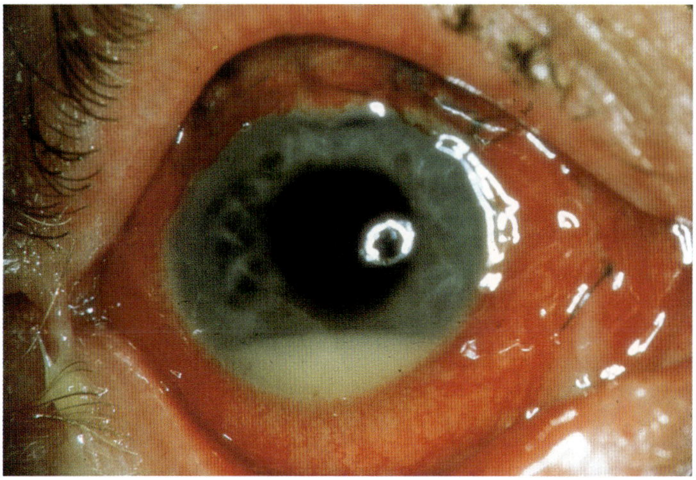

Figure 11-18 Endophthalmitis. *(Courtesy of Karla J. Johns, MD.)*

associated with decreased vision, little or no pain, and a nidus of the infectious agent within the eye. The chronic form is associated with organisms of lower pathogenicity; the most common are *P acnes, S epidermidis,* and fungi. (See also BCSC Section 9, *Uveitis and Intraocular Inflammation,* and Section 12, *Retina and Vitreous.*)

In the Endophthalmitis Vitrectomy Study (EVS), most cases of endophthalmitis presented within 3–10 days of surgery, with a median of 6 days, and 25% presented without pain. Later onset also occurred; 22% of cases presented 2–6 weeks after surgery. The most common bacterial causes in that study were gram-positive coagulase-negative *S epidermidis* (70%), *Staphylococcus aureus* (9.9%), *Streptococcus* species (9.0%), other gram-positive bacteria (3.1%), *Enterococcus* species (2.2%), and gram-negative bacteria (5.9%). Most infections are caused by organisms similar to the patients' own periocular bacterial flora. Drug-resistant strains are becoming more common.

Endophthalmitis Vitrectomy Study Group. Results of the Endophthalmitis Vitrectomy Study: a randomized trial of immediate vitrectomy and of intravenous antibiotics for the treatment of postoperative bacterial endophthalmitis. *Arch Ophthalmol.* 1995;113(12):1479–1496.

Treatment

The recommended approach to the management of postoperative endophthalmitis is based on the results of the EVS. As soon as a clinical diagnosis of endophthalmitis is suspected, assessment of visual acuity will help direct management decisions. Immediate pars plana vitrectomy and antibiotic injections are indicated when the patient's visual acuity is light perception. When the visual acuity is hand motions or better, a less-invasive anterior chamber and/or vitreous biopsy for cultures with immediate subsequent intravitreal injection of antibiotics is indicated (a "tap-and-inject" procedure).

A tap-and-inject procedure can be performed in the office under sterile conditions. Because clinical features do not distinguish between gram-positive and gram-negative organisms, the mainstay of treatment remains broad-spectrum intravitreal antibiotics for both classes of bacteria. Currently, vancomycin 1 mg and ceftazidime 2.25 mg are preferred, with amikacin 0.4 mg administered for cephalosporin-allergic patients. Topical cycloplegic and corticosteroid drops may be helpful. Although oral or intravenous antibiotics, fortified topical or subconjunctival antibiotics, and intravitreal corticosteroids are sometimes used, they were not beneficial in a controlled study.

Chronic or delayed-onset endophthalmitis is also best treated with vitreous biopsy and intraocular antibiotics. However, because of sequestration of infectious material in the capsular bag or vitreous, a vitrectomy and posterior capsulectomy or even IOL exchange is often necessary to remove the nidus of infection.

Retinal Complications

Cystoid Macular Edema

Cystoid macular edema (CME), also known as *Irvine-Gass syndrome,* is a common cause of decreased vision after cataract surgery. Although the exact pathogenesis of CME is

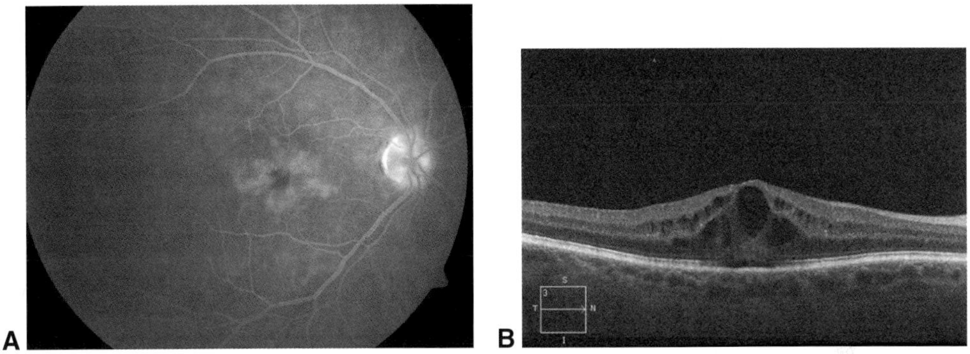

Figure 11-19 Cystoid macular edema (CME). **A,** Fluorescein angiogram demonstrates late pooling of dye in a petaloid pattern in the macula and staining of the optic nerve head. **B,** Spectral-domain optical coherence tomography scan shows diffuse retinal thickening with cystic areas of low reflectivity predominantly in the inner nuclear and outer plexiform layers. *(Courtesy of Thomas L. Beardsley, MD.)*

unknown, the final common pathway appears to be increased perifoveal capillary permeability with accumulation of fluid in the inner nuclear and outer plexiform layers. CME is often associated with intraocular inflammation and may be mediated through the release of prostaglandins and leukotrienes.

CME may be recognized by an otherwise unexplained reduction in vision, by the characteristic petaloid appearance of cystic spaces in the macula on ophthalmoscopy or fluorescein angiography (Fig 11-19A), or by cystic areas of low reflectivity and retinal thickening on OCT (Fig 11-19B). Most affected patients are asymptomatic, although there may be some loss of contrast sensitivity even in the absence of reduced Snellen visual acuity. In addition, patients with angiographic CME after phacoemulsification score substantially lower in logMAR (logarithm of the minimum angle of resolution) visual acuity than do patients with no CME, even though their Snellen visual acuities remain better than 20/40. Table 11-4 summarizes the incidence of CME according to the type of cataract surgery and the basis of diagnosis of CME.

The incidence of both angiographic and clinical CME peaks 6–10 weeks after surgery. Spontaneous resolution occurs in approximately 95% of uncomplicated cases, usually within 3–12 months. In rare cases, CME may develop many years after surgery, especially in association with delayed postoperative rupture of the anterior vitreous face. CME has also been associated with the use of topical epinephrine and dipivefrin for the treatment of aphakic glaucoma. Prostaglandin analogues have been associated with reversible CME in eyes that have undergone recent intraocular surgery, although a causal relationship has not been established. The risk is believed to be greater in the absence of an intact posterior capsule. Table 11-5 lists risk factors for CME.

The risk of early postoperative CME is reduced with prophylactic postoperative use of topical corticosteroids and NSAID drops. An American Academy of Ophthalmology report found that topical NSAIDs after cataract surgery were effective in reducing the incidence of CME and hastened postoperative visual recovery in the short term. However, level 1 evidence that NSAID therapy prevents vision loss from CME at 3 months or longer after cataract surgery is lacking.

Table 11-4 Incidence of CME According to Basis of CME Diagnosis and Type of Surgery

	Basis of CME Diagnosis		
Surgical Procedure	CME on IFVA	Increased Macular Thickness on OCT	VA ≤20/40 and CME (on OCT or IFVA)
ICCE	40%–70%	No data	2%–10%
ECCE/phacoemulsification	1%–19%	≤41%	1%–2% for ECCE with intact posterior capsule 0.10%–2.35% for phacoemulsification with intact posterior capsule

CME = cystoid macular edema; ECCE = extracapsular cataract extraction; ICCE = intracapsular cataract extraction; IVFA = intravenous fluorescein angiography; OCT = optical coherence tomography; VA = visual acuity.

Table 11-5 Risk Factors for Cystoid Macular Edema

Preoperative	Surgical and Postoperative
Uveitis	Posterior capsule rupture
Epiretinal membrane	Vitreous loss
Vitreomacular traction	Iris manipulation
Diabetes mellitus	Prolonged surgical time
Diabetic retinopathy	Improper intraocular lens positioning
Retinal vein occlusion	Retained lens fragments
Retinitis pigmentosa	Poorly controlled postoperative inflammation
Previous occurrence of cystoid macular edema	Transient or prolonged hypotony

Medical treatment of chronic postoperative CME typically begins with a course of anti-inflammatory drugs such as topical corticosteroids and/or NSAIDs. A prospective randomized clinical trial of chronic CME found that combination therapy with ketorolac 0.5% and prednisolone acetate 1.0% 4 times a day was more effective than either drug alone in improving visual acuity. Topical anti-inflammatory therapy may take 3–6 months to resolve chronic CME, and the condition may recur after cessation of therapy. Sub-Tenon steroid injection or intravitreal injections of corticosteroids alone or via a sustained drug-delivery system may be effective. In refractory cases, systemic carbonic anhydrase inhibitors may be beneficial. Intravitreal vascular endothelial growth factor inhibitors have been successful in chronic CME cases that do not respond to conventional treatment.

When the inciting source of chronic CME can be defined and the edema fails to respond to medical therapy, surgical therapy may be indicated. Any retained lens fragments should be removed. Nd:YAG laser vitreolysis or vitrectomy can be used to remove vitreous adhering to the cataract incision and relieve iris deformity or vitreomacular traction. If the IOL is malpositioned and contributing to chronic uveitis, repositioning or exchange may be helpful. For further discussion of CME, see BCSC Section 12, *Retina and Vitreous.*

Kim SJ, Schoenberger SD, Thorne JE, Ehlers JP, Yeh S, Bakri SJ. Topical nonsteroidal anti-inflammatory drugs and cataract surgery: a report by the American Academy of Ophthalmology. *Ophthalmology.* 2015;122(11):2159–2168.

Wielders LHP, Schouten JSAG, Winkens B, et al; ESCRS PREMED Study Group. Randomized controlled European multicenter trial on the prevention of cystoid macular edema after cataract surgery in diabetics: ESCRS PREMED Study Report 2. *J Cataract Refract Surg.* 2018;44(7):836–847.

Hemorrhagic Occlusive Retinal Vasculitis

Hemorrhagic occlusive retinal vasculitis (HORV) is a rare but serious complication characterized by delayed-onset painless vision loss, mild anterior chamber and vitreous inflammation, retinal ischemia with sectoral hemorrhages in areas of ischemia, and predilection for venules and peripheral involvement. The disease was first reported as a complication associated with intraoperative use of intraocular vancomycin in 2015. The mechanism of HORV is presumed to be a delayed hypersensitivity immune response occurring 1–21 days after surgery. Because of the delayed onset, some patients have experienced bilateral HORV, with the second eye undergoing cataract surgery before the first eye exhibited signs of HORV.

Outcomes are poor despite aggressive corticosteroid therapy and other treatments, with 1 series reporting that 61% of eyes had visual acuity ≤20/200 and 22% had no light perception. When choosing an appropriate antibiotic for intraocular prophylaxis, it is important for the surgeon to consider this rare but severe complication of intraocular vancomycin.

Witkin AJ, Chang DF, Jumper JM, et al. Vancomycin-associated hemorrhagic occlusive retinal vasculitis: clinical characteristics of 36 eyes. *Ophthalmology.* 2017;124(5):583–595.

Retinal Light Toxicity

Prolonged exposure to the illuminating filament of an operating microscope can increase the risk of CME or a burn to the retinal pigment epithelium (RPE). The risk of an RPE burn is particularly high during cataract surgery, when the filtering effects of the natural lens (cataract) are removed, exposing the vulnerable RPE to unfiltered blue light and near-ultraviolet radiation. If a burn occurs, a central or paracentral scotoma may result. Minimizing retinal exposure to the operating microscope light, filtering light wavelengths below 515 nm, and, when possible, using pupillary shields and oblique lighting reduce the risk of this complication.

Delayed Suprachoroidal Hemorrhage

For a discussion of *intraoperative* suprachoroidal hemorrhage, please see Chapter 10. Delayed suprachoroidal hemorrhage may occur in the early postoperative period, presenting with sudden onset of pain, loss of vision, and shallowing of the anterior chamber. Predisposing factors for postoperative choroidal hemorrhage or effusion include prolonged hypotony, wound leak, unrecognized scleral perforation, trauma, uveitis, cyclodialysis, and excessive filtration. This condition is far more common after glaucoma filtering procedures than routine cataract surgery and may also arise after laser photocoagulation or cryotherapy.

When an incision remains intact and the IOP can be controlled medically, limited suprachoroidal hemorrhage may be observed and frequently will resolve spontaneously. If the incision is not intact, surgical revision may be sufficient to allow the hemorrhage to resolve. Medical management consists of systemic corticosteroids, topical and oral ocular hypotensive agents for elevated IOP, topical cycloplegia, and close observation. Surgical drainage of the suprachoroidal space is indicated when there is a flat anterior chamber, medically uncontrolled glaucoma, or persistent or adherent (kissing) choroidal detachments.

Retinal Detachment

The incidence of pseudophakic rhegmatogenous retinal detachment (RRD) has been reported as 0.2%–3.6%, depending on follow-up time and patient demographics. RRD occurs most frequently within 1 year of cataract surgery or 6 months after posterior capsulotomy. During the first postoperative year after phacoemulsification, the incidence of RRD ranges from 0.6% to 1.7%. The incidence of RRD is lower with small-incision phacoemulsification surgery than with large-incision ECCE and ICCE.

For all age groups and both sexes, eyes that have undergone cataract surgery have an approximately fourfold-higher risk of RRD than fellow phakic eyes. Uncomplicated cataract surgery and laser posterior capsulotomy are risk factors for RRD in part because they are risk factors for early onset of PVD. Myopic eyes have a much higher risk of RRD whether pseudophakic or phakic, and this risk rises with each additional millimeter of axial length. Whether phakic or pseudophakic, additional risk factors for RRD include axial myopia (6- to 10-times-greater risk with axial length >25 mm), younger age (4-times-greater risk with age <60 years), male sex, lattice degeneration of the retina, a previous retinal tear or detachment in the surgical eye, a history of retinal detachment in the fellow eye, and a family history of retinal detachment.

After cataract surgery complicated by posterior capsule rupture, the risk of postoperative RRD is increased at least tenfold compared with pseudophakic eyes with an intact capsule. Some studies have reported that Nd:YAG laser posterior capsulotomy increases the risk for RRD, whereas other studies found no evidence of increased risk with capsulotomy. Neither the size of the capsulotomy nor the total energy delivered is thought to increase risk.

Pars plana vitrectomy with or without a scleral buckle is most commonly used to repair RRD; the success rate is approximately 85% with 1 operation and ultimately 98% with multiple procedures. (See also BCSC Section 12, *Retina and Vitreous.*)

Bjerrum SS, Mikkelsen KL, La Cour M. Risk of pseudophakic retinal detachment in 202,226 patients using the fellow nonoperated eye as reference. *Ophthalmology.* 2013;120(12): 2573–2579.

Clark A, Morlet N, Ng JQ, Preen DB, Semmens JB. Risk for retinal detachment after phacoemulsification: a whole-population study of cataract surgery outcomes. *Arch Ophthalmol.* 2012;130(7):882–888.

CHAPTER 12

Preparing for Cataract Surgery in Special Situations

This chapter includes related videos. Go to www.aao.org/bcscvideo_section11 or scan the QR codes in the text to access this content.

Highlights

- Unique considerations are needed for patients with psychological disorders, systemic diseases, external ocular abnormalities, corneal pathologies, glaucoma, uveitis, or retinal conditions.
- Cataract surgeons need to be prepared for nonroutine procedures in eyes compromised by limited visualization of the lens, loss of integrity of the lens or capsule, zonular weakness, trauma, or extremely long or short axial length.
- Minimally invasive procedures allow for glaucoma treatment at the time of cataract extraction.
- An emphasis on preoperative planning, the use of emerging technological devices during surgery, and appropriate intraocular lens calculation help enable a safe and successful surgery, even in a challenging situation.

A complete discussion of the indications for and technique of cataract surgery in the pediatric age group is presented in BCSC Section 6, *Pediatric Ophthalmology and Strabismus.*

Psychosocial Considerations

Claustrophobia

Patients with claustrophobia may find it helpful to be given details about the operating room and sterile-draping requirements prior to surgery. The medical team can make accommodations for a patient who becomes anxious and extremely uncomfortable when confined to a small space or when covered by a surgical drape over the head. The anesthetist can titrate intravenous sedation and hold the patient's hand to provide comfort and reassurance. When feasible, the surgeon can supplement topical or local ocular anesthesia with soothing vocal support (ie, a "vocal local"). Options for reducing the sensation of claustrophobia and avoiding retention of carbon dioxide under the drape include placing a suction catheter under the drape, tenting open the side of the drape, or placing an elevated Mayo stand over the patient's torso. Using a transparent drape also can help mitigate claustrophobia. General anesthesia can be given when these measures are not adequate.

Neurocognitive and Neurodevelopmental Disorders

When dementia or other central nervous system impairment interferes with a patient's ability to communicate symptoms of cataract, the patient's functional deficit must be evaluated by other methods, such as discussion with surrogates about the patient's capacity to carry out activities of daily living. To estimate the visual impairment resulting from the cataract, the surgeon may have to rely on objective findings, such as degradation of the red reflex, slit-lamp abnormalities, and visualization of the retina, rather than subjective measurements of visual acuity. The patient's ability to tolerate sedation and draping throughout surgery must be appraised, and general anesthesia can be considered for the patient who cannot cooperate. When general anesthesia is required, the surgeon also may consider cataract extraction bilaterally in the same surgical session. In general, the decision to proceed with cataract extraction in complex cases is based on the following aims:

- potentially rehabilitating vision
- improving visualization of the fundus to monitor and treat retinal disease
- enhancing quality of life

Patient Communication During Eye Surgery

All patients benefit from a preoperative discussion of the surgical experience, especially those with hearing loss and those who speak a language different from the surgical team. For patients with bilateral hearing aids, the ipsilateral hearing aid often is removed to avoid the risk of water damage during surgery. Patients may wear their hearing aid in the ear contralateral to the eye being treated to allow communication. Moreover, the ipsilateral hearing aid can remain in place if it is covered carefully by multiple layers of occlusive dressing. The surgeon, anesthetist, and patient can determine how best to communicate in the operating room. Simple hand signals between the patient and the anesthetist can be effective. If the patient is very anxious and cannot communicate adequately, general anesthesia could be considered instead of topical or local anesthesia. However, light sedation combined with peribulbar or retrobulbar block often can allow for a safe procedure with decreased risk of postoperative delirium.

Systemic Considerations

Medical Status

Medical evaluation by the patient's primary care physician may be part of the preoperative planning process. Conditions such as hypertension and diabetes mellitus should be stabilized. Patients often are required to fast prior to surgery; insulin or oral hypoglycemic medication may need to be adjusted in diabetic patients. For these patients, it is preferable to schedule procedures early in the day to minimize large fluctuations in blood glucose levels.

In patients with lung disease, pulmonary function should be optimized prior to and during surgery; for instance, patients may be permitted to bring their inhalers into the operating room. Patients with lung disease may be prone to coughing, which can damage ocular structures during surgery and threaten wound security. Medication can be used to control coughing, and the patient can be advised to tell the surgeon of any need to cough. With small-incision surgery, the risk of such intraoperative complications can be reduced and wound security enhanced. Patients with chronic obstructive pulmonary disease (COPD), bronchitis, congestive heart failure, or obesity may benefit from being placed in the reverse Trendelenburg position to reduce venous congestion in the head and neck and lessen the risk of vitreous loss and choroidal hemorrhage.

Patients with severe arthritis may have difficulty lying comfortably during surgery. The surgical table can be adjusted, and pillows can be added to provide comfort without interfering with surgical access to the eye. Patients with ankylosing spondylitis and cervical immobility present an extreme challenge in surgical positioning (Fig 12-1); if no systemic medical contraindications exist and if adequate access cannot be attained otherwise, general anesthesia can be considered.

Patients with prostate conditions and those with hypertension may be on α-antagonist medication. The surgeon may encounter intraoperative floppy iris syndrome (IFIS) in these patients. Although no benefit has been shown for discontinuing the medication prior to surgery, special caution is warranted, and surgical modifications may be indicated (eg, intracameral lidocaine with epinephrine or pupillary expansion devices). For further discussion of ocular surgery in patients with systemic disease, see BCSC Section 1, *Update on General Medicine.*

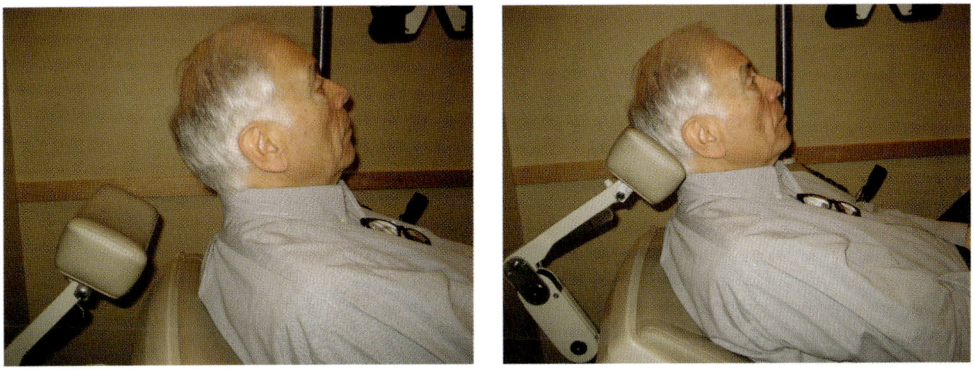

Figure 12-1 Inflammatory systemic disease. Individuals with ankylosing spondylitis, such as the patient shown in these photos, often have cervical immobility. Evaluating patients in the office examination chair allows the surgeon to anticipate accommodations necessary for carrying out surgery safely and comfortably for both patient and surgeon in the operating room. This patient requires adjustment of the headrest to provide adequate support of his head and neck. *(Courtesy of Lisa F. Rosenberg, MD.)*

Anticoagulation Therapy or Bleeding Disorders

In patients receiving anticoagulation therapy, clear corneal cataract surgery performed with topical anesthesia is not associated with an increased risk of vision-threatening hemorrhagic complications. Minor bleeding problems, such as eyelid ecchymosis, hyphema, and subconjunctival hemorrhage, are more common with anticoagulant use, but these are transient and self-limited. If a retrobulbar block is used, the risk of retrobulbar hemorrhage is higher in patients on anticoagulants. It is important to weigh the systemic risks of discontinuing anticoagulation or antiplatelet therapy with the surgical risks of continuing therapy. When warfarin is continued, the international normalized ratio (INR) is typically maintained within the therapeutic range.

If anticoagulation therapy is to be discontinued or adjusted for surgery, coordination with the prescribing physician is recommended. Discontinuation of anticoagulants is recommended in patients who have previously experienced a suprachoroidal hemorrhage because these patients are predisposed to recurrent bleeding. Time to restoration of normal coagulation is variable and depends on the specific anticoagulant in use; warfarin usually requires 3–5 days. Platelet function resumes 10–21 days after stopping antiplatelet therapy. Typically, it is recommended that patients restart anticoagulant or antiplatelet therapy within the first postoperative day. It is important to ask the patient about the use of all medications, including nonprescription items that may contain aspirin, vitamin E, or vitamin K, which could affect coagulation status. Table 12-1 presents a list of anticoagulant and antiplatelet agents approved by the US Food and Drug Administration (FDA).

In the absence of hypotony or hemorrhagic complications, anticoagulation therapy may be safely resumed following the first postoperative visit. The patient's coagulation profile should be reviewed preoperatively for systemic conditions that might alter clotting ability. For further discussion of ocular hemorrhage, see Chapter 10.

Grzybowski A, Ascaso FJ, Kupidura-Majewski K, Packer M. Continuation of anticoagulant and antiplatelet therapy during phacoemulsification cataract surgery. *Curr Opin Ophthalmol.* 2015;26(1):28–33.

Table 12-1 Anticoagulant and Antiplatelet Medications Approved by the US FDA[a]

Anticoagulants	Antiplatelet Agents
Apixaban (Eliquis)	Anagrelide (Agrylin)
Dabigatran (Pradaxa)	Aspirin/dipyridamole (Aggrenox)
Edoxaban (Savaysa)	Cilostazol (Pletal)
Enoxaparin (Lovenox)	Clopidogrel (Plavix)
Fondaparinux (Arixtra)	Dipyridamole (Persantine)
Rivaroxaban (Xarelto)	Prasugrel (Effient)
Warfarin (Coumadin)	Ticagrelor (Brilinta)
	Ticlopidine (Ticlid)
	Vorapaxar (Zontivity)

FDA = Food and Drug Administration.
[a]Approved as of 2019.

External Ocular Abnormalities

Blepharitis and Acne Rosacea

To reduce bacterial colony counts on the ocular surface, preoperative control of blepharitis, which is particularly common in patients with acne rosacea, is recommended. Uncontrolled blepharitis that causes irritation and an unhealthy tear film may adversely affect the quality of the patient's vision after cataract surgery. Treatments for anterior blepharitis include hot compresses and eyelid scrubs. The mainstay of therapy for meibomian gland dysfunction involves saponification of inspissated meibomian secretions with systemic tetracycline, doxycycline, or minocycline. Topical ointments poorly penetrate meibomian orifices, but newer topical eyedrops, such as azithromycin, reduce bacterial flora at the surface of the meibomian glands. Thermal pulsation or devices that clean the eyelid margin may improve eyelid hygiene preoperatively in severe cases. For a detailed description of the signs and symptoms of blepharitis, see BCSC Section 8, *External Disease and Cornea.*

Packer M, Chang DF, Dewey SH, et al. Prevention, diagnosis, and management of acute postoperative bacterial endophthalmitis. *J Cataract Refract Surg.* 2011;37(9):1699–1714.

Wykoff CC, Parrott MB, Flynn HW Jr, Shi W, Miller D, Alfonso EC. Nosocomial acute-onset postoperative endophthalmitis at a university teaching hospital (2002–2009). *Am J Ophthalmol.* 2010;150(3):392–398.

Keratoconjunctivitis Sicca

Optimizing therapy for dry eye disease (keratoconjunctivitis sicca, also known as dysfunctional tear syndrome) before cataract surgery improves visual outcomes. This can be especially important in patients who desire excellent refractive outcomes with the placement of premium intraocular lenses (IOLs), such as toric and multifocal lenses. There are numerous aqueous-layer supportive treatments, allowing for customization to the patient, including

- topical preserved and nonpreserved liquid tear preparations, gels, and ointments
- topical cyclosporine or lifitegrast
- punctal plugs

For additional detail on dry eye therapy, see BCSC Section 8, *External Disease and Cornea.*

During the procedure, the surgeon can prevent desiccation of the corneal epithelium by frequently hydrating the area with irrigating solution or by coating the cornea with a topical ophthalmic viscosurgical device (OVD). Visual recovery may be delayed if the dry eye condition is exacerbated; for such patients, preoperative or postoperative placement of punctal plugs can be helpful.

Patients with dry eyes associated with collagen vascular disease, rheumatoid arthritis, Sjögren syndrome, mucous membrane pemphigoid, or Stevens-Johnson syndrome present a special challenge to the cataract surgeon. Close observation of these patients in the weeks following surgery is warranted to identify and treat toxic keratoconjunctivitis and corneal ulceration resulting from collagenase activation secondary to postoperative corticosteroid therapy. If prescribed, topical nonsteroidal anti-inflammatory drugs (NSAIDs) should be used with caution because of the increased risk of corneal melting. In extreme cases, persistent epithelial defects with stromal loss may require a bandage (therapeutic) contact lens, tarsorrhaphy, or an amniotic membrane transplant.

Mucous Membrane Pemphigoid

Eyes with mucous membrane pemphigoid are severely dry due to scarring of the meibomian glands and accessory lacrimal glands that results in occlusion of the lacrimal gland orifices. Corneal haze or opacification impairs the surgeon's view into the anterior segment intraoperatively. Extensive symblepharon or ankyloblepharon may limit positioning and exposure of the eye during surgery. The eyelid speculum should be placed carefully to avoid traction and pressure on the globe.

Exposure Keratitis and Cranial Nerve VII Palsy

Patients with paralytic or mechanical eyelid abnormalities may have significant corneal dryness, which may be exacerbated by cataract surgery. Administration of topical anesthetics preoperatively may desiccate the corneal epithelium. A peribulbar or retrobulbar block can produce a neurotrophic cornea that persists for hours after surgery; a large corneal abrasion may also develop, unless a pressure patch is applied. Lubrication with antibiotic ointment may be necessary in the early postoperative period to facilitate healing of the epithelial surface and to control pain from an abrasion. Extended-wear therapeutic contact lenses can promote rapid healing of the epithelium and can be employed as a moisture chamber in cases of exposure keratitis, in conjunction with preventive local antibiotic treatment and patient adherence.

Corneal Pathologies

Corneal Disease

The cornea has the most refractive power of any structure in the eye. Preoperatively, the surgeon evaluates the cornea for abnormalities that might impair vision and diminish the expected improvement in vision:

- corneal scars
- tear film abnormalities (these should be addressed as described in the previous section Blepharitis and Acne Rosacea)
- epithelial basement membrane dystrophy
- irregular astigmatism (this can be assessed by corneal topography and masked by a gas-permeable trial contact lens to determine the effect on vision impairment)

Corneal irregularities affect the accuracy of keratometry and lead to erroneous calculation of lens power. In an eye with epithelial basement membrane dystrophy, epithelial debridement may help produce a smoother corneal surface (Fig 12-2). After debridement, it is necessary to wait a few weeks before repeating keratometry so the corneal surface can

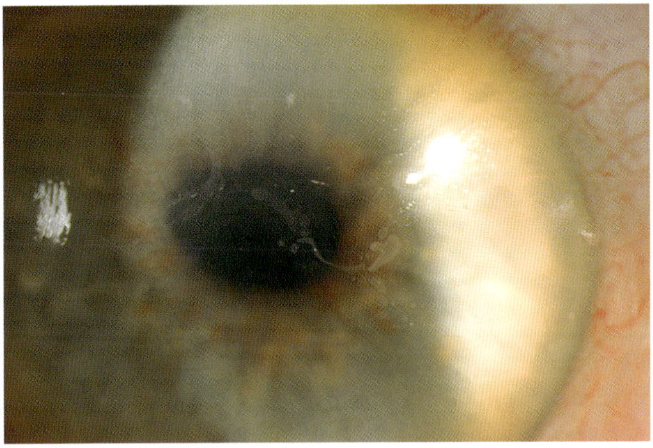

Figure 12-2 Irregular corneal astigmatism occurs in patients with epithelial basement membrane dystrophy. This corneal condition can further decrease vision in a patient with cataract-related vision impairment, in which case the vision improvement after cataract surgery might be less than expected. *(Courtesy of Christopher J. Rapuano, MD.)*

become smooth and stable. Mild corneal stromal opacities are unlikely to reduce vision in the presence of a pristine anterior refractive surface.

In patients with a history of herpes simplex virus (HSV) infection, epithelial or stromal keratitis may be exacerbated after cataract surgery. Although the Herpetic Eye Disease Study (HEDS) did not specifically address HSV following surgery, the results did show that prophylactic treatment with oral acyclovir (400 mg, twice daily) reduces the incidence of recurrent HSV keratitis. Because recurrent stromal keratitis may result in loss of visual acuity, many ophthalmologists use oral acyclovir, famciclovir, or valacyclovir perioperatively and observe the patient closely for recurrent keratitis postoperatively.

Cataract surgery in patients with keratoconus poses a challenge in IOL calculation. These patients have increased potential for unexpected refractive outcomes, given the irregular astigmatism and potentially abnormal keratometry values. Preoperatively, it is important to inform patients with significant keratoconus that they likely will need contact lens correction of the irregular astigmatism after cataract surgery. The surgeon can attempt to stabilize the keratoconus, if possible (eg, with collagen crosslinking) to predict the refractive outcome more accurately.

Cataract and Keratoplasty

When both cataract and corneal opacity contribute to a patient's vision loss, the surgeon has 3 options:

1. Remove the cataract first.
2. Repair the cornea first.
3. Combine the procedures.

Removing the cataract first requires adequate visualization of the anterior segment. It may be possible to remove the cataract and monitor the patient for worsening corneal opacity; however, eyes that exhibit corneal endothelial dysfunction are at higher risk of corneal decompensation following cataract surgery. Signs and symptoms of corneal endothelial dysfunction are microcystic edema, stromal thickening, low cell count on specular microscopy, and/or diurnal fluctuations in vision with prolonged blurred vision upon waking. Keratoplasty is indicated in these eyes.

A penetrating keratoplasty (PKP) or an endothelial keratoplasty (EK) may be performed, either as primary surgery or as part of a combined procedure with cataract extraction (ie, a triple procedure). The advantages of performing keratoplasty as a stand-alone procedure include less postoperative inflammation and more reliable keratometry readings for future calculation of IOL power. In patients with primarily corneal endothelial disease, the advantages of EK over PKP include faster rehabilitation and more dependable keratometry readings with which to calculate IOL power, although a hyperopic shift from 0.50 D to 1.50 D may be encountered.

A triple procedure (combined keratoplasty [PKP or EK], cataract extraction, and IOL implantation) may be chosen if both the cataract and the corneal disease are significant and the patient would benefit from concurrent treatment. Advantages of the triple procedure include a single visit to the operating room, which reduces the attendant perioperative surgical risks, and relatively rapid rehabilitation. Disadvantages of PKP with cataract surgery are decreased predictability of IOL calculation and a period of "open sky"; that is, exposure of the intraocular contents while the cataract is removed and the IOL is placed, prior to replacement of the corneal button. IOL power calculation may be less reliable for eyes that have undergone PKP than for those that have undergone EK.

In conjunction with cataract surgery, the advantages of EK (vs PKP) include the following:

- faster corneal rehabilitation
- higher likelihood of regular astigmatism postsurgically
- relative ease of regrafting

The disadvantages of EK (versus PK) in conjunction with cataract surgery include the following:

- potential for damage to grafted corneal endothelium resulting from the additional entry into the anterior chamber (AC)
- possible disruption of the graft

Patients with EK often have hyperopic shifts from their corneal surgeries; therefore, when this procedure is combined with cataract surgery, it is preferable to aim for a slightly myopic correction. Cornea surgeons often find EK easier to perform in a pseudophakic eye than in a phakic eye. (For a detailed discussion of keratoplasty procedures, see BCSC Section 8, *External Disease and Cornea.*)

Even if the cataract is not the primary source of vision impairment, it may be advisable to extract it at time of corneal surgery because of the eventual need for cataract removal, the possible progression of cataract due to prolonged postoperative corticosteroid therapy, and the risk of additional damage to the corneal endothelium during secondary surgery.

Hwang RY, Gauthier DJ, Wallace D, Afshari NA. Refractive changes after Descemet stripping endothelial keratoplasty: a simplified mathematical model. *Invest Ophthalmol Vis.* 2011; 52(2):1043–1054.

Cataract Following Keratoplasty

Cataract formation soon after keratoplasty may be caused by lens trauma during the transplantation procedure or by prolonged corticosteroid use to prevent graft rejection. It is preferable to delay cataract surgery in an eye with a history of PKP until the corneal contour and surface are stable and reliable keratometry readings are obtained. The probability of graft survival 5 years after cataract surgery is at least 80%; nevertheless, a corneal graft may not survive even routine cataract surgery.

Preoperatively, the surgeon evaluates the corneal graft for thickening and anticipated reduced intraoperative clarity through the graft. A scleral tunnel approach has the benefits of being farther from the corneal transplant and minimizing endothelial trauma during surgery. The risk of postoperative graft failure is lowest when the corneal endothelium is protected with a dispersive OVD during surgery and when postoperative inflammation is aggressively treated.

Selecting the IOL power before the cornea is fully healed can lead to implantation of an incorrectly powered IOL and symptomatic anisometropia. Posterior chamber lenses are preferred because they minimize contact between the optic and the corneal endothelium. If capsular support is inadequate for IOL placement in the capsular bag (ie, "in-the-bag"), a posterior chamber scleral fixation or iris suture may be placed. If the additional manipulation required for a sutured lens poses a risk of excessive endothelial trauma, insertion of a flexible anterior chamber IOL (ACIOL) is an option. A modified IOL target may be considered in patients who have had previous corneal transplantation and are undergoing cataract surgery. The goal of this is to balance the 2 eyes.

Cataract Following Refractive Surgery

Patients who have undergone corneal refractive surgery and later develop a visually significant cataract present several unique challenges. Measurement of corneal power after refractive surgery is problematic, requiring multiple instruments and/or formulas to try to determine the new corneal power. Moreover, accurate axial length measurement (eg, with optical biometry) is required. Advanced IOL calculations are used to determine the appropriate power. (For a detailed discussion of IOL power calculation, see Chapter 7 in this volume and BCSC Section 13, *Refractive Surgery*.) Irregular astigmatism resulting from a refractive surgical procedure may compromise the ultimate vision outcome after cataract removal (Fig 12-3). Because unanticipated postoperative refractive results may occur, it is important to inform the patient about the limits of precision in lens power calculation and the possible requirement for postsurgical refractive correction to obtain optimal vision.

In general, postoperative hyperopia is more commonly encountered after cataract surgery in patients who have undergone previous refractive surgery. The corneal refractive incisions in eyes that have undergone radial keratotomy (RK) often swell after cataract surgery, thereby flattening the cornea and inducing hyperopia. Swelling may require more

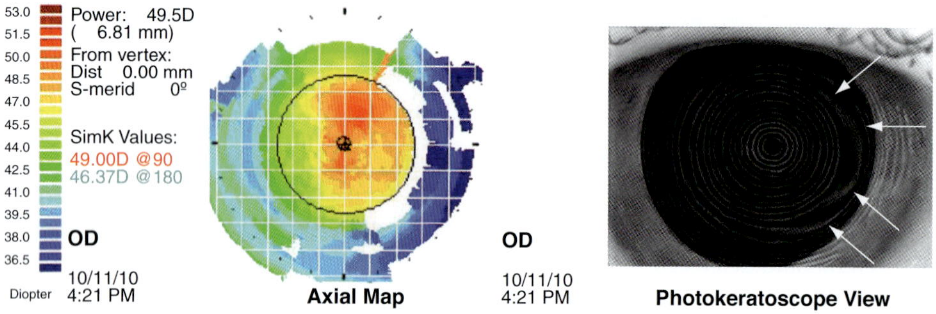

Figure 12-3 Accurate lens implant power is difficult to determine when the corneal surface is abnormal, as shown here by an irregular corneal topographic map *(left)* and distorted corneal rings *(right, arrows)*. *(Courtesy of Lisa F. Rosenberg, MD.)*

than 3 months to resolve. If a clear corneal incision is chosen, it should be placed between the RK incisions. Violating a prior RK incision can destabilize the wound, causing it to pull apart. The presence of multiple deep RK incisions or unstable wounds increases the likelihood of AC shallowing during cataract surgery and makes final closure of the wound difficult. Unless adequate clearance between RK incisions can be ensured with a clear corneal approach, a scleral tunnel incision is preferable to reduce the likelihood of violating an RK incision.

In eyes that have undergone laser in situ keratomileusis (LASIK), the surgeon should make the clear corneal cataract incisions posterior enough and avoid a long tunnel that could disrupt the LASIK flap. Corneal swelling after LASIK may require more than 1 month to resolve. Cataract surgery in eyes that have undergone photorefractive keratectomy (PRK) does not present the same type of technical challenges of surgery in post-LASIK eyes.

Because patients who have undergone refractive surgery may have corneal aberrations from the initial surgery, it is important to carefully assess the use of multifocal, extended depth of focus, or toric lenses.

Compromised Visualization of the Lens

Small Pupil

Operating through a small pupil may increase the risk of intraoperative complications. It is important to note the maximum pharmacologic pupil dilation in the preoperative evaluation. A small pupil that is minimally responsive to dilating agents may be widened intraoperatively. The pupil can be bimanually stretched with Kuglen or Lester hooks, the iris can be tethered with hooks (Fig 12-4), or pupil-expansion devices can be employed (Fig 12-5). Viscodilation with a high-viscosity OVD is another method for pupil enlargement. These maneuvers break posterior synechiae and release the pupillary sphincter. However, with excessive manipulation of the iris, the risk of postoperative inflammation

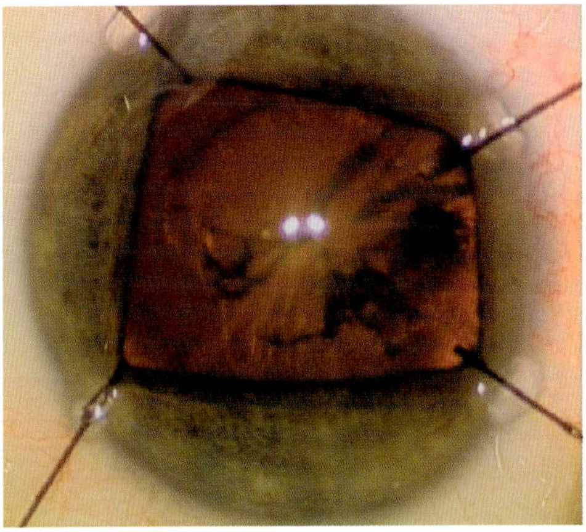

Figure 12-4 A pupil that dilates insufficiently to allow access to the lens may be widened with iris hooks. In this case, 4 hooks are placed to expose the lens for surgery. *(Courtesy of Lisa F. Rosenberg, MD.)*

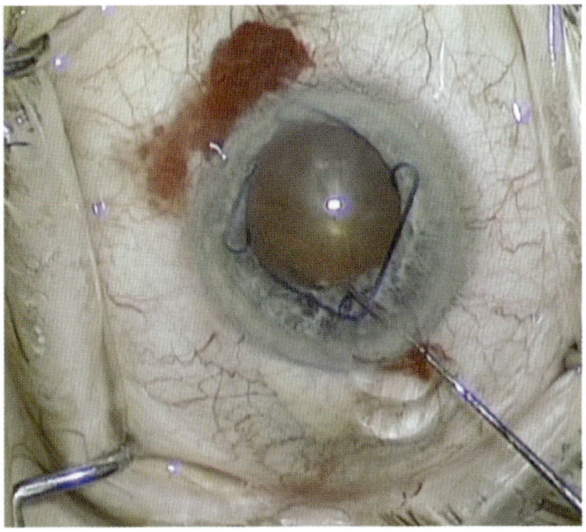

Figure 12-5 A Malyugin ring is positioned at the pupillary margin circumferentially. *(Courtesy of Steven Vold, MD.)*

increases. Also, because the iris tends to be flaccid and floppy after manual stretching and release, it is more likely to be damaged by the phaco tip.

To enlarge a small pupil resulting from IFIS, most surgeons prefer to use pupil-expansion devices because unless the pupil is held open mechanically, progressive miosis of the floppy iris tends to occur as the surgery proceeds (Video 12-1). IFIS is a common cause of small pupils; as discussed in detail in Chapter 10, planned adjustments can be considered.

VIDEO 12-1 Malyugin ring insertion.
Courtesy of Boris Malyugin, MD, PhD.
Go to www.aao.org/bcscvideo_section11 to access all videos in Section 11.

Poor Red Reflex

As discussed in Chapter 8, creation of a continuous curvilinear capsulorrhexis (CCC) is a key component of safe phacoemulsification. An abnormal red reflex makes it difficult for the surgeon to discriminate the capsular edge, thus increasing the risk of an incomplete or errant capsulorrhexis. In an eye with dense brunescent or cortical cataract, the capsule is prone to radial tears. The tears result from vaulting of the anterior capsule, caused by increased lens thickness and cortical hydration. Corneal scars compromise the surgeon's view of the capsule and make intraocular manipulation treacherous. These challenges can be addressed by staining the capsule with trypan blue (Fig 12-6).

Prior to capsulotomy, AC fluid can be replaced with air, and a small amount of OVD can be used to occlude the paracentesis site. Alternatively, a high-viscosity OVD can be

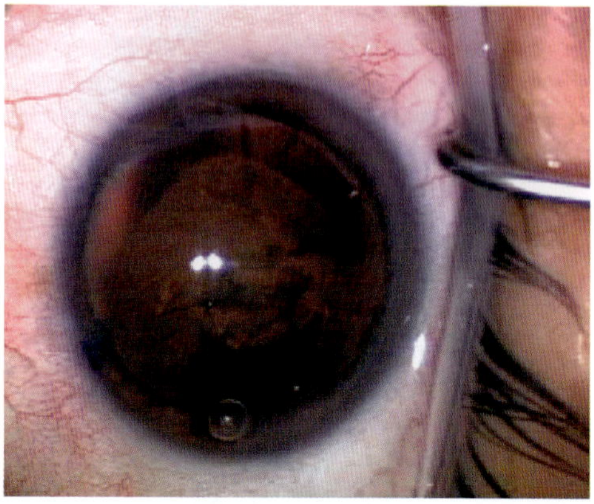

Figure 12-6 The anterior capsule is stained lightly with trypan blue, thereby aiding visualization of the capsule during creation of a capsulorrhexis. This technique is helpful in eyes with dense brunescent or cortical cataracts that interfere with the red reflex. *(Courtesy of Lisa F. Rosenberg, MD.)*

instilled to fill approximately two-thirds of the anterior chamber. The surgeon then injects trypan blue through a 27-gauge blunt cannula, starting as far away from the paracentesis incision as possible to deliver the dye directly to the capsule. In the presence of a healthy endothelium, the trypan blue can be injected without prior air or viscoelastic injection. Usually, the dye is then rinsed from the AC with balanced salt solution and replaced with a high-viscosity OVD, under which the stained anterior capsule is easily visible. The high-viscosity OVD exerts pressure on the anterior capsule, maintaining chamber depth and flattening the capsule to prevent radial extension of the capsular tear. A CCC is then created (Video 12-2).

VIDEO 12-2 Capsule staining with trypan blue dye.
Courtesy of Lisa Park, MD.

Jacobs DS, Cox TA, Wagoner MD, Ariyasu RG, Karp CL; American Academy of Ophthalmology; Ophthalmic Technology Assessment Committee Anterior Segment Panel. Capsule staining as an adjunct to cataract surgery: a report from the American Academy of Ophthalmology. *Ophthalmology.* 2006;113(4):707–713.

Altered Lens and Zonular Anatomy

Intumescent Cataract

A cataract that is swollen with cortical material and often envelops a hard nucleus floating within the capsular bag is described as *intumescent.* This type of cataract presents specific challenges during phacoemulsification cataract surgery. Intumescent cataracts have weak zonular fibers and fragile capsules. Because intumescence creates positive pressure in the capsular bag, the initial incision in the capsule may extend peripherally (Video 12-3; also see the sidebar).

VIDEO 12-3 Intumescent mature cataract.
Courtesy of Virgilio Centurion, MD, and Juan Carlos Caballero, MD.

PROPOSED INTERVENTIONS TO REDUCE THE INTRAOPERATIVE COMPLICATIONS ASSOCIATED WITH INTUMESCENT CATARACT

1. Stain the capsule with trypan blue and fill the AC with a high-viscosity OVD (as described in the previous section Poor Red Reflex).
2. Prior to capsulotomy, place a 25- or 27-gauge needle attached to a syringe at the center of the anterior capsule. While suction is applied, use the needle to pierce the anterior capsule, and aspirate the milky cortex. This decompresses the lens to avoid radial extension of the CCC.
3. Use a cystotome attached to the OVD syringe during creation of the CCC to enable injection of additional OVDs, which will clear away the milky egress.
4. Use caution during phacoemulsification, because the freely mobile lens, without an epinuclear barrier, makes segmentation challenging.

Advanced Cataract

In eyes with dense, brunescent cataracts, surgical manipulation increases the risks of iris trauma, zonular tearing, capsular rupture, vitreous loss, and the dropping of lens fragments into the posterior segment. The increased ultrasound energy required for phacoemulsification of dense lenses increases the risk of endothelial trauma and wound burn. Creation of a larger capsulorrhexis is helpful because it allows the surgeon to perform the maneuvers that are necessary to minimize these complications. Thorough hydrodissection and hydrodelineation of the nucleus facilitate smooth rotation during phacoemulsification. When an initial groove is made in the hard nucleus, it is important that the surgeon make a deep and even pass. The aim is to crack the nucleus without leaving interdigitations, which would interfere with removal and potentially result in rupture of the posterior capsule. Viscodissection helps separate sticky cortical attachments that impede rotation. If the surgeon uses excessive mechanical force on a nucleus that does not freely rotate, zonular dialysis may result from transmittal of that force to the capsular bag. Mechanical segmentation techniques for nucleus disassembly, such as vertical and horizontal chopping, require less ultrasound energy and may induce less zonular stress than the "divide and conquer" method (see Chapter 8). Familiarity with multiple techniques, and the ability to switch from 1 technique to another as the situation requires, enables the surgeon to minimize complications.

If phacoemulsification ceases to be appropriate for lens removal, conversion to an extracapsular technique can be considered. The surgeon may proceed through the corneal incision, enlarging it to permit passage of the cataract and lens implant. Alternatively, the surgeon may close the corneal wound and make a new, larger corneoscleral incision. Often, a corneoscleral incision is more stable than a large corneal wound and induces less astigmatism postoperatively.

Iris Coloboma and Corectopia

Zonular dehiscence or absence commonly occurs in the area of iris coloboma (Fig 12-7A) or a misshapen pupil. Pharmacologic dilation can be carried out to assess the extent of zonular abnormality. Iris hooks can be used intraoperatively to pull a flaccid iris out of the way. A capsular tension ring (CTR) that incorporates a coloboma diaphragm (Fig 12-7B) helps stabilize the capsular bag and serves as an artificial iris diaphragm. The surgeon also has the option of repairing the coloboma with a suture at the conclusion of the case. When the iris defect is sufficiently large to indicate the use of a prosthesis, the surgeon can implant an artificial iris.

Posterior Polar Cataract

A weak or absent area of the posterior lens capsule in the region of a posterior polar opacity places the eye at increased risk of capsular rupture during surgery. Accordingly, the surgeon should avoid exerting excessive pressure within the capsular bag or on the posterior capsule. Complete hydrodissection is also avoided because of possible tearing of the capsule directly under the opacity. Instead, the following procedure is undertaken:

1. Deliver small volumes of fluid around the cortex up to, but not across, the opacity.
2. Perform gentle hydrodelineation, leaving a generous amount of epinuclear bowl in which to mobilize the nucleus and protect the capsule.
3. Maintain the AC depth and limit fluctuations in IOP by low irrigation and aspiration.

After the nucleus is removed, OVD is used for viscodissection of the epinucleus from the capsular bag. The posterior polar opacity is removed last; viscodissection can be performed for this step as well. If the central portion of the posterior capsule is missing,

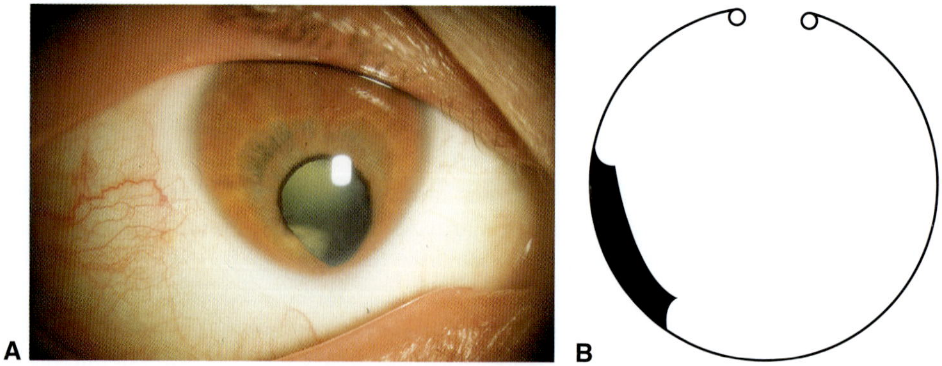

Figure 12-7 Zonular dehiscence or absence is common in iris coloboma. **A,** Coloboma of the iris with nuclear cataract. Absent or abnormal zonular fibers correlate with the area of the iris defect. A preoperative evaluation of associated posterior segment abnormalities is an important way to assess vision potential. **B,** Capsular tension ring with coloboma diaphragm. *Note:* This device is not approved by the US Food and Drug Administration; compassionate use is available. *(Part A courtesy of Robert S. Feder, MD; part B illustration by Natalie A. Afshari, MD.)*

filling the capsular bag with OVD before removing the irrigating phaco handpiece from the eye will stabilize the chamber for lens insertion. Alternatively, if the posterior polar opacity is very adherent, it can be left in place, assessed for its impact on vision postoperatively, and treated with laser capsulotomy, if indicated. After the IOL is placed in the capsular bag in an uncomplicated procedure, movement of the bag can be minimized with slow and gentle OVD removal.

Zonular Dehiscence With Lens Subluxation or Dislocation

Common causes of zonular incompetence include pseudoexfoliation syndrome (Fig 12-8), ocular trauma, prior vitrectomy, prior trabeculectomy, and high myopia. Marfan syndrome, Ehlers-Danlos syndrome, homocystinuria, hyperlysinemia, and Weill-Marchesani syndrome are less-common sources of inadequate zonular support. Iridodonesis, detected at the slit lamp, is often an initial finding that signals zonular weakness or absence. If the entire lens becomes dislocated into the posterior segment, surgical removal of the lens may not be necessary, unless uveitis develops. In some eyes, the remaining zonular fibers tether the lens within the anterior vitreous such that when the patient sits upright at the slit lamp, the lens seems accessible for extraction. However, when that patient is supine during surgery, the lens tilts backward, out of the surgeon's reach. Thus, when iridodonesis or phacodonesis is detected preoperatively, it is helpful to confirm lens position with the patient supine during the preoperative examination.

Zonular status may be determined by direct visualization of the lens equator through a widely dilated pupil or by use of a goniolens to visualize zonular fibers behind the dilated pupil. If zonular disruption is extensive preoperatively, the surgeon may consider removal

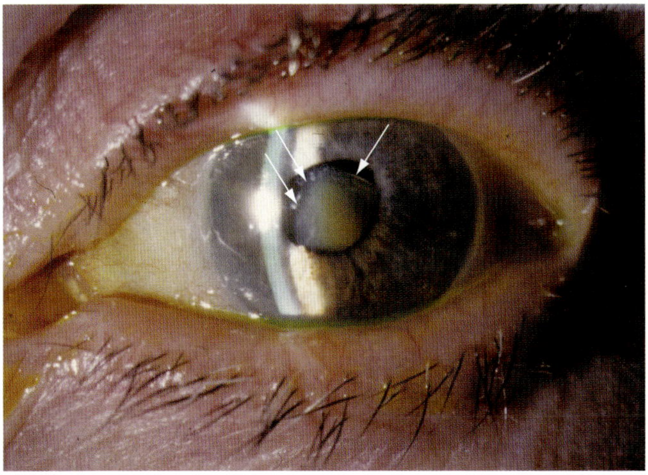

Figure 12-8 Subluxed lens. This lens with pseudoexfoliation is displaced inferiorly because zonular fibers at the superior edge of the lens are stretched, damaged, or broken. *Arrows* indicate the superior edge of the inferiorly displaced lens. Cataract surgery on a displaced lens requires meticulous preoperative planning to minimize surgical complications. *(Courtesy of Lisa F. Rosenberg, MD.)*

of the cataract using one of the following:

- extracapsular cataract extraction (ECCE)
- intracapsular cataract extraction (ICCE)
- phacoemulsification with capsular hooks followed by suturing a capsular segment to stabilize the capsule during and after surgery (see the Appendix)

Zonular incompetence becomes apparent intraoperatively with phacodonesis, decentration of the capsular bag, and sometimes vitreous prolapse into the AC. If phacodonesis prevents the use of a CCC or if zonular disruption is extensive, the surgeon may convert from phacoemulsification to ECCE or ICCE. Otherwise, phacoemulsification can proceed safely with application of the same measures recommended in the Advanced Cataract section, earlier in this chapter. Reducing the flow rate diminishes turbulence and fluctuation in AC depth, lowering the risk of vitreous prolapse through the area of zonular absence. A larger capsulorrhexis enables easier separation of lens components within the capsular bag. Thorough hydrodissection and hydrodelineation of the nucleus facilitate smooth rotation during phacoemulsification. Viscodissection helps separate cortical attachments that may impede rotation. Excessive mechanical maneuvers in the nucleus, cortical aspiration, and inadvertent aspiration of the anterior capsule edge contribute to further zonular compromise. Viscodissection of cortical remnants and IOL insertion prior to complete cortical removal are maneuvers that help maintain capsular integrity. Tangential, rather than radial, removal of cortex from the bag minimizes zonular stress. Pars plana lensectomy may be preferred to lens extraction in cases of severe zonular loss and in the absence of contraindicating ocular comorbidities.

If capsular support is insufficient for safe phacoemulsification, capsular hooks, a CTR, or CTR segments can be used (Videos 12-4, 12-5). Capsular hooks (Fig 12-9) support the anterior capsule edge in the area of weakened zonular fibers. They are placed through paracentesis incisions, and adjustment of tension on each hook centers the capsule for phacoemulsification. CTRs provide support by exerting an outward force against the capsule equator in areas of absent or weakened zonular fibers.

VIDEO 12-4 Insertion of capsular tension ring.
Courtesy of David F. Chang, MD.

VIDEO 12-5 Capsule hooks and capsular tension ring.
Courtesy of David F. Chang, MD.

Radial tension may further extend the capsular defect. Therefore, placement of either capsular hooks or a CTR may be cautiously considered if the anterior capsule is torn radially or if the capsulorrhexis is interrupted. The ring can be used in patients with posterior capsule defects as long as the anterior rhexis remains continuous; its use is controversial in the presence of a noncontinuous rhexis. With a CTR in position, the surgeon can proceed to nuclear and cortical removal more safely and can place the chosen IOL in the capsular bag (ie, an "in-the-bag" IOL). Insufficient zonular support can also be managed with a

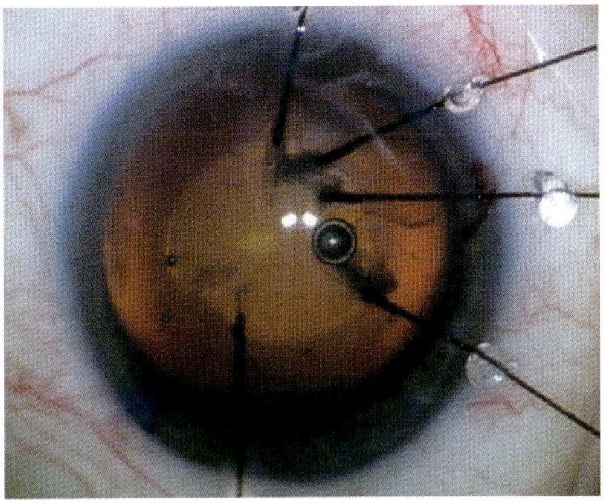

Figure 12-9 Hooks are placed around the anterior capsule edge to stabilize the capsular bag during phacoemulsification in this eye with a subluxed lens. Trypan blue is used to aid visualization of the capsular edge. *(Courtesy of Lisa F. Rosenberg, MD.)*

modified CTR or CTR segment sutured to the scleral wall. If there is severe instability, the help of a vitreoretinal surgeon may be enlisted to employ a pars plana approach.

If zonular support is insufficient to use a 1-piece IOL in the capsular bag, the surgeon can choose from the following options:

- a 3-piece IOL with the haptics placed in the location of zonular weakness
- a 3-piece IOL placed in the ciliary sulcus (with or without optic capture)
- a transscleral-fixated or iris-fixated posterior chamber IOL (PCIOL)
- an ACIOL

It is preferable to avoid the use of premium IOLs, such as multifocal and toric lenses, in eyes with capsular decentration or significant potential for decentration.

Crandall AS, Slade DS. Placement of endocapsular IOLs in eyes with zonular compromise. *Focal Points: Clinical Modules for Ophthalmologists.* American Academy of Ophthalmology; 2014, module 7.

Pseudoexfoliation Syndrome

Eyes with pseudoexfoliation are characterized by poor pupillary dilation and weakened zonular fibers. These findings increase the likelihood of intraoperative complications such as lens dislocation, capsular rupture, and vitreous loss. Safe cataract surgery in these eyes involves the same techniques as in eyes with advanced cataract and zonular dehiscence (discussed earlier in this chapter). Progressive capsular contraction, or capsular phimosis, is common in eyes with pseudoexfoliation. Dislocation of the implant into the vitreous is also possible. Careful consideration of the style and placement of the chosen lens implant is important. Capsular contraction is less likely with a 3-piece lens placed inside the capsular bag. If capsular phimosis occurs, a Nd:YAG laser may be used to create radial incisions in the anterior capsule to release tension on the zonular fibers and maintain the lens centrally.

Cataract in Aniridia

The lens capsule in patients with aniridia is thin and fragile, which makes performing a capsulorrhexis more challenging. Ideally, the edge of a well-centered capsulorrhexis overlaps the optic edge by 1 mm. Corneal haze and neovascularization are common in these eyes because of stem cell deficiency; capsular staining may aid visualization through the cornea during creation of an adequately sized capsular opening. Use of a high-viscosity OVD also optimizes visualization while stabilizing the capsular surface. The surgeon should avoid working inside the capsular bag, which could place tension on the capsular rim. Low infusion helps reduce turbulence and capsular fluctuation. The capsule in aniridic eyes acts as a pseudoiris when it opacifies.

Conditions Associated With Extremes in Axial Length

High Myopia

When the surgeon introduces the phaco tip into the anterior chamber of a highly myopic eye, the chamber may deepen dramatically, making lens manipulation difficult. To avoid extensive deepening of the anterior chamber, the surgeon is advised to lower the irrigation bottle and increase the flow rate before entering the eye with the phaco tip. Placing a second instrument between the iris and the anterior capsule prior to turning on infusion may prevent excess deepening. Despite this maneuver, high-myopic eyes are susceptible to lens–iris diaphragm retropulsion syndrome (LIDRS), wherein 360° of iridocapsular contact occurs, causing reverse pupillary block, pupillary dilation, and pain. A defect or laxity in the zonular fibers predisposes myopic eyes to LIDRS. Manual separation of the iris from the anterior capsule rim using a sideport instrument corrects the situation (see Chapter 10).

It is important to calculate IOL power preoperatively for myopic eyes to determine whether a special-order IOL, such as a plano-power or minus-power implant, is required. It is preferable that the patient receive an IOL when possible; the lens implant serves as a barrier to movement of the vitreous base and associated traction on the retina. Because myopic eyes are at increased risk of retinal detachment postoperatively, acrylic lens implants are favored when there is a strong possibility that the patient will later undergo a vitreoretinal surgery. During vitreoretinal surgery involving an open posterior capsule, silicone IOLs develop condensation that compromises visualization into the eye. Silicone lenses have also been observed to migrate through the capsular opening into the vitreous.

To avoid unexpected difficulty with glasses postoperatively, it is helpful to discuss anisometropia with patients who have high myopia and do not wear a contact lens in the other eye.

High Hyperopia and Nanophthalmos

An eye with cataract and high hyperopia often has a shallow AC and is prone to uveal prolapse, iris damage, and excessive corneal endothelial trauma during cataract surgery. Deepening of the AC and protection of intraocular tissue can be achieved with a high-viscosity OVD, a low aspiration rate, and elevation of the irrigation bottle prior to insertion of the phaco tip. Mannitol may be administered preoperatively to dehydrate the vitreous volume in a patient with no systemic contraindications. Iris prolapse is avoided by entering through an anterior corneal incision and by taking care not to overfill the eye with OVDs. If all these measures fail to provide sufficient AC volume for cataract removal, a small amount of liquid vitreous can be withdrawn using a 25-gauge needle or a vitrectomy handpiece through a pars plana puncture.

Nanophthalmos is a rare condition in which the eye is extremely short and the ratio of lens volume to eye volume is larger than normal. Diagnostic criteria vary, but these eyes generally have shallow anterior chambers, narrow angles, and thickened sclerae, with little room for the surgeon to maneuver. Axial length is shortened by at least 2 standard deviations below age-matched controls—usually to 20 mm or less. Small-incision bimanual surgery may be considered for these eyes. Because nanophthalmic eyes are at high risk of uveal effusion, precautions include the following measures:

- Maintaining positive pressure in the AC and limiting the length of the procedure help prevent intraoperative uveal effusion.
- Scleral windows can be considered as a prophylactic measure.
- Suturing the wound helps prevent hypotony and consequent uveal effusion postoperatively.

Hypotony

A shortened axial length with choroidal thickening is often accompanied by chronic hypotony and posterior scleral flattening. Hypotony makes biometry technically challenging and complicates calculation of IOL power. The clinician should attempt to determine the cause of hypotony and undertake specific treatment before cataract surgery. If the cataract obscures examination of the posterior segment, B-scan ultrasonography is helpful in revealing posterior segment pathology. A cyclodialysis cleft or retinal detachment requires a more extensive procedure when combined with cataract surgery. Severe hypotony or prephthisis is a poor prognostic indicator for improvement in vision after cataract extraction.

Glaucoma

Assessment

When cataract surgery is being considered in a patient with glaucoma, it is important to assess how well the glaucoma is controlled preoperatively. It can be challenging to predict the visual outcome in an eye with both cataract and glaucoma because both conditions can contribute to blurred vision, and the patient's visual symptoms may not be exclusively attributable to 1 condition or the other. An advanced visual field defect may limit vision improvement after cataract surgery. In contrast, an advanced cataract may exaggerate a mild visual field abnormality (Fig 12-10). Surgical options include cataract surgery alone, combined cataract and glaucoma surgery, and staged procedures of glaucoma surgery (eg, trabeculectomy or drainage device) followed by cataract surgery in a subsequent session. Uncomplicated phacoemulsification alone may lower the long-term IOP by 10%–34%. Minimally invasive glaucoma surgery (MIGS) can be combined with cataract extraction to further reduce IOP in a blebless, conjunctiva-sparing manner. Small-incision cataract

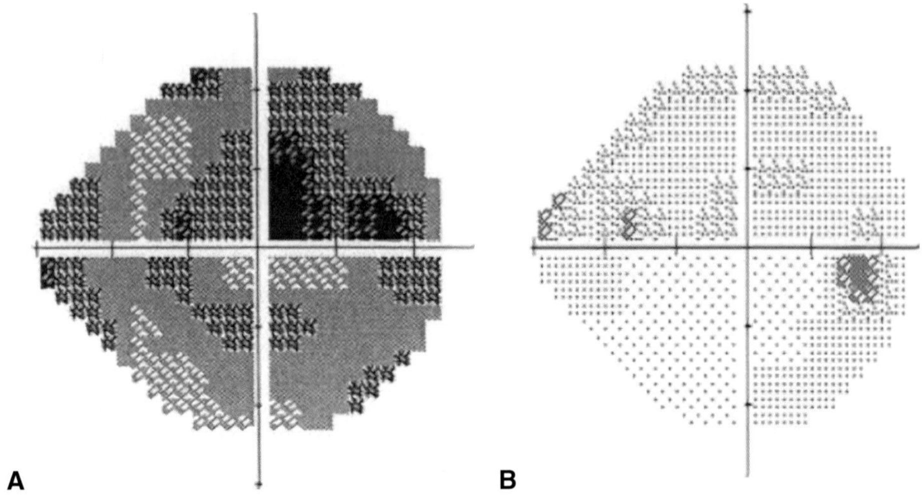

Figure 12-10 Visual field before and after cataract surgery. Media opacity, such as cataract, can impair the visual field. **A,** An abnormal Humphrey visual field in a glaucoma patient with a dense cataract. **B,** Improved Humphrey visual field following cataract removal and lens implantation. *(Courtesy of Lisa F. Rosenberg, MD.)*

surgery with a clear corneal approach minimizes conjunctival damage; this is essential if filtering surgery is required in the future. In an eye with a functioning filtering bleb, a small incision in a temporal or superotemporal location makes cataract surgery straightforward and is less likely to compromise IOP control. Issues influencing determination of the surgical approach include

- preoperative IOP
- desired postoperative IOP
- degree of damage to the optic nerve and visual field
- number of medications required to control IOP
- expected patient adherence to the medication regimen
- potential adverse effects of the medications
- potential impact on quality of life

Surgical decision making in the glaucomatous eye and combined cataract and glaucoma surgery are discussed in BCSC Section 10, *Glaucoma.*

Most surgical challenges in eyes with both glaucoma and cataract are not unique. For instance, zonular compromise and phacodonesis can complicate capsulorrhexis creation and lens removal in eyes with traumatic or pseudoexfoliation glaucoma. When a patent peripheral iridotomy (PI) is performed, the surgeon may inadvertently hydrate the vitreous; and caution is advised while injecting dye into the AC to avoid vitreous staining by injecting dye through the PI. Uveitic glaucoma and miotic therapy may limit pupillary dilation and increase the risk of postoperative macular edema. After surgery, the IOP can increase, owing to retained OVDs or inflammation, and pressures rise to a higher level in glaucomatous eyes with reduced outflow through the trabecular meshwork.

The use of topical prostaglandin medication may be associated with postoperative cystoid macular edema (CME), although there are few proven cases. In part, this is because clinically significant CME after uncomplicated phacoemulsification occurs only in rare instances. In cases of early postoperative CME, discontinuation of the prostaglandin is advisable to determine whether this medication is contributing to the edema.

Cataract Surgery in an Eye With a Functioning Filter

Small-incision cataract surgery can be performed in glaucomatous eyes without affecting the results of the previous filtering surgery. With a temporal corneal incision, the surgeon avoids the superior conjunctiva and the site in which filtering surgery was conducted. If conversion to an extracapsular technique is indicated (eg, in extreme phacodonesis with zonular instability or in capsular rupture with vitreous present in the AC), the surgeon may extend the clear corneal or scleral incision to permit removal of the crystalline lens. Closure of the temporal incision and creation of a larger corneoscleral incision superiorly can minimize astigmatism but also may compromise an existing filter. Aggressive control of postoperative inflammation is vital to ensure continued bleb function.

Francis BA, Singh K, Lin SC, et al. Novel glaucoma procedures: a report by the American Academy of Ophthalmology. *Ophthalmology.* 2011;118(7):1466–1480.

Combining Minimally Invasive Glaucoma Surgery With Cataract Surgery

MIGS comprises a diverse group of IOP-lowering procedures that have a better safety profile than do trabeculectomy and glaucoma drainage devices. Performing MIGS at the time of cataract extraction can benefit patients with mild to moderate glaucoma, especially those who cannot adhere to or tolerate IOP-lowering eyedrops. Even a modest pressure decrease following a combined MIGS/cataract surgery may lead to future dependency on fewer classes of eyedrops. This translates to improvement in quality of life.

Surgeons performing MIGS may utilize FDA-approved ab interno trabeculectomy devices, such as blades (eg, Trabectome [Kahook]), Schlemm canal implants (eg, iStent [Glaukos]), the Hydrus Microstent (Ivantis), and subconjunctival-space implants (eg, Xen Gel Stent [Allergan]).

Results of the HORIZON randomized multicenter clinical study showed significant IOP reduction and decreased medication use among patients with mild-to-moderate primary open angle glaucoma who received the Hydrus stent in combination with phacoemulsification, compared with patients who underwent phacoemulsification alone. Safety profiles were similar for the 2 arms. The iStent in combination with phacoemulsification also resulted in significant IOP reduction and decreased need for glaucoma medications versus phacoemulsification alone. The market withdrawal of the CyPass Micro-Stent (Alcon) because of increased endothelial cell loss in patients who received this device at time of cataract surgery emphasizes the importance of long-term clinical trials to evaluate the safety of relatively new devices.

Arriola-Villalobos P, Martínez-de-la-Casa JM, Díaz-Valle D, et al. Combined iStent trabecular micro-bypass stent implantation and phacoemulsification for coexistent open-angle glaucoma and cataract: a long-term study. *Br J Ophthalmol.* 2012;96(5):645–649.

Francis BA, Minckler D, Dustin L, et al. Combined cataract extraction and trabeculotomy by the internal approach for coexisting cataract and open-angle glaucoma: initial results. *J Cataract Refract Surg*. 2008;34(7):1096–1103.

Helmut H, Ahmed IK, Grisanti S, et al. Early postoperative safety and surgical outcomes after implantation of a suprachoroidal micro-stent for the treatment of open-angle glaucoma concomitant with cataract surgery. *J Cataract Refract Surg*. 2013;39(3):431–437.

Maeda M, Watanabe M, Ichikawa K. Evaluation of trabectome in open-angle glaucoma. *J Glaucoma*. 2013;22(3):205–208.

Malvankar-Mehta MS, Iordanous Y, Chen YN, et al. iStent with phacoemulsification versus phacoemulsification alone for patients with glaucoma and cataract: a meta-analysis. *PLoS One*. 2015;10(7):e0131770.

Samuelson TW, Chang DF, Marquis R, et al; HORIZON Investigators. A Schlemm canal microstent for intraocular pressure reduction in primary open-angle glaucoma and cataract: the HORIZON study. *Ophthalmology*. 2019;126(1):29–37.

Uveitis

Chronic or recurrent uveitis and the corticosteroid therapy used to manage it contribute to cataract formation. Decreased vision due to cataract must be differentiated from that caused by coexisting macular edema or posterior segment pathology. Fluorescein angiography (FA) or optical coherence tomography (OCT) can be used preoperatively to identify CME. Complications can be minimized when inflammation has been controlled for several months before surgery and is treated aggressively after surgery. Topical and oral corticosteroids are the mainstay of therapy; topical NSAIDs and cytotoxic agents may be used to supplement treatment.

To minimize risk of scleral or corneal necrosis, it is important to preoperatively control ocular inflammation, such as scleritis and uveitis associated with connective-tissue or inflammatory diseases. The ophthalmologist can work with other physicians involved in the patient's care to monitor therapy with systemic corticosteroids and immunosuppressive agents.

Uveitic eyes may dilate poorly and require expansion and lysis of iridolenticular adhesions, similar to eyes with small pupils. The pupillary membrane should be incised and stripped to avoid interference with the capsulorrhexis. Vigorous stretching and manipulation of the pupil can lead to bleeding of the iris and fibrinous inflammation postoperatively. Meticulous cleanup of cortical material can help prevent exuberant postoperative inflammation. The use of prostaglandins for IOP control postoperatively is controversial because of the potentially increased risk of CME. Although there is no evidence for stopping prostaglandin analogue use pre- or postsurgically, caution is warranted in the use of these medications in complex eyes with retinal comorbidities that undergo cataract surgery.

Insertion of a silicone lens implant is discouraged because inflammatory precipitates can collect on the lens surface (Fig 12-11). Instead, acrylic PCIOLs placed in the capsular bag are well tolerated. When complications arise and a lens cannot be inserted into the capsular bag, the surgeon may decide against placing a lens in the ciliary sulcus or implanting an AC lens. Other options include leaving the eye aphakic or using

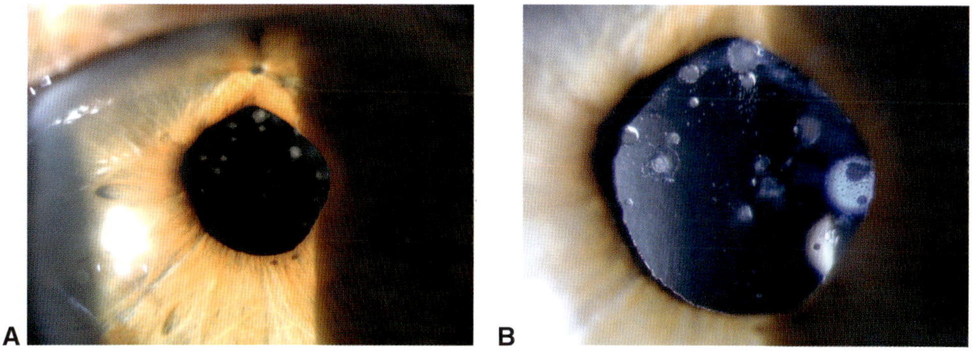

Figure 12-11 Low-power **(A)** and high-power **(B)** views of a silicone intraocular lens with keratic precipitates. *(Courtesy of Steven Vold, MD; photography by Matthew Poe.)*

a scleral-fixated lens. In uveitis associated with membrane formation, repeated Nd:YAG procedures may be necessary to clear the lens surface. (See also BCSC Section 9, *Uveitis and Ocular Inflammation.*)

Abela-Formanek C, Amon M, Kahraman G, Schauersberger J, Dunavoelgyi R. Biocompatibility of hydrophilic acrylic, hydrophobic acrylic, and silicone intraocular lenses in eyes with uveitis having cataract surgery: long-term follow-up. *J Cataract Refract Surg.* 2011;37(1):104–112.

Hernstadt DJ, Hosain R. Effect of prostaglandin analogue use on the development of cystoid macular edema after phacoemulsification using STROBE statement methodology. *J Cataract Refract Surg.* 2017;43(4):564–569.

Retinal Conditions

Retinal Disease

The ocular records of a patient with retinal disease may indicate his or her visual acuity before the onset of cataract. Macular function tests, such as the macular photostress test or the potential acuity test (see Chapter 6), can be employed to help predict the visual outcome in patients with retinal disease. The clinician must interpret test results with caution because poor or equivocal test performance does not rule out a benefit from cataract removal. OCT and FA can be used to detect the presence of diabetic or hypertensive retinopathy, degenerative changes, macular distortion, and leakage of fluid into the foveal area. Proper management of patient expectations is crucial in vision-threatening retinal disease.

If diabetic macular edema is present and the view of the retina is adequate preoperatively, the clinician may consider focal laser treatment or intravitreal injection of steroids or anti–vascular endothelial growth factor (anti-VEGF) medications. Ideally, cataract surgery is delayed until the macular edema has resolved; this may take several months. The clinician also may consider perioperative administration of topical NSAIDs. Researchers have found that this may decrease the incidence of postoperative CME and that NSAIDs are beneficial in preventing macular edema in patients with diabetes mellitus.

Patients known to have peripheral vitreoretinopathy should be examined by a retina specialist to determine whether pretreatment with laser or cryotherapy would help reduce the risk of retinal tears or detachment. After prophylactic treatment, a period of a few weeks may elapse before elective cataract surgery. (See also BCSC Section 12, *Retina and Vitreous.*)

If visualization of the retina is restricted by a small pupil, cataract surgery can provide an opportunity to enlarge the pupil using stretch maneuvers, iris hooks, expansion devices, or multiple sphincterotomies. In addition, a generous anterior capsulotomy with complete cortical cleanup can enhance the view of the retinal periphery after surgery.

When safe, it is preferable that the patient receive a PCIOL. A silicone IOL should be avoided in a patient for whom vitrectomy is anticipated because condensation on the posterior surface of the implant limits visibility during pars plana vitrectomy.

Eriksson U, Alm A, Bjärnhall G, Granstam E, Matsson AW. Macular edema and visual outcome following cataract surgery in patients with diabetic retinopathy and controls. *Graefes Arch Clin Exp Ophthalmol.* 2011;249(3):349–359.

Shah AS, Chen SH. Cataract surgery and diabetes. *Curr Opin Ophthalmol.* 2010;21(1):4–9.

Cataract Following Pars Plana Vitrectomy

Nuclear cataract formation is common after pars plana vitrectomy, especially in patients older than 50 years. The use of silicone oil during retinal surgery typically yields posterior subcapsular opacification. Posterior plaque may also be seen after pars plana vitrectomy. In the absence of a vitreous cushion, the posterior capsule becomes more mobile. Thus, careful attention to fluctuations in AC depth is important, to avoid a surge upon breaking vacuum when a piece of lens is aspirated (see Chapters 8 and 10). Lowering the irrigation bottle and decreasing the fluid flow rate prior to placing the phaco tip inside the eye are helpful. These maneuvers are also recommended when zonular integrity is altered as a result of prior retinal surgery or preexisting ocular disease. Note that overfilling the anterior chamber with OVDs can cause zonular stretch and breakage. Extra caution is also necessary to prevent pieces of the lens from being lost during hydrodissection in case an inadvertent capsular break had occurred during the retinal surgery. A large capsulorrhexis allows prolapse of the nucleus during hydrodissection for an iris-plane phaco chop. If the surgeon selects an extracapsular surgical technique instead of phacoemulsification, the absence of vitreous reduces posterior pressure to aid lens expression. Alternatively, after capsulorrhexis and hydrodissection of the nucleus from its cortical attachments, the nucleus can be removed using a lens loop or irrigating vectis. Patients who receive intravitreal injections also may have an inadvertent opening of the posterior capsule; these patients may be treated similarly to postvitrectomy patients (described previously).

Cataract With Intraocular Silicone Oil

In an eye with silicone oil, the cataract usually is very soft. It is important to avoid pressurizing the eye with excessive OVDs or a high infusion pressure of balanced salt solution. During cataract surgery, silicone oil can migrate through a break in the zonular fibers if the AC is overfilled with OVDs. This can be counteracted with the use of low-flow irrigation or decreased aspiration rate during surgery. Droplets of silicone oil that were not apparent in the AC during surgery might become visible postoperatively. A few droplets are usually not toxic to the cornea. Silicone lens implants are contraindicated in these eyes because silicone oil adheres to the implant surface. The surgeon can create an inferior iridotomy if a patent one is not already present. (See Chapter 7 for a discussion of IOL calculations in eyes with silicone oil.)

Ocular Trauma

Ocular Assessment

When a patient presents with a history of ocular trauma sufficient to cause a dense cataract, it is important to evaluate the other anterior segment structures, which also may be affected. If the corneal endothelium, zonular fibers, or anterior chamber angle have sustained damage, adjustments in surgical technique are needed. Gonioscopy is essential when planning IOL placement, and the surgeon should exercise great care when evaluating ocular findings and determining the potential for visual recovery (discussed in Chapter 6). Cataract may occur acutely after substantial trauma (see Chapter 5). A slowly progressive cataract after ocular trauma can be monitored while intraocular inflammation and other comorbidities are treated.

Visualization During Surgery

Corneal laceration and edema can impair the view into the eye such that phacoemulsification cannot be performed safely. Instead, an extracapsular approach may be advisable. Hemorrhage during surgery can further reduce visualization of the anterior segment. The surgeon may use OVDs and inject air intracamerally to occlude vessels and marginalize bleeding. If visualization remains inadequate, the surgeon should close the wound and delay the operation.

Inflammation

Acute and chronic inflammation are common sequelae of ocular trauma. Severe uveitis may mimic infectious endophthalmitis. Fibrin membranes on the iris lead to synechiae formation, pupil seclusion, and miosis; these are treated with pupil-enlarging maneuvers (described previously in the section Small Pupil). In an inflamed eye, a peripheral iridotomy can help prevent pupillary block glaucoma. Inflamed uveal tissue bleeds upon the slightest manipulation. OVDs should be used liberally to protect the corneal endothelium and to improve visualization into the anterior segment. Postoperative IOP elevation is typical and is exacerbated by the use of OVDs. Control of inflammation warrants cycloplegia as well as intensive topical and possibly oral corticosteroid therapy.

Retained Foreign Matter

A foreign body in the AC may be easier to see when the patient is seated upright at the slit lamp rather than positioned supine under the operating microscope. Irrigating solutions may dislodge a foreign body from its preoperative location. When an intraocular foreign body is suspected to be located in the posterior segment, indirect ophthalmoscopy is a viable option, provided ocular media are sufficiently clear. When the view is obscured by cataract or hemorrhage, a computed tomography (CT) scan, x-ray, or ultrasonogram can help the clinician determine the presence and location of the foreign body. Magnetic resonance imaging (MRI) is contraindicated if the foreign body is potentially metallic. A dense cataract may be removed by either a pars plana or an anterior approach, followed by pars plana vitrectomy and removal of the foreign body.

Cataract in an Eye With Damage to Other Ocular Tissues

Iris trauma commonly coexists with traumatic cataract (Fig 12-12). Sphincter ruptures result in irregular pupil size and shape. The surgeon can repair iridodialysis at the time of cataract removal by suturing the iris root to the scleral spur. Though not apparent on slit-lamp examination, corneal endothelial damage can be significant and may not manifest until after surgery, when severe corneal edema occurs. Preoperative specular microscopy can be helpful in determining the status of the corneal endothelium and its ability to withstand cataract surgery. Trauma sufficient to cause iris tears and cataract warrants careful inspection for zonular damage and insult to the posterior segment. If a retinal detachment is present, cataract removal may be necessary to allow adequate visualization for subsequent surgical repair.

Removal of Traumatic Cataract

A traumatic cataract may leak lens protein into the aqueous and vitreous, inciting uveitis and glaucoma. If cortical material is identified in the AC or if a mature cataract interferes with the diagnosis and treatment of injuries in the posterior segment, prompt

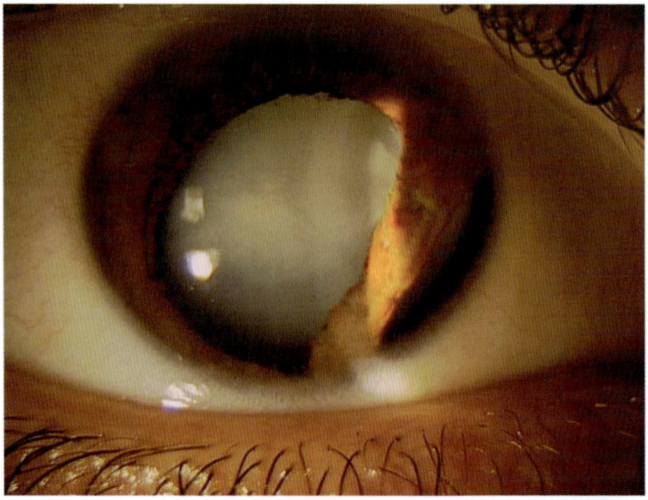

Figure 12-12 Traumatic cataract and iridodialysis secondary to a paintball injury. *(Courtesy of Mark H. Blecher, MD.)*

removal of the cataract is warranted. Rupture of the capsule causes rapid hydration of the lens cortex, leading to formation of a milky-white cataract. This type of cataract is usually soft and can be aspirated through the large port of the irrigating/aspirating handpiece. It is important to be aware of the possibility of preexisting capsular rupture, which may not be visible on preoperative examination. In these cases, hydrodissection is best performed slowly to minimize the possibility of extending a capsular break and causing the lens to fall into the posterior segment.

If a hard nuclear cataract was present before the trauma, the surgeon employs techniques for cataract removal (described in the earlier section Zonular Dehiscence With Lens Subluxation or Dislocation). An OVD can be used to provide a tamponade to anterior vitreous movement in areas of zonular incompetence. If vitreous has migrated into the anterior chamber, an anterior vitrectomy is performed before removing the lens to avoid vitreous manipulation and retinal traction.

When the nucleus is substantially subluxed and vitreous fills much of the AC, the surgeon can consider a pars plana lensectomy, in collaboration with a retinal surgeon (see BCSC Section 12, *Retina and Vitreous*).

Vision Rehabilitation

After ocular trauma, primary implantation of a posterior chamber lens is recommended, provided intraocular inflammation and hemorrhage are minimal and the view of anterior segment structures is good. An ACIOL or fixated posterior chamber lens may be necessary if there is inadequate capsular support for a PCIOL. In rare situations, the surgeon may decide against placing an IOL primarily and instead insert an IOL as a secondary procedure after sufficient evaluation of the anterior segment and anterior angle anatomy. Even less commonly, the eye may be left aphakic and managed with a contact lens. Scarring from a corneal laceration changes the contour of the cornea, and inaccurate keratometry and biometry measurements can result in erroneous IOL power selection, increasing the risk of postoperative anisometropia. A rigid contact lens may be required to mask irregular astigmatism from a corneal scar.

IOL Selection After Trauma

The clinician tailors the lens implant to the patient's ocular anatomy and to the desired postoperative outcome. In patients with a history of uveitis, hydrophobic acrylic IOLs are preferred to silicone lens implants because vision-impairing inflammatory debris is more likely to collect on the surface of silicone lens implants (see Fig 12-11). Silicone lens implants are also not preferred in eyes that are likely to undergo vitreoretinal surgery in the future. In eyes that have more than 4 clock-hours of inadequate zonular support but an intact anterior capsule, a 3-piece posterior chamber lens may be placed in the ciliary sulcus. If there is no capsular support, a 3-piece lens may be fixated to the scleral wall. AC lenses are designed to be sufficiently flexible for open-angle glaucomatous eyes. Ultimately, the choice of IOL is determined by the surgeon's experience with lens options and implantation methods.

APPENDIX

Historical Development of Cataract Surgery and Non-Phacoemulsification Cataract Surgery Techniques

This appendix includes related videos. Go to www.aao.org/bcscvideo_section11 or scan the QR codes in the text to access this content.

Highlights

- Cataract surgery is not a modern invention; it has an ancient lineage and likely was first performed by a bold surgeon over 2500 years ago.
- Cataract surgery has undergone considerable evolution, in concert with other developments in engineering and medicine, which have resulted in more successful surgeries with fewer complications.
- Phacoemulsification for cataract has become the dominant surgical technique in developed areas; however, in less-developed areas manual small-incision extracapsular cataract surgery (MSICS) is performed frequently and at a fraction of the cost, with comparable vision outcomes.

A Brief History of Cataract Surgery

Ancient and medieval therapy for cataract included couching, a technique whose history dates to approximately the fifth century BCE. Used throughout the Roman Empire, Europe, India, and sub-Saharan Africa, couching was performed on mature cataracts. With the patient in a seated position, the surgeon quickly inserted a needle posterior to the corneoscleral junction and pushed the lens inferiorly (Fig A-1) into the vitreous cavity. Although the lens no longer occluded the visual axis, it remained in the eye.

By 1600, anatomists had correctly identified the position of the crystalline lens (see the Introduction, Fig I-3), and understood cataract as opacification of the lens. By the 17th century, a better understanding of the anatomy led to a fundamental improvement in technique. Jacques Daviel (1696–1762) is credited with introducing a method to extract

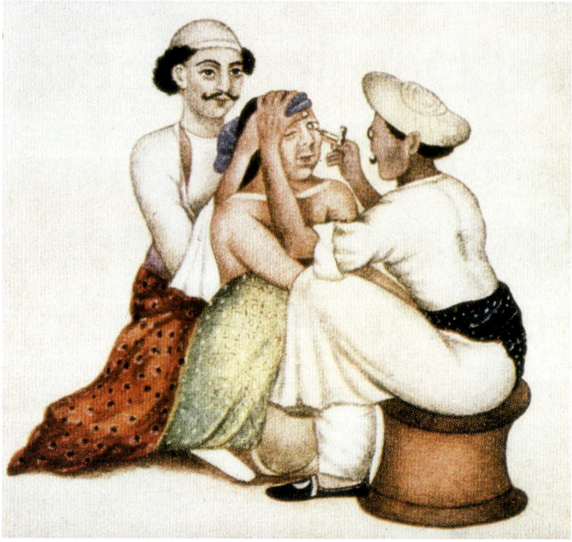

Figure A-1 Couching. *(Reproduced from Duke-Elder S.* Diseases of the Lens and Vitreous; Glaucoma and Hypotony. *Mosby; 1969.* System of Ophthalmology; *vol II.)*

the cataract rather than simply displacing it from the visual axis. His method involved creating an incision through the inferior cornea, enlarging the wound with scissors, incising the lens capsule, expressing the nucleus, and removing the cortex by curettage, leaving the capsular bag in place (Fig A-2). This technique, called extracapsular cataract extraction (ECCE), became the new standard of care. Because of the large incision size used, early ECCE was complicated by problems with wound healing, vitreous and uveal prolapse, and infection. In addition, lens remnant–induced inflammation and capsular opacification were common, and secondary discission of pupillary membranes was often necessary.

Subsequently, Albrecht von Graefe advanced this technique by developing a corneal knife that created a cleaner incision and led to improved wound healing. The development of fine suture material, the invention of the binocular operating microscope, and the introduction of effective sterilization techniques reduced surgical complications. Variations on manual ECCE are widely used by surgeons in many countries today.

Removal of a cataract via intracapsular cataract extraction (ICCE) was first performed by Samuel Sharp in 1753. Today, this procedure is rarely performed, but its use may still be indicated, for example, in cases of traumatic cataract, when the zonule is disrupted. In ICCE, the lens is removed through a limbal incision with its capsule intact by disrupting the zonular fibers that attach the lens to the ciliary body. Various instruments were developed to grasp and extract the lens, including toothless forceps and suction cup–like devices called erysiphakes. Although ICCE avoids one likely complication of ECCE, in which the posterior capsule opacifies following surgery, it introduces a higher risk of vitreous prolapse and requires the placement of an anterior chamber intraocular lens (ACIOL) or an intraocular lens (IOL) attached to the iris or sclera, because there is no possibility

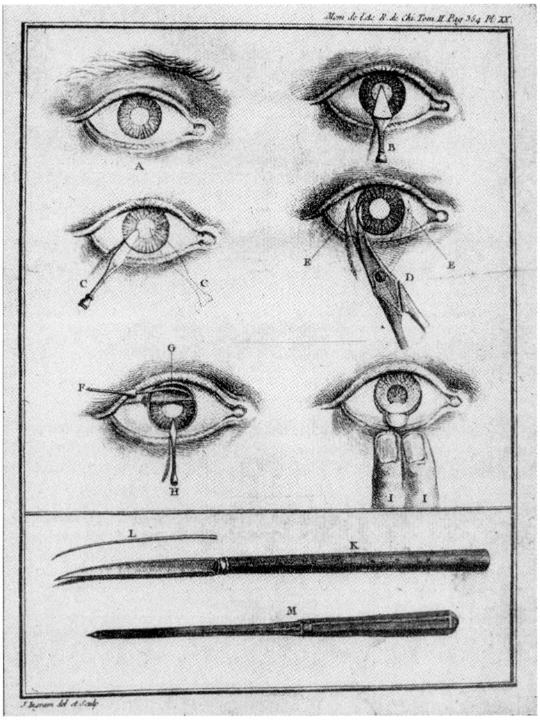

Figure A-2 A new method to cure cataract by extracting the crystalline lens. *(Reproduced from Louis M, et al.* Memoires de l'Académie Royale de Chirurgie. *Théophile Barrois Lejeune; 1787.)*

of capsular support. Twentieth-century advances in ICCE included chemical dissolution of zonular fibers with α-chymotrypsin, reported by Barraquer in 1957, and use of the cryoprobe, introduced by Kelman in 1962. ICCE remained the most widely used method for cataract surgery in the United States until the late 1970s, when ECCE, and later phacoemulsification, predominated.

Today, phacoemulsification is the preferred method of cataract extraction for most surgeons in highly developed areas. This technique is described in detail and illustrated in Chapter 8 of this volume. However, not every cataract is a good candidate for removal by phacoemulsification, and the costly phacoemulsification unit may not be available to all surgeons. Therefore, it is useful for all surgeons, even those practicing in developed areas, to learn techniques that do not require phacoemulsification. Some of these techniques are older, typically used only in special circumstances or in complicated cases. Other techniques, for example, manual small-incision cataract surgery (MSICS), are now used widely by surgeons operating in countries without access to the latest technology or the logistical support phacoemulsification requires (eg, disposable tubing and electricity). Among skilled surgeons, vision outcomes with MSICS have been demonstrated to be similar to phacoemulsification, but the costs associated with MSICS are lower.

Non-Phacoemulsification Methods for Cataract Extraction

Standard Extracapsular Cataract Extraction

Some patients present with cataracts judged to be too dense to safely employ phacoemulsification. Other patients have damaged corneas that may not permit adequate visualization for the usual cataract surgery techniques. For such patients, standard extracapsular surgery (Video A-1) may be the best option, depending on the surgeon's preference.

VIDEO A-1 Standard extracapsular cataract surgery.
Courtesy of Yen Cheng Hsia, MD, and Cynthia S. Chiu, MD.
Go to www.aao.org/bcscvideo_section11 to access all videos in Section 11.

Patient preparation

After informed consent is obtained, the operative site is marked, and the pupil is maximally dilated. A "time-out" is performed to ensure that the surgical team is prepared for the correct surgical procedure on the correct patient, with the correct implant (surgical planning is discussed in more detail in Chapter 7). After anesthesia (typically a retrobulbar block) has been administered and the eye has been prepared and draped in sterile fashion, an eyelid speculum is placed.

Incision

A fornix-based conjunctival flap is made superiorly, followed by cauterization of the scleral bed. The initial incision usually consists of a limbal groove, fashioned with a round-tipped steel blade, sharp microknife, or diamond knife. Some surgeons prefer a slightly more posterior incision with anterior dissection, creating a scleral flap or tunnel. Nucleus expression requires a limbal chord length of 8–12 mm, smaller than the incision required for ICCE. A stab incision is made under the flap into the anterior chamber in preparation for anterior capsulotomy, and the cystotome is inserted to begin the procedure. The anterior chamber depth is usually stabilized with ophthalmic viscosurgical devices (OVDs).

Anterior capsulotomy

An anterior capsulotomy allows the surgeon to remove the cataract with enough capsular support to stabilize the IOL, once implanted, within the capsular bag. The surgeon initiates a continuous curvilinear capsulorrhexis (CCC) by making a puncture in the anterior capsule using a cystotome needle or capsulorrhexis forceps with special tips for grasping and tearing. The edge of this tear is then grasped with forceps and pulled around smoothly, removing a circular portion of the anterior capsule. The CCC used for ECCE needs to be larger (>6 mm) than the CCC created for routine phacoemulsification (approximately 5 mm) to allow for safe expression of an intact nucleus. Expression of a large or dense nucleus may require relaxing incisions in the CCC in order to avoid uncontrolled traumatic tears in the capsulorrhexis, which can lead to rupture of the posterior capsule. Alternatively, a cystotome needle may be used to make a series of connected punctures or small tears in a circular pattern (*can-opener capsulotomy;* Fig A-3). After the capsulotomy is completed, the initial limbal or scleral incision is widened to allow safe passage of the nucleus through the incision.

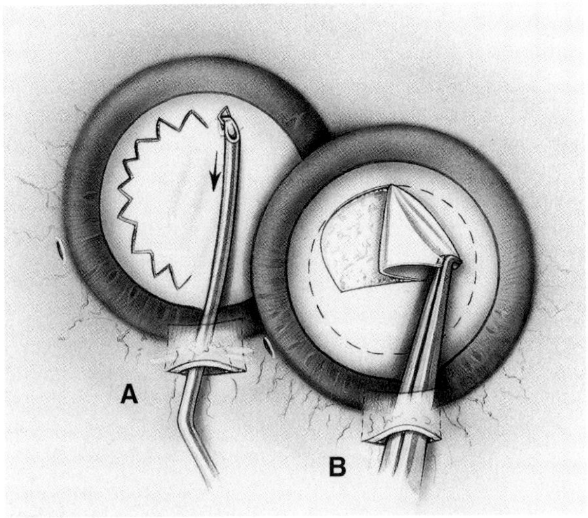

Figure A-3 Anterior capsulotomy techniques. **A,** In a can-opener incision, punctures are made peripherally and pulled centrally so that the torn edges connect. Each puncture site has the potential for a radial tear if stressed. **B,** In a capsulorrhexis, tearing is begun within the area to be excised and finished from the outside in. When stress lines in the free flap appear between forceps and the tear site, best control is maintained by regrasping the flap near the tear site. "Positive vitreous pressure" makes the tear travel peripherally; filling the anterior chamber with an ophthalmic viscosurgical device will counteract the posterior vitreous pressure and make it easier to complete the capsulorrhexis tear. *(Reproduced from Johnson SH. Phacoemulsification.* Focal Points: Clinical Modules for Ophthalmologists. *American Academy of Ophthalmology; 1994, module 6. Illustration by Christine Gralapp.)*

Nucleus removal

Manual expression of the nucleus involves pressing on the inferior limbus to tip the superior pole of the nucleus up and out of the capsular bag. Applying additional counterpressure on the globe by using an instrument to indent the sclera posterior to the limbus, 180° away from the incision, expresses the nucleus from the anterior chamber. The surgeon removes the nucleus by loosening and elevating it from the capsule with the use of a hook or irrigating cannula and then supporting it on a lens loop, spoon, or vectis that will subsequently be used to slide or irrigate the nucleus out of the chamber.

The incision is partially sutured to allow deepening of the anterior chamber with irrigation. Using the irrigation/aspiration equipment or a Simcoe cannula (Fig A-4), the surgeon then aspirates the lens cortex.

IOL insertion

Prior to IOL insertion, the anterior chamber is usually filled with an OVD. An appropriate posterior chamber IOL (PCIOL) may be inserted into the ciliary sulcus or into the capsular bag. Sulcus fixation typically requires an IOL with a larger overall diameter (at least 13 mm) and a large-diameter optic (at least 6 mm), which is more forgiving in case of postoperative decentration.

To insert the IOL into the capsular bag, an OVD is injected into the bag, with care taken to separate the anterior capsule flap completely from the posterior capsule. Direct visualization of haptic placement in the capsular bag during IOL insertion is critical.

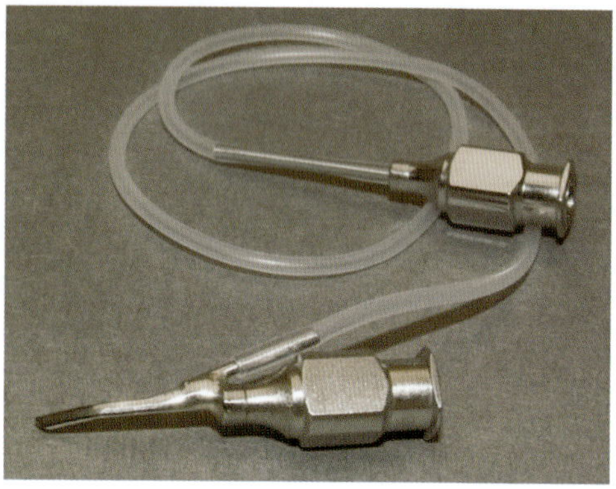

Figure A-4 Simcoe irrigating/aspirating cannula. *(Courtesy of Carol Everhart Roper.)*

Closure

The ECCE incision is typically closed with multiple interrupted sutures of 10-0 nylon. Proper suture tension helps reduce postoperative astigmatism: loose sutures induce corneal flattening, whereas tight sutures cause corneal steepening in the axis of the suture. The refraction is typically stable by the fourth to sixth postoperative week, after which spectacles may be prescribed. If a significant amount of postoperative astigmatism is present in the axis of tight sutures, the clinician may selectively remove the sutures, as guided by wound stability, keratometry readings, or corneal topography measurements.

Manual Small-Incision Cataract Surgery

Manual small-incision cataract surgery (MSICS; Video A-2) is a variation of ECCE, first described by Blumenthal in 1994. MSICS uses surgical instruments similar to those employed in standard ECCE, as well as a binocular operating microscope, but MSICS does not require access to other electronic instrumentation and is faster to complete, making it particularly useful in areas of the world in need of high-volume, low-cost cataract extraction.

VIDEO A-2 Manual small-incision cataract surgery.
Courtesy of Charles Cole, MD; video by Grace Sun, MD.

The primary differences between ECCE and MSICS are that, in the latter, a smaller corneal incision and mechanical fragmentation of the nucleus for delivery may be used. The scleral incision is made 1.5–2.0 mm posterior to the limbus in the form of a straight or frown-shaped groove 6–7 mm in length. Using a crescent blade, the surgeon tunnels this incision forward 1.5 mm, into clear cornea. The tunnel is shaped like a trapezoid, such that the internal incision is wider than the external scleral incision. This construction allows for delivery of the nucleus, which can be divided into smaller segments prior to removal, while generally maintaining a self-sealing external incision. A small, or soft, nucleus may be expressed intact with a Simcoe cannula (see Fig A-4), vectis, or lens loop. A large or dense nucleus may require bimanual fragmentation prior to delivery.

Aspiration of cortex is performed using the Simcoe cannula. A rigid 6-mm polymethyl methacrylate (PMMA) lens is then placed into the capsular bag. A properly constructed wound should be self-sealing. If necessary, the wound may be closed with 10-0 nylon sutures to prevent wound leakage.

Studies have shown that, in comparison to ECCE, MSICS allows a higher surgical volume and faster vision recovery, and it results in less postoperative astigmatism and better uncorrected visual acuity. Vision outcomes and complication rates for MSICS are similar to those for phacoemulsification performed in developed areas.

Tabin GC, Feilmeier MR. Cataract surgery in the developing world. *Focal Points: Clinical Modules for Ophthalmologists.* American Academy of Ophthalmology; 2011, module 9.

Intracapsular Cataract Extraction

Patient preparation

The preparation for planned ICCE (Video A-3) is similar to that for ECCE. If retrobulbar anesthesia is used, preoperative orbital massage by digital pressure or a compressive device may be employed to decrease the pressure effect from the increased orbital volume produced by this anesthetic. Some surgeons use mannitol to decrease the orbital and vitreous volume. Mannitol should be used with caution in elderly patients and those with congestive heart failure, diabetes mellitus, or renal compromise.

VIDEO A-3 Intracapsular cataract surgery.
Courtesy of John A Hovanesian, MD.

Exposure of the globe

After the skin and ocular surface have been prepared and the eye is draped, an eyelid speculum is placed. A bridle suture is usually required to hold the eye in a slight downward position. The surgeon can accomplish this step by placing a 6-0 silk suture beneath the superior rectus tendon or within sclera and securing the suture to the superior drape.

Incision

The surgeon creates a fornix-based conjunctival flap and then uses cautery to achieve hemostasis. A scleral support ring may be necessary in young patients or in those with high myopia to avoid scleral collapse when the lens is extracted. In patients with deep-set eyes, the ring may be needed to improve exposure.

Incision placement varies according to surgeon preference and the patient's anatomy. More anterior or corneal incisions may be of shorter chord length and result in less bleeding. However, closure of such incisions induces corneal steepening in the meridian of the incision. Incisions that are more posterior heal faster and, when covered by a conjunctival flap, are more comfortable for the patient. Posterior incisions induce less astigmatism and are less damaging to the corneal endothelium, but they cause more bleeding.

Sutures are preplaced across the incision and looped out of the way; their presence allows rapid closure of the eye in case of choroidal hemorrhage, Valsalva maneuver, or other causes of positive posterior pressure. An additional suture may be placed through the anterior lip of the incision only; this will allow the surgical assistant to elevate the cornea to facilitate delivery of the cataractous lens later on.

Iridectomy and lens delivery

An iridectomy is performed at this point during the procedure. If the eye has a small pupil after dilation, the surgeon may consider performing sector iridectomy, radial iridectomy, or multiple sphincterotomies or using iris hooks to expand the pupil.

α-Chymotrypsin, if available, can be injected via a cannula through the pupillary space into the posterior chamber to dissolve the zonular fibers. An iris retractor can be used to expose the superior surface of the lens. A cellulose sponge is employed to dry the anterior lens capsule. Next, the surgeon positions a cryoprobe, a hollow metal-tipped probe that is cooled by compressed nitrous oxide, on the lens surface. Once an ice ball has formed and the lens has adhered to the probe (Fig A-5), gentle to-and-fro maneuvers are used to deliver the lens. At this point, the anterior cornea lip should be elevated, to ensure the cryoprobe does not touch the cornea. An iris retractor or cellulose sponge can be used to strip the vitreous from the posterior surface of the lens during delivery. Vitreous loss, combined with the larger incision of intracapsular surgery, contributes to posterior scleral collapse. Thus, the surgeon should anticipate the need for management of vitreous loss. An anterior vitrectomy unit can be used for controlled removal of vitreous. In addition, cellulose sponges may be used to engage vitreous, which can then be cut with Vannas scissors; this process should be repeated until all externalized vitreous has been removed.

Next, a lens implant may be inserted, or the patient may be left aphakic. An anterior chamber lens can be inserted after instillation of acetylcholine or carbachol. Other lens implant options include posterior chamber lenses with iris or scleral fixation.

The surgeon then uses sutures to close the incision while an OVD or balanced salt solution is utilized to keep the anterior chamber formed. The conjunctival flap is secured. Subconjunctival or sub-Tenon injection of antibiotics or corticosteroids can be given at this point. A patch and shield should be applied.

Postoperative course

The postoperative course for ICCE is generally similar to that for ECCE. If the eye has been left aphakic, visual acuity can be estimated with a +10.00 to +12.00 diopter (D) lens.

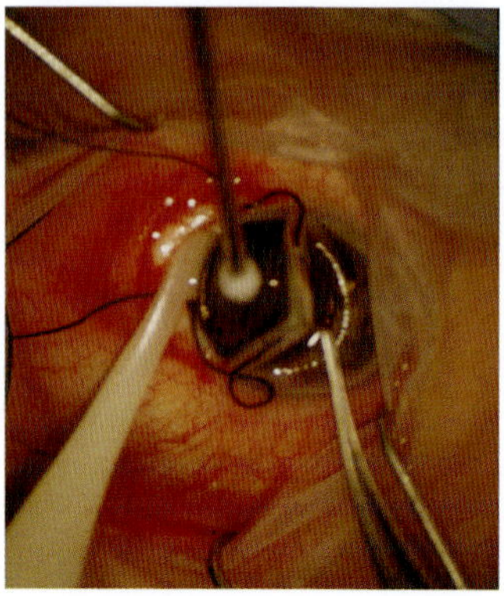

Figure A-5 Cryoextraction of cataract (intracapsular cataract extraction). The lens is being lifted out of the eye. *(Courtesy of Lisa F. Rosenberg, MD.)*

The surgeon should monitor the appearance of the cornea, the integrity of the wound, the depth of the anterior chamber, the degree of inflammatory reaction, and the intraocular pressure (IOP). Visualizing the posterior segment is important for evaluation of vitreous clarity and position and for detecting any retinal or optic nerve pathology.

It is not unusual to see mild eyelid edema and erythema. The upper eyelid may be moderately ptotic. The conjunctiva is often mildly hyperemic, and subconjunctival hemorrhage may be present. The cornea should be clear, but some superior corneal edema is often present from the bending of the cornea during lens extraction. This edema generally resolves during the first postoperative week. The anterior chamber should have normal depth with mild to moderate cellular reaction. The pupil should be round and the iridectomy, patent.

The postoperative course is typically characterized by steady improvement in vision and comfort. Topical antibiotics, nonsteroidal anti-inflammatory drugs, and corticosteroids are often used during the first postoperative weeks. The refraction generally becomes stable 6–12 weeks after intracapsular surgery, depending on the wound-closure technique employed. It usually takes longer to achieve a stable refraction after ICCE than after ECCE or other procedures, because of the larger incision required for ICCE.

IOLs: Historical Perspectives and Lens Modifications

Historical Perspectives

Before 1949, cataract surgery resulted in aphakia, and patients were destined (unless they had high myopia) to wear high-hyperopic spectacles, which were heavy and caused image magnification and distortion of peripheral vision. When they became available, scleral contact lenses and eventually corneal contact lenses could be used instead.

IOL implantation began in 1949. Harold Ridley, an English ophthalmologist, observed that PMMA fragments from airplane cockpit windshields were well tolerated in the anterior segment of the eyes of injured World War II pilots. After performing an ECCE on a 45-year-old woman, Ridley placed a disc-shaped PMMA lens into the posterior chamber of her eye (Fig A-6).

Ridley's lens corrected aphakic vision, but a high incidence of postoperative complications such as glaucoma, uveitis, and dislocation caused him to abandon his design. Ridley showed foresight in 3 important areas:

1. He constructed his original lens of PMMA, a biologically inert, optically clear material in a biconvex design.
2. He used extracapsular surgery for cataract removal, preserving the capsule to support an IOL.
3. He placed the lens in the posterior chamber.

Ridley set the stage for a period of advances in cataract surgery that continues to this day. Although his work was considered highly controversial at the time, he ultimately received a knighthood and numerous professional accolades for his important contributions to cataract surgery.

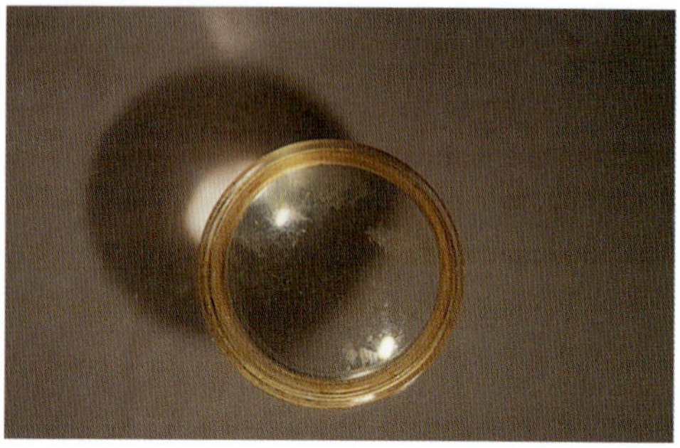

Figure A-6 Photograph of the original Ridley lens, which was first implanted by Harold Ridley in November 1949. *(Courtesy of Robert C. Drews, MD.)*

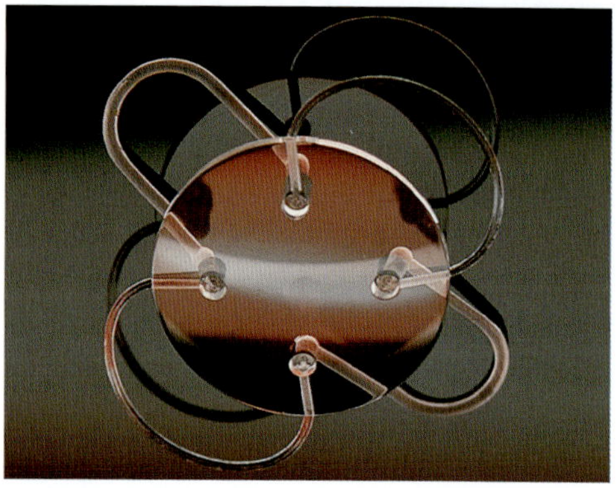

Figure A-7 Original iris-fixated lens designed by Fyodorov, as made in the United States; 2 looped haptics were placed posterior to the iris, and the optic and 2 opposing loops were placed anterior to the iris. *(Courtesy of Robert C. Drews, MD.)*

The extracapsular cataract surgery of the 1950s was crude by modern standards and was generally associated with retained lens cortex, which caused fibrosis and adhesions between iris and capsule. ICCE eliminated residual cortical material and became the preferred procedure. Because ICCE was more commonly performed in the early days of lens implantation, IOLs of that period featured optics with loops, struts, or holes for the sutures required for fixation to the iris for support (Fig A-7).

The anterior chamber angle was an alternate site for IOL support. The first ACIOLs, created by Joaquin Barraquer, Benedetto Strampelli, and others, were crude and ultimately required explantation because of severe inflammatory reactions. Matching the length of the lens to the width of the anterior chamber was difficult. The IOL length was selected by estimating the anterior chamber width on the basis of the horizontal corneal diameter. Because such estimation is inexact even with modern instruments, complications arose. Oversized lenses and closed-loop IOLs caused pupillary distortion and contributed to development of uveitis-glaucoma-hyphema (UGH) syndrome. ACIOLs that were too short would spin, decenter, and come into contact with the corneal endothelium.

Complications associated with rigid ACIOLs spurred the development of flexible, open-loop ACIOLs with 4-point fixation. These modifications dramatically improved clinical outcomes and allowed ACIOLs to remain an acceptable treatment option for cases with compromised capsular support or for secondary IOL insertion (see Chapter 8, Fig 8-16).

Posterior Chamber IOLs and Other Lens Modifications

With advances in cataract surgery technology, the desire to place the IOL in the lens capsule spurred research into posterior chamber lens implantation. Steven Shearing modified a flexible version of a 3-piece IOL with closed loops by opening the loops and inserting the haptics into the capsular bag for posterior chamber placement. Subsequent, successful modifications of this lens by Shearing, Jerry Pierce, and Robert Sinskey allowed ECCE with PCIOL implantation to become the standard for modern cataract surgery at that time.

Thomas Mazzocco is generally credited for developing the foldable IOL. His plate-style lens design influenced the design of modern phakic refractive IOLs (see BCSC Section 13, *Refractive Surgery*). Foldable versions of the Shearing-style lens soon followed (see Chapter 8, Fig 8-15). The obvious advantage of the foldable-lens design is that it allows implantation of the IOL through a smaller incision, reducing the frequency of wound-related complications and postoperative astigmatism. The availability of a small-incision lens influenced many ECCE surgeons' decision to adopt phacoemulsification as their primary technique.

See Chapters 8 and 9 in this volume, as well as BCSC Section 3, *Clinical Optics and Vision Rehabilitation*, for discussions of currently used IOL implants.

Additional Materials and Resources

Related Academy Materials

The American Academy of Ophthalmology is dedicated to providing a wealth of high-quality clinical education resources for ophthalmologists.

Print Publications and Electronic Products

For a complete listing of Academy products related to topics covered in this BCSC Section, visit our online store at https://store.aao.org/clinical-education/topic/cataract-anterior-segment.html. Or call Customer Service at 866.561.8558 (toll free, US only) or +1 415.561.8540, Monday through Friday, between 8:00 a.m. and 5:00 p.m. (PST).

Online Resources

Visit the Ophthalmic News and Education (ONE®) Network at https://www.aao.org/cataract-anterior-segment to find relevant videos, online courses, journal articles, practice guidelines, self-assessment quizzes, images, and more. The ONE Network is a free Academy-member benefit.

Access free, trusted articles and content with the Academy's collaborative online encyclopedia, EyeWiki, at aao.org/eyewiki.

Get mobile access to the *Wills Eye Manual*, watch the latest 1-minute videos, and set up alerts for clinical updates relevant to you with the AAO Ophthalmic Education App. Download today: Search for "AAO Ophthalmic Education" in the Apple app store or in Google Play.

Basic Texts and Additional Resources

Agarwal S, Agarwal A, Agarwal A, eds. *Phacoemulsification*. 3rd ed. Taylor & Francis; 2004.

Apple DJ, Auffarth GU, Peng Q, Visessook N. *Foldable Intraocular Lenses: Evolution, Clinicopathologic Correlations, and Complications*. Slack; 2000.

Bahadur GG, Sinskey RM. *Manual of Cataract Surgery*. 2nd ed. Butterworth-Heinemann; 2000.

Blumenthal M, Kansas P. *Small Incision Manual Cataract Surgery*. Highlights of Ophthalmology International; 2004.

Buratto L, Werner L, Zanini M, Apple DJ. *Phacoemulsification: Principles and Techniques*. 2nd ed. Slack; 2003.

Chang D. *Phaco Chop and Advanced Phaco Techniques: Strategies for Complicated Cataracts*. 2nd ed. Slack; 2013.

Fishkind WJ, ed. *Phacoemulsification and Intraocular Lens Implantation: Mastering Techniques and Complications in Cataract Surgery*. 2nd ed. Thieme; 2017.

Fry LL, Garg A, Guitérrez-Camona F, Pandey SK, Tabin G, eds. *Clinical Practice in Small Incision Cataract Surgery*. Taylor & Francis; 2004.

Garg A, Fine IH, Alió JL, et al, eds. *Mastering the Techniques of Advanced Phaco Surgery.* Jaypee Brothers Medical Publishers; 2008.
Henderson BA, ed. *Essentials of Cataract Surgery.* 2nd ed. Slack; 2014.
Jaffe NS, Jaffe MS, Jaffe GF. *Cataract Surgery and Its Complications.* 6th ed. Mosby; 1998.
Kohnen T, Koch DD, eds. *Essentials in Ophthalmology—Cataract and Refractive Surgery.* Springer-Verlag; 2006.
Olsen RJ, Jin GJC, Ahmed IK, Crandall AS, Cionni RJ, Jones JJ. *Cataract Surgery from Routine to Complex: A Practical Guide.* Slack; 2011.
Pineda R, Espaillat A, Perez VL, Rowe S. T*he Complicated Cataract: The Massachusetts Eye and Ear Infirmary Phacoemulsification Practice Handbook.* Slack; 2001.
Seibel BS. *Phacodynamics: Mastering the Tools and Techniques of Phacoemulsification Surgery.* 4th ed. Slack; 2004.
Steinert RF, ed. *Cataract Surgery.* 3rd ed. Elsevier; 2010.
Tasman W, Jaeger EA, eds. *Duane's Ophthalmology on DVD-ROM.* Lippincott Williams & Wilkins; 2012.
Wilson ME Jr, Trivedi RH, eds. *Pediatric Cataract Surgery: Techniques, Complications, and Management.* 2nd ed. Lippincott Williams & Wilkins; 2014.

Requesting Continuing Medical Education Credit

The American Academy of Ophthalmology is accredited by the Accreditation Council for Continuing Medical Education (ACCME) to provide continuing medical education for physicians.

The American Academy of Ophthalmology designates this enduring material for a maximum of 10 *AMA PRA Category 1 Credits*™. Physicians should claim only the credit commensurate with the extent of their participation in the activity.

To claim *AMA PRA Category 1 Credits*™ upon completion of this activity, learners must demonstrate appropriate knowledge and participation in the activity by taking the posttest for Section 11 and achieving a score of 80% or higher.

This activity meets the Self-Assessment CME requirements defined by the American Board of Ophthalmology (ABO). Please be advised that the ABO is not an accrediting body for purposes of any CME program. ABO does not sponsor this or any outside activity, and ABO does not endorse any particular CME activity. Complete information regarding the ABO Self-Assessment CME Maintenance of Certification requirements is available at https://abop.org/maintain-certification/cme-self-assessment/.

To take the posttest and request CME credit online:

1. Go to www.aao.org/cme-central and log in.
2. Click on "Claim CME Credit and View My CME Transcript" and then "Report AAO Credits."
3. Select the appropriate media type and then the Academy activity. You will be directed to the posttest.
4. Once you have passed the test with a score of 80% or higher, you will be directed to your transcript. *If you are not an Academy member, you will be able to print out a certificate of participation once you have passed the test.*

CME expiration date: June 1, 2023. *AMA PRA Category 1 Credits*™ may be claimed only once between June 1, 2020, and the expiration date.

For assistance, contact the Academy's Customer Service department at 866.561.8558 (US only) or +1 415.561.8540 between 8:00 a.m. and 5:00 p.m. (PST), Monday through Friday, or send an e-mail to customer_service@aao.org.

Study Questions

Please note that these questions are not part of your CME reporting process. They are provided here for your own educational use and identification of any professional practice gaps. The required CME posttest is available online (see "Requesting Continuing Medical Education Credit"). Following the questions are answers with discussions. Although a concerted effort has been made to avoid ambiguity and redundancy in these questions, the authors recognize that differences of opinion may occur regarding the "best" answer. The discussions are provided to demonstrate the rationale used to derive the answer. They may also be helpful in confirming that your approach to the problem was correct or, if necessary, in fixing the principle in your memory. The Section 11 faculty thanks the Resident Self-Assessment Committee for drafting these self-assessment questions and the discussions that follow.

1. What systemic disorder increases the likelihood of developing a posterior subcapsular cataract (PSC)?
   a. benign essential hypertension
   b. diabetes mellitus
   c. hypercholesterolemia
   d. ischemic cardiovascular disease

2. How is metabolic waste removed from the crystalline lens?
   a. It is broken down by lysosomes.
   b. It is removed by the venous system of the lens.
   c. It is stored in the lens and not removed, contributing to the increase in lens size throughout life.
   d. It is removed via the aqueous humor.

3. What common role do superoxide dismutase, catalase, and glutathione peroxidase play in lens physiology?
   a. adjustment of pH to act as a buffer
   b. control of enzymatic functions in glucose metabolism
   c. conversion of water-soluble to water-insoluble proteins
   d. protection against oxidative and free radical damage

4. What carbohydrate metabolism–related change occurs in the lens in the presence of high levels of glucose?
   a. Aldose reductase activity increases.
   b. Glucose that is not phosphorylated to glucose-6-phosphate (G6P) enters the Krebs cycle.
   c. Hexokinase activity increases until all glucose is phosphorylated.
   d. Sorbitol is produced and then eliminated from the lens via diffusion through the capsule into the anterior chamber.

5. The lens has higher levels of what electrolyte in comparison to the surrounding aqueous and vitreous humors?
   a. chloride ions (Cl^-)
   b. potassium ions (K^+)
   c. sodium ions (Na^+)
   d. water (H^+/OH^-)

6. With what congenital disorder is microspherophakia associated?
   a. Axenfeld anomaly
   b. Axenfeld-Rieger syndrome
   c. galactosemia
   d. Weill-Marchesani syndrome

7. What is the most common cause of acquired ectopia lentis?
   a. aniridia
   b. homocystinuria
   c. Marfan syndrome
   d. trauma

8. A patient presents with a mature lens and secondary angle-closure glaucoma without evidence of pupillary block. What is the most likely diagnosis?
   a. lens particle glaucoma
   b. phacoantigenic uveitis
   c. phacolytic glaucoma
   d. phacomorphic glaucoma

9. Glaukomflecken are seen on exam. What is the histologic finding and most likely clinical scenario?
   a. endothelial cells associated with Cogan-Reese syndrome
   b. gray-white fibrillar material from pseudoexfoliative glaucoma
   c. macrophages engorged with phagocytosed proteinaceous, eosinophilic lens material from phacolytic glaucoma
   d. necrotic lens epithelial cells (LECs) and degenerated subepithelial cortex following angle-closure glaucoma

10. A 14-year-old African American girl with atopic dermatitis has been maintained on topical corticosteroids, phototherapy, and antihistamines. Her best-corrected visual acuity (BCVA) is 20/100. What is the most likely cause of her decreased vision?

a. anterior subcapsular cataract
b. PSC
c. steroid-induced glaucoma
d. ultraviolet (UV) corneal burn

11. Determining axial length with an immersion technique or contact applanation is most appropriate in what setting?
    a. dense vitreous hemorrhage
    b. history of corneal refractive surgery
    c. patient with aphakia
    d. posterior chamber filled with silicone oil

12. While examining a patient for cataract surgery, the ophthalmologist notes that although the cornea is clear, there are significant cornea guttae. How would the ophthalmologist manage this patient intraoperatively?
    a. Increase the use of cohesive ophthalmic viscosurgical devices (OVDs) during phacoemulsification.
    b. Increase the use of dispersive OVDs during phacoemulsification.
    c. Perform vigorous hydrodissection to prolapse the lens into the anterior chamber and minimize the amount of energy needed to create a groove in the nucleus.
    d. Prepare for possible penetrating keratoplasty by having cornea tissue available in the operating room.

13. What adjustment in intraocular lens (IOL) power needs to be made if a planned in-the-bag IOL is put into the sulcus with optic capture?
    a. Decrease the power of the IOL.
    b. Increase the power of the IOL.
    c. Do not change the power of the IOL.
    d. Change the power of the IOL only if the patient does not have an intact posterior capsule.

14. A peristaltic or flow pump is a type of aspiration system within a phacoemulsification machine that performs what function in relation to control of aspiration flow rate (AFR) and vacuum?
    a. directly controls AFR and indirectly produces the vacuum level
    b. directly controls AFR and directly produces the vacuum level
    c. directly controls the level of vacuum in the tubing and indirectly controls the AFR
    d. directly controls the level of vacuum in the tubing and directly controls the AFR

15. During cataract surgery, there is a large break in the posterior capsule. The surgeon decides to place an IOL in the ciliary sulcus. Why should a 3-piece IOL be used instead of a single-piece acrylic IOL?
    a. The larger haptics on the single-piece acrylic IOL can make contact with uveal tissues and lead to uveitis-glaucoma-hyphema (UGH) syndrome.
    b. The larger haptics on the single-piece acrylic IOL can make contact with and weaken the zonular fibers, potentially causing dislocation of the IOL.
    c. Placement of a single-piece acrylic IOL in the sulcus will lead to excess myopic shift due to the planar nature of that IOL, as opposed to the posterior vaulting of a 3-piece IOL.
    d. The planar nature of the single-piece acrylic lens makes it difficult to perform optic capture within the capsulorrhexis when the IOL is placed in the ciliary sulcus.

16. What factor may reduce posterior capsular opacification (PCO) following implantation of an acrylic foldable IOL?
    a. avoidance of hydrodissection of the cortex
    b. capsulorrhexis larger than the unfolded lens optic
    c. sulcus haptic placement
    d. truncated or square-edge optic design

17. What examination finding separates postoperative capsular block syndrome from aqueous misdirection?
    a. elevated intraocular pressure (IOP)
    b. peripheral choroidal detachment
    c. space between IOL and posterior capsule
    d. uniformly shallow anterior chamber

18. An ophthalmologist is performing a routine phacoemulsification when she notes that the remaining half of the nucleus has suddenly dropped through an open posterior capsule and appears to be suspended on the anterior vitreous face. What is the best next step?
    a. immediate withdrawal of the phaco instrument and any secondary instrument from the eye
    b. injection of OVD to stabilize the anterior chamber
    c. lollipopping the nucleus with the phaco tip in order to pull it into the anterior chamber
    d. vigorous irrigation with a balanced salt solution to swill the remaining nucleus into the anterior chamber

19. During phacoemulsification, the surgeon notes loss of anterior chamber depth, the eye becomes firm, and the patient reports feeling pain. What should the surgeon do next?
    a. Ask the anesthesiologist to increase the patient's IV pain medication.
    b. Decrease the infusion pressure and increase the aspiration rate.
    c. Prepare for a pars plana vitrectomy.
    d. Suture the wounds closed and examine the fundus.

20. An eye with extreme increased axial length may be susceptible to what intraoperative issue?
    a. higher risk of endothelial damage
    b. higher risk of iris prolapse
    c. higher risk of wound burn
    d. lens–iris diaphragm retropulsion syndrome (LIDRS)

21. If vitreous prolapse occurs, what is the recommended technique for anterior vitreous removal by an anterior segment surgeon?
    a. coaxial anterior vitrectomy through the main corneal incision
    b. complete vitrectomy and lensectomy through 2 pars plana incisions
    c. manual externalization and cutting of vitreous through the main corneal incision
    d. 2-port bimanual anterior vitrectomy with instruments through new limbal incisions or cutting instrument through pars plana

22. After cataract surgery, a patient presents with a shallow anterior chamber and high IOP. A laser peripheral iridotomy fails to deepen the chamber or lower the IOP. What is the next appropriate treatment?
    a. cyclophotocoagulation
    b. cycloplegia and aqueous suppression
    c. surgical vitrectomy
    d. topical miotics and a second laser peripheral iridotomy

23. What clinical finding can help distinguish toxic anterior segment syndrome (TASS) from infectious endophthalmitis?
    a. anterior chamber inflammation
    b. corneal edema
    c. severity of visual acuity loss
    d. time of onset of symptoms after surgery

24. What type of IOL implant is most likely to cause negative dysphotopsia?
    a. anterior chamber IOL (ACIOL)
    b. decentered multifocal IOL (MFIOL)
    c. square-edge posterior chamber IOL (PCIOL) in the bag
    d. sulcus-fixated 1-piece acrylic IOL

25. What intraoperative occurrence may increase the incidence of cystoid macular edema (CME) after otherwise uncomplicated cataract surgery?
    a. forceps delivery of a foldable IOL
    b. implantation of an MFIOL
    c. prolonged surgical time
    d. temporal, clear corneal incision

26. What criterion determines the type of intervention that should be performed for post–cataract extraction endophthalmitis, based on the results of the Endophthalmitis Vitrectomy Study (EVS)?
    a. amount of time that has passed since surgery
    b. degree of inflammation in the vitreous
    c. presence of intact posterior capsule
    d. visual acuity

27. What technique helps maintain corneal clarity after cataract surgery in an eye that has previously undergone penetrating keratoplasty?
    a. minimizing OVD use during surgery
    b. operating while corneal sutures are still in place
    c. placing an ACIOL
    d. using a scleral tunnel approach

28. During phacoemulsification, the surgeon realizes that zonular dialysis of 3 clock-hours (90°) is present. How should the surgeon proceed?
    a. Increase the bottle height and flow rate to maintain adequate anterior chamber depth.
    b. Close the corneal incision and convert to an extracapsular cataract extraction with a superior corneoscleral incision.
    c. Proceed with phacoemulsification and place an ACIOL.
    d. Place a capsular tension ring (CTR) or capsular hooks, complete phacoemulsification, and insert a PCIOL.

29. What complication is common in cataract surgery in a patient with nanophthalmos?
    a. endophthalmitis
    b. irregular astigmatism
    c. rhegmatogenous retinal detachment
    d. uveal effusion

30. For a patient with mild glaucoma and a visually significant cataract, what is the average extent of IOP lowering that may be expected from performing phacoemulsification and IOL implantation on an eye with high IOP?
    a. <10%
    b. 10%–30%
    c. 30%–45%
    d. >45%

Answers

1. **b.** Diabetes mellitus is associated with accelerated development of all age-related lens changes, including posterior subcapsular cataracts (PSCs). The proposed pathophysiologic reasons for these changes are multifactorial, including increased lens hydration from sorbitol accumulation, glycation of lens proteins, and increased oxidative stress. Systemic hypertension, hypercholesterolemia, and ischemic cardiovascular disease are not associated with increased risk for developing PSCs, although these conditions may be relevant for evaluation of general health and for preoperative planning for cataract surgery.
2. **d.** After fetal development, the lens has no blood supply or organelles and depends on the aqueous humor for removal of metabolic waste. Changes in lens size occur throughout life as the lens epithelial cells (LECs) at the equator continue to divide.
3. **d.** Superoxide dismutase, catalase, and glutathione perioxidase work together to destroy the superoxide anion (O^{-}_{2}), protecting the lens against oxidative and free radical damage. There are no known repair mechanisms for free radical damage to proteins or membrane lipids in the lens cortex. Glutathione acts as a major free radical scavenger along with vitamin E and ascorbic acid in the lens. These 3 enzymes have no effect on the pH of the lens and do not participate in the carbohydrate metabolism of the lens. Conversion from water-soluble to water-insoluble proteins appears to be a natural (age-related) process in lens fiber maturation and does not involve an enzymatic function.
4. **a.** When glucose concentration increases in the lens, the sorbitol pathway is activated; aldose reductase, which is the key enzyme in this pathway, is increased. The hexokinase reaction is the rate-limiting step in glucose phosphorylation. Sorbitol is retained in the lens because of poor permeability, promoting lens opacification.
5. **b.** The lens has higher concentrations of potassium ions (K^+) and amino acids than the surrounding aqueous and vitreous humors. Because it is dehydrated, it has lower concentrations of water (H^+/OH^-; remember that the lens swells when the capsule is violated). The lens also has lower concentrations of sodium ions (Na^+) and chloride ions (Cl^-) compared with the surrounding aqueous and vitreous. Recall that the Na^+/K^+-ATPase is located on the anterior lens capsule and creates a gradient of elevated intralenticular K^+ and elevated extralenticular Na^+.
6. **d.** Microspherophakia, a developmental abnormality in which the lens is small in diameter and spherical, is most often associated with Weill-Marchesani syndrome. It can also be associated with a variety of diseases, including Peters anomaly, Marfan syndrome, Alport syndrome, Lowe syndrome, and congenital rubella. It is not associated with Axenfeld-Rieger syndrome, galactosemia, or Axenfeld anomaly.
7. **d.** Trauma is the most common cause of acquired lens displacement. Aniridia is associated with lens opacities, poor zonular integrity, and ectopia lentis, but it is an uncommon panocular syndrome. Marfan syndrome and homocystinuria are also associated with ectopia lentis, but they are inherited disorders and less common than trauma as etiology for lens displacement.
8. **c.** Phacolytic glaucoma occurs when denatured lens protein leaks through an intact but permeable capsule. The trabecular meshwork becomes clogged with lens protein and engorged macrophages. Lens particle glaucoma is associated with a penetrating lens injury or surgery. In phacoantigenic uveitis, leaking of lens protein produces a granulomatous

inflammatory reaction. In phacomorphic glaucoma, the mature lens causes pupillary block and secondary angle closure.

9. **d.** Glaukomflecken are composed of necrotic LECs and degenerated subepithelial cortex that result from prolonged elevated intraocular pressure (IOP), as in acute angle-closure glaucoma. Glaukomflecken are not associated with the other findings and scenarios presented. Pseudoexfoliation syndrome is a systemic condition that is characterized by the production and progressive accumulation of a fibrillar material in tissues throughout the anterior segment and in the connective tissue of various visceral organs.

10. **a.** Atopic dermatitis is associated with cataract formation in up to 38% of affected patients. The cataracts are most often bilateral, anterior subcapsular opacities that resemble shield-like plaques and usually develop in the second or third decade of life. Steroid-induced glaucoma and PSC may be associated with topical corticosteroids, but these are less likely. Ultraviolet (UV) corneal burn is a rare complication of phototherapy when adequate safeguards are in place.

11. **a.** To obtain accurate measurements, optical biometers require adequate clarity of the cornea, aqueous, lens, and vitreous. In eyes with significant corneal scarring, PSCs, or vitreous hemorrhage, biometry may not be obtainable, and an immersion technique or contact applanation would be more appropriate. Biometry calculations must be adjusted when there are alterations in the average velocity through the ocular media, such as in patients with aphakia or silicone oil in the posterior chamber. However, accurate measurements can still be achieved if these factors are considered.

12. **b.** Protecting the corneal endothelium with a coating agent, or a dispersive ophthalmic viscosurgical device (OVD), would be recommended for an eye with cornea guttae. A cohesive agent, while maintaining space, would be easily expelled from the eye during phacoemulsification. Prolapsing the lens into a supracapsular position for phacoemulsification would not necessarily be helpful, because the phaco tip would then be closer to the endothelium. Unless corneal edema is observed preoperatively, the surgeon would not plan for a keratoplasty until some months postoperatively.

13. **c.** The intended anatomic location of the lens within the eye has an impact on the lens power selected. As the lens moves forward from in-the-bag placement to sulcus placement to anterior chamber placement, the distance from the retina increases and the power required for the implant decreases. As a general rule, an anterior chamber intraocular lens (ACIOL) will be approximately 3.00 diopters (D) lower in power than a planned in-the-bag posterior chamber IOL (PCIOL). However, no adjustment is needed if the lens is placed in the sulcus and optic capture is performed, because the optic is effectively in the bag.

14. **a.** A peristaltic pump directly creates flow with a set of rollers that move along flexible tubing, pushing fluid through the tubing. The pressure differential between the lower-pressure aspiration tubing and the higher-pressure anterior chamber creates a relative vacuum. Although a vacuum limit is set on the machine, the peristaltic pump does not directly produce the level of vacuum. Rather, it controls the aspiration flow rate (AFR), which indirectly produces vacuum. In contrast, a Venturi (or vacuum) pump directly creates the vacuum based on the Venturi effect. Direct control of vacuum level in the pump cassette then indirectly produces flow (while the aspiration port is not occluded) by "pulling" on the fluid in the aspiration tubing. In the absence of significant occlusion, higher vacuum levels produce a faster AFR.

15. **a.** A single-piece acrylic intraocular lens (IOL) has large haptics that can make contact with uveal tissues, causing uveitis-glaucoma-hyphema (UGH) syndrome. Damage to the zonular fibers and late dislocation due to the haptics have not been reported. Single-piece acrylic IOLs are planar and not posteriorly vaulted like 3-piece IOLs. However, any IOL placed in the sulcus without optic capture will have more effective refracting power. Therefore, the power of the IOL should be decreased. If the surgeon is planning to capture the optic in the capsulorrhexis, the IOL power should not be changed. Single-piece acrylic IOLs are very flexible, and optic capture could easily be performed. Because of the issue of the haptics in the sulcus, however, it is not advisable to do so. Some surgeons have described a "reverse optic capture," where the single-piece acrylic haptics are placed into the capsular bag and the optic is brought forward through the capsulorrhexis. This is useful if the capsule is broken, but the surgeon would still want to use the single-piece acrylic IOL, such as in cases when a multifocal IOL (MFIOL) was planned. Reverse optic capture has also been described as a technique to reduce negative dysphotopsia after cataract surgery.
16. **d.** Use of a truncated or square-edge optic design decreases the incidence of posterior capsular opacification (PCO). The design of this optic is thought to exert a mechanical barrier effect, create contact inhibition of migrating LECs at the capsular bend, and place higher pressure on the posterior capsule. These effects prevent growth and migration of LECs and thus reduce the incidence of PCO. Avoiding hydrodissection of the cortex makes cortical cleanup more difficult, likely increasing the risk of PCO. A large capsulorrhexis increases wrinkling and opacification of the posterior capsule, which has been demonstrated in multiple studies. Ciliary sulcus placement of the IOL haptics increases the risk and incidence of PCO.
17. **c.** Postoperative capsular block syndrome is caused by trapped viscoelastic or aqueous fluid behind an IOL in an intact capsular bag, leading to a large space between the IOL and the posterior capsule. The posterior capsular distention pushes the IOL forward, uniformly shallows the anterior chamber, and causes a myopic refractive shift. The anterior chamber narrowing can lead to a rise in IOP. Aqueous misdirection also leads to a uniformly shallow anterior chamber with an anteriorly displaced IOL. This condition can also cause elevated IOP. Neither aqueous misdirection nor capsular block syndrome is associated with peripheral choroidal detachment.
18. **b.** If capsule rupture occurs during phacoemulsification, lens fragments may enter the posterior segment. At the time of posterior capsule rupture, the surgeon should stabilize the anterior chamber by reducing the high fluid flow and vacuum levels and by compartmentalizing the vitreous with OVD before removing the phaco instrument. The surgeon should avoid immediate withdrawal of the phaco instrument from the eye, because that would result in an outward pressure gradient, bringing more vitreous forward into the anterior chamber and outward toward the incisions. OVD can also be introduced posterior to a suspended nuclear fragment in an effort to float it anteriorly. Insertion of a second instrument or lens glide behind the nuclear remnant may help prevent the remnant from being dislocated into the vitreous, whereas attempts to impale the nuclear fragment with the phaco tip may force the fragment posteriorly by either the tip or the irrigation, as might also occur if attempting to swill the fragment with vigorous balanced salt solution irrigation. Lollipopping the nuclear fragment with the phaco tip may force it back and may transect the fragment, exposing the aspiration port and increasing the risk of aspirating vitreous.

19. **d.** With a suprachoroidal hemorrhage, the eye typically becomes very firm, and the patient becomes agitated and reports having pain. The surgeon should immediately close the incisions and confirm the diagnosis by examining the fundus with an indirect ophthalmoscope or fundus lens. If the hemorrhage or effusion is significant, the operation should be postponed.

20. **d.** Eyes with very high axial lengths are at risk for lens–iris diaphragm retropulsion syndrome (LIDRS), in which a reverse pupillary block occurs, and the anterior chamber becomes very deep, causing pain. Eyes with lax zonular fibers are more prone to this issue. Lifting the iris off the capsule with a second instrument and lowering the infusion bottle might help correct this problem. Endothelial damage and iris prolapse are more commonly associated with small eyes. Wound burn is more associated with dense nuclei.

21. **d.** The surgeon should avoid manually externalizing and cutting vitreous through the incision. A 2-port bimanual anterior vitrectomy can be performed with separate infusion and aspirating/cutting instruments inserted through new, properly sized limbal incisions. Alternatively, the aspiration/cutting instrument may be placed through a pars plana incision while irrigation is continued through the limbus. This directs flow posteriorly and reduces the amount of vitreous that migrates into the anterior segment, thereby decreasing vitreoretinal traction. Coaxial anterior vitrectomy is no longer recommended.

22. **b.** Malignant glaucoma (also known as ciliary block glaucoma, aqueous misdirection, or vitreous block) results from ciliolenticular block induced by anterior movement of the lens–iris diaphragm, poor vitreous fluid conductivity, and choroidal expansion. These factors result in a shallow anterior chamber and secondary elevation of IOP as a consequence of angle obstruction. IOP remains elevated despite the presence of a patent iridectomy or iridotomy. Medical treatment consists of cycloplegia and aqueous suppression. Use of miotics is not recommended because they can worsen malignant glaucoma by exacerbating anterior displacement of the lens–iris interface. Surgical intervention consists of Nd:YAG laser irido-zonulo-hyaloidotomy and *occasionally* vitrectomy to disrupt the anterior vitreous face and vitreous–ciliary body interface.

23. **d.** Toxic anterior segment syndrome (TASS) generally presents within hours of surgery, whereas infectious endophthalmitis typically develops 2 to 7 days postoperatively. Both entities can cause severe vision loss, corneal edema, and anterior chamber inflammation, even hypopyon.

24. **c.** Negative dysphotopsia is caused by the shadow (penumbra) cast on the nasal retina as light rays entering the eye from the temporal periphery interact with the nasal edge of a well-centered IOL in the capsular bag. It is seen with all types of IOLs placed in the capsular bag but is most common with smaller, square-edge optic designs. Negative dysphotopsia does not occur with ACIOLs. Decentered PCIOLs of all types are associated with positive dysphotopsias. A 1-piece acrylic IOL in the ciliary sulcus increases the risk of UGH syndrome but not negative dysphotopsia.

25. **c.** Intraoperative factors that place a patient at risk for postoperative cystoid macular edema (CME) (Irvine-Gass syndrome) include vitreomacular traction, posterior capsular rupture, vitreous loss, iris prolapse, transient or prolonged hypotony, improper IOL positioning, and prolonged surgical time. Other risk factors include poorly controlled postoperative inflammation, uveitis, preexisting epiretinal membrane, diabetes mellitus, previous retinal vein occlusion, retinitis pigmentosa, and a previous occurrence of CME. Clear corneal incision, implantation of an MFIOL, and use of forceps to place an IOL do not increase the risk of CME.

26. **d.** As a result of the Endophthalmitis Vitrectomy Study (EVS), immediate pars plana vitrectomy and antibiotic injections are recommended when the patient's visual acuity is light perception. When the visual acuity is hand motions or better, a less-invasive anterior chamber and vitreous biopsy for cultures, with subsequent intravitreal injection of antibiotics, may be sufficient. Time passed since surgery, degree of vitreous inflammation, and presence of intact posterior capsule were not used in the determination for management option in the EVS study.
27. **d.** A scleral tunnel approach minimizes endothelial injury during cataract surgery. OVD usage protects the endothelium during surgery, therefore OVDs should be used liberally. Ideally, cataract surgery should be delayed until all penetrating keratoplasty sutures have been removed. PCIOLs are preferred because they minimize contact between the optic and the endothelium.
28. **d.** For a patient with 90° of zonular dialysis, management consists of continued phacoemulsification and capsular tension ring (CTR) placement. The timing of the CTR placement depends on the extent of the zonular compromise and the surgeon's preference. Placement of the CTR before completion of phacoemulsification stabilizes the capsule or further lens manipulation and extraction but makes cortical aspiration more difficult. Thorough cortical aspiration is easier if CTR placement is delayed until just before IOL insertion. However, there is a risk of extending the zonular dialysis if phacoemulsification is performed without adequate capsule support. The flow rate and bottle height should not be increased, because doing so could cause vitreous to prolapse through the dialysis and into the anterior chamber. OVD may be used as a tamponade against the forward movement of vitreous in the area of the dialysis. Unless the situation deteriorates further, neither conversion to extracapsular cataract extraction nor use of an ACIOL would be necessary.
29. **d.** Nanophthalmos is a rare condition in which the eye is extremely short (axial length <20 mm) and the ratio of lens volume to eye volume is higher than normal. These eyes have shallow anterior chambers, narrow angles, and thickened sclerae, with little room for the surgeon to maneuver. Small-incision bimanual surgery is an alternative technique to consider. Intraoperative or postoperative uveal effusion is a unique hazard in nanophthalmic eyes. Maintaining positive pressure in the anterior chamber and limiting the length of the procedure help prevent intraoperative uveal effusion. Scleral windows should be considered as a prophylactic measure to treat uveal effusion. A sutured wound prevents hypotony from contributing to this complication postoperatively. Endophthalmitis, irregular astigmatism, and rhegmatogenous retinal detachments are not common complications in these patients.
30. **b.** Uncomplicated phacoemulsification surgery lowers IOP between 10% and 34%, on average, in some eyes. It can therefore be considered as a stand-alone procedure in eyes with early to moderate glaucoma. For more advanced cases of glaucoma and visually significant cataract, adjunctive filtration procedures may need to be considered at the time of cataract surgery. Staged procedures can also be considered (either cataract or glaucoma procedure first, then the second procedure at later date). Factors to consider when deciding types and order of procedures include IOP goal, level of severity of glaucoma/visual field damage, patient adherence, adverse effects/number of medications, and effect on quality of life.

Index

(*f* = figure; *t* = table)